Recent Results in Cancer Research 130

W. Hinkelbein G. Bruggmoser H. Frommhold
M. Wannenmacher (Eds.)

Acute and Long-Term Side-Effects of Radiotherapy

Biological Basis and Clinical Relevance

With 64 Figures and 47 Tables

Springer-Verlag
Berlin Heidelberg New York
London Paris Tokyo
Hong Kong Barcelona
Budapest

PD Dr. Wolfgang Hinkelbein
Dr. Gregor Bruggmoser
Prof. Dr. Hermann Frommhold
Radiologische Universitätsklinik
Abteilung Strahlentherapie
Hugstetter Strasse 55
W-7800 Freiburg, Germany

Prof. Dr. Michael Wannenmacher
Radiologische Universitätsklinik
Abteilung Radiologie
Im Neuenheimer Feld 400
W-6900 Heidelberg, Germany

ISBN-13:978-3-642-84894-0 e-ISBN-13:978-3-642-84892-6
DOI: 10.1007/978-3-642-84892-6

Library of Congress Cataloging-in-Publication Data. Acute and long-term side-effects of radiotherapy : biological basis and clinical relevance / W. Hinkelbein . . . [et al.]. p. cm. – (Recent results in cancer research : 130) Includes bibliographical references and index. ISBN-13:978-3-642-84894-0 1. Cancer – Radiotherapy – Side effects. 2. Radiotherapy – Side effects. I. Hinkelbein, W. (Wolfgang), 1948– . II. Series. [DNLM: 1. Radiotherapy – adverse effects. 2. Radiation Effects. 3. Radiation Injuries. W1 RE106P v.130 / WN 250 A189 1993] RC271.R3A27 1993 616.99'40642 – dc20 93-18099

Typesetting by Best-set Typesetter Ltd., Hong Kong
19/3130/SPS-5 4 3 2 1 0 – Printed on acid-free paper

Preface

In the radiation treatment of solid tumors as practiced today, radiotolerance in the surrounding tissues and organs is an important dose-limiting factor and so it determines the rate of local failure. Therefore it is very useful for clinicians and scientists to discuss experimental data with respect to their clinical relevance, as they did in November 1991 in Freiburg, Germany. Most of the papers presented at the symposium are summarized in this book.

This volume gives an up-to-date overview of both the present scientific basis and clinical experience of how normal tissues respond to curative radiotherapy. The basic principles of early and late normal tissue injuries are summarized with regard to the impact on the microvasculature, dose per fraction, repopulation, and repair. Experimental data and the clinical effects of irradiation on mucosa and skin, muscle, and the urinary bladder are discussed, covering questions of IORT and combined radiochemotherapy. Another topic is the effect of radiation on the lung and heart, including experimental study reports, aspects of diagnosis and prognosis, and TBI to condition patients for bone marrow transplantation. Radiation-induced sequelae in the CNS and the eye is another interesting field, with its special problems of myelopathy after hyperfractionated accelerated radiotherapy, stereotactic implants, and brain dysfunction in children, and acute and long-term neuropsychological effects. Particular problems in pediatric radiotherapy and a contribution pertaining to the incidence of second malignancies in patients with Hodgkin's disease complete this volume.

This scientific exchange should be continued, which hopefully will help us to reduce normal tissue damage without decreasing tumor radiation doses in the future.

Freiburg, January 1993

W. Hinkelbein
G. Bruggmoser

Contents

*List of Contributors**

* The address of the principal author is given on the first page of each contribution.

[1] Page on which contribution begins.

Reinhold, H. S. *1*
Ritter, J. *251*
Robbins, M. E. C. *1*
Roes, F. *259*
Rossi, R. *259*
Schaefer, U. W. *133*
Schäffer, G. *269*
Schellong, G. *259*
Schraube, R. *219*
Schultz-Hector, S. *145*
Schwarz, R. *103*
Sigmund, G. *123*
Slanina, J. *123, 269*
Steinberg, F. *109, 133*
Streffer, C. *133*
Turesson, I. *49*
Van Dyk, J. *189*
Von Eiff, M. *251*
Von Lengerke, H.-J. *251, 259*
Wagensommer C. *219*
Wannenmacher, M. *219*
Whitehouse, E. M. *1*
Wiegel, T. *103*
Wong, C. S. *189*
Wuismann, P. *251*

I. Basic Principles

Microvasculature and Radiation Damage

J.W. Hopewell[1], W. Calvo[2], R. Jaenke[3], H.S. Reinhold[4], M.E.C. Robbins[1], and E.M. Whitehouse[1]

[1] CRC Normal Tissue Radiobiology Research Group, Research Institute (University of Oxford), Churchill Hospital, Oxford, UK
[2] Institut für Arbeits- und Sozialmedizin der Universität Ulm, Fed. Rep. of Germany
[3] Department of Pathology, Colorado State University, Fort Collins, CO 80523, USA
[4] TNO Radiobiological Institute, Rijswijk, The Netherlands

Introduction

The association between late damage in irradiated tissues and the vasculature was reported shortly after the discovery of X-rays. Gross blood vessel abnormalities were a consistent finding in radiation-damaged tissues (Gassmann 1899; Mühsam 1904). Since then there have been numerous pathology reports emphasizing the significance of vascular damage in association with late radiation effects. This led to a hypothesis, to a major degree conceived by Rubin and Casarett (1968), that the vascular system was the main target for late radiation damage in normal tissues, the effects seen being related to vascular insufficiency. Although the validity of this hypothesis has been correctly challenged (Withers et al. 1980), there is still sufficient evidence to implicate the slowly dividing cells in the walls of blood vessels as the target cell populations in the pathogenesis of late radiation effects. Most recently, research related to radiation effects on the vasculature has focused on radiation-induced modifications in endothelial cell clonogenic survival and time-related changes in endothelial cell number. In addition, within the last decade, modifications in endothelial cell function have become more fully understood. Some of the most recent findings have raised the possibility of treating the endothelial-cell-mediated effects, leading to the amelioration of late radiation damage in normal tissues.

Radiation Effects on Endothelial Cells

Cell Survival Assays

For a cell to be considered to be reproductively viable after irradiation it must usually be shown to produce a progeny of at least 50 cells: a clone. Attempts to assess the clonogenic reproductive survival of endothelial cells in vivo have been made complex by the way the vasculature responds to a proliferative stimulus. Although the capillary sprouts produced in response to a stimulus may develop from a single viable endothelial cell, these sprouts rapidly anastomose to produce a neovascular network (Reinhold 1972). In a neovascular network it is not possible to count the capillary sprouts that would identify survival in truly clonogenic endothelial cells. As a result of this, assays of endothelial cell survival that have involved the application of a proliferative stimulus for a week or more (Fike and Gillette 1978; Reinhold and Buisman 1973) have measured changes in capillary density and not the number of endothelial cells or cell colonies directly.

The dose–effect curves obtained from such assays suggest the D_0 value for endothelial cells to be in the range 1.7–2.65 Gy (Hopewell 1983), similar to those for most mammalian cells and for endothelial cells assayed in vitro (Reinhold et al. 1991). Much higher D_0 values were obtained in two studies (Hopewell and Patterson 1972; Reinhold 1974) where capillary sprouts were counted, either directly or indirectly, although counting had to be carried out from 2 to 5 days after the first application of a proliferative stimulus. The shallow dose–effect curves, which were consistent with D_0 values of 9.0 Gy and 10.3 Gy, were thought to indicate subclonogenic endothelial cell proliferation (Reinhold et al. 1985). The terminal slopes of these dose–effect curves suggested only a change in effect of about 3%–5% per 1 Gy increment in dose.

Cell Numbers

There have been relatively few studies that have examined both the dose- and time-related changes in the density of endothelial cells after irradiation. Moreover, these studies have been carried out in simple vascular structures such as the mesentery of the mouse (Hirst et al. 1980) or in the vessels of the choroid plexus (Calvo et al. 1987) of the rat brain. Both studies indicated that the numbers of endothelial cells lining the walls of blood vessels declined rapidly in the first 3–9 weeks after irradiation with single doses of 17.5–30 Gy. This phenomenon was most adequately explained by a population of endothelial cells with a growth fraction of 1%–2% rapidly cycling cells, rather than a population in which all cells were cycling very slowly (Hirst et al. 1980). The half time for the loss of endothelial cell nuclei from the choroid plexus after single doses of 17.5–25 Gy was 8.4 ± 0.6

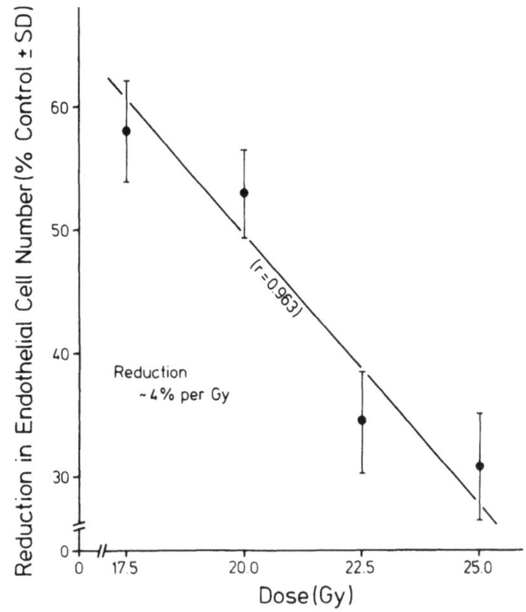

Fig. 1. Dose-related changes in the maximum reduction in the relative number of endothelial cell nuclei in the vessels of the choroid plexus of the rat brain 26–52 weeks after single doses of irradiation. Error bars indicate ±SE. (From Hopewell et al. 1989, with permission)

weeks, range 6.7–9.6 weeks (Hopewell et al. 1989). In both vascular systems there was either direct or indirect evidence of an attempt at repopulation by surviving endothelial cells (Hirst et al. 1980; Calvo et al. 1987). These time-related changes in endothelial cell number in these simple vascular models are broadly in keeping with those found in more complex tissues, such as the vasculature of the dermis in the pig (Archambeau et al. 1984). In this tissue there was also evidence of increased proliferation by surviving endothelial cells, which was sometimes very extensive, leading to the physical occlusion of blood vessels by "clones" of cells (Hopewell 1983).

The maximum reduction in the density of endothelial cell nuclei in the choroid plexus of the irradiated rat brain indicated a very shallow dose–effect relationship (Fig. 1). The slope of the linear regression line fit to the data points suggested a change in effect of about 4% per Gray, similar to that reported above. This has been interpreted as an indication of the dose–response relationship for subclonogenic proliferation in endothelial cells.

Cell Function

In recent years there has been a marked and rapid expansion in knowledge as to the complex functions carried out by endothelial cells, the important molecules they synthesize, and their interactions with the blood and the cells and matrix of the subendothelium (Jaffe 1987). The importance of these direct effects of radiation on endothelial cell functions and/or changes in function resulting from endothelial cell loss are still not fully understood (Fajardo 1989; Pearson 1991). The endothelial cell functions that may have the most bearing on our understanding of the late radiation response of normal tissues are related to coagulation, inflammation, the immune response, and specific metabolic activities.

Endothelial cells produce and express angiotensin-converting enzyme (ACE) on their surfaces and its expression has been shown to decline progressively with time after irradiation in the lung (Ward et al. 1983). This effect parallels the decrease in pulmonary arterial perfusion. The latency associated with a 50% reduction in ACE activity was approximately 8 weeks after 25 Gy, and at 2 and 6 months after irradiation the dose-related reduction in ACE activity was represented by a change in effect of about 4% per Gray (Fig. 2). The observed decrease in ACE activity may be a direct result of radiation injury to the pulmonary endothelium or it may simply reflect the loss of endothelial cells. The changes in the time- and dose-related response in the severity of this effect, when compared directly with that for the loss of endothelial cells in other systems (Hopewell et al. 1989), would indicate the latter to be true. This suggestion is also consistent with electron microscopic evidence suggesting endothelial cell lethality for times greater than 30 days after irradiation. In addition to this dose-related decline in ACE activity (Ward et al. 1987) there was a comparable reduction in plasminogen activator (PLA) activity and increases in the production of prostacyclin (PGI_2) and thromboxane (TXA_2) (Ward et al. 1983).

Studies on the effects of radiation on PGI_2 production both "in vitro" and "in vivo" and its relationship to TXA_2 production infer an imbalance in the PGI_2/TXA_2 ratio (Allen et al. 1981; Sinzinger et al. 1984), excess levels of TXA_2 being associated with vasoconstriction and proaggregatory changes. The endothelium can also express prothrombotic activity, abetted by the presence of cytokines or pathological factors which include oxygen-derived free radicals (Boisseau 1991). This results in the increased expression of adhesion molecules, such as ELAM-1 (endothelial leukocyte adhesion molecule) and ICAM-1 (intracellular adhesion molecule), on the cell surface which increase the attachment of leukocytes and lymphocytes to the endothelium, respectively. The nature of these interactions has recently been uncovered but appears to have considerable pathophysiological significance (Lipowski et al. 1988; Dinerman and Mehta 1990; Pober and Cotran 1991).

An increased expression (upregulation) of adhesion molecules by endothelial cells, as has been reported for endothelial cells irradiated "in vitro" (Dunn et al. 1986; Matzner et al. 1988), may help to explain some recent observations in irradiated tissues. Investigations in the glomerulus of the irradiated kidney of pigs have indicated an increased accumulation of leukocytes some 6–9 weeks after irradiation. The results of electron microscopic studies have clearly illustrated the close interaction, possibly adhesion, between the leukocytes and the endothelium (Fig. 3). At longer time

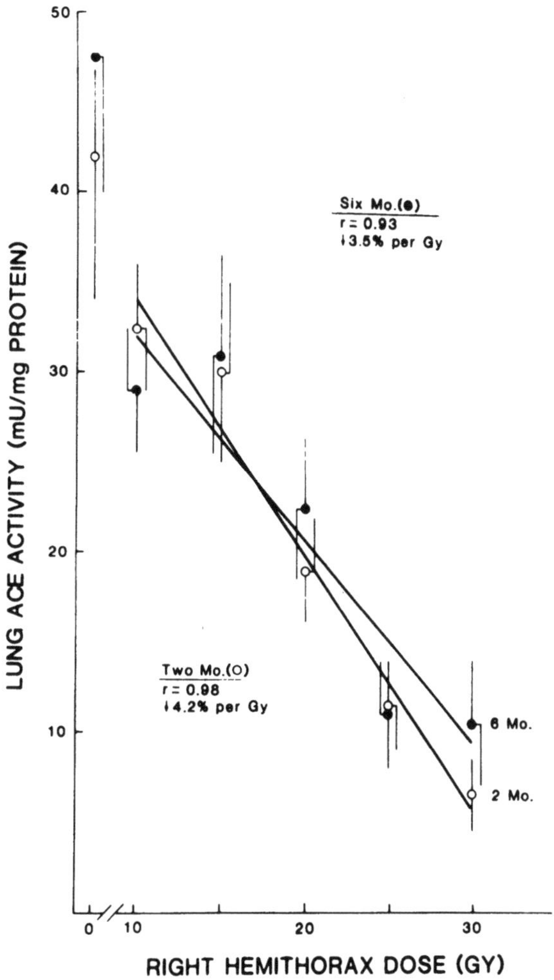

Fig. 2. Dose-related changes in the ACE activity in the right lung of the rat at 2 months (*open circles*) and 6 months (*filled circles*) after irradiation with single doses of X-rays. Error bars indicate ±SE. (Redrawn from Ward et al. 1985)

intervals after irradiation leukocytes are found in the subendothelial space. The endothelium is also separated from the basement membrane and the space filled with an amorphous material (Fig. 4), resulting in a marked reduction in glomerular capillary lumina.

In other studies designed to examine the effects of radiation on the spinal cord of pigs, observations made with respect to the main inferior artery are of specific interest. The adhesion of leukocytes to the endothelium was noted approximately 8 weeks after irradiation with single doses of 25.0–29.0 Gy of ^{60}Co γ-rays (Fig. 5). At later times there was an infiltration of leukocytes into the subendothelial space and the deposition of amorphous

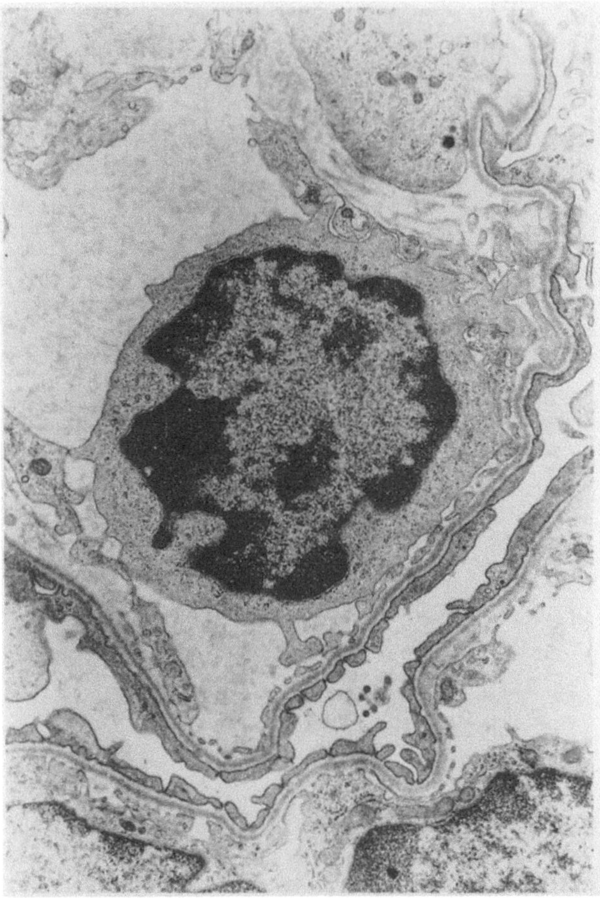

Fig. 3. The close association between a leukocyte present within the glomerular capillary lumen and the endothelia; note the foot processes emanating from the leukocyte. Electron micrograph taken from a renal biopsy obtained 9 weeks after the irradiation of both kidneys of a mature pig with a single dose of 9.8 Gy of γ-rays. (×4200)

material and loose connective tissue between the endothelium and the internal elastic lamina (Fig. 6). At 3–6 months after irradiation the lumen of vessels may be occluded to a varying degree (Fig. 7) by cells. This has been referred to as myointimal proliferation in pathology reports of radiation-induced damage to medium-sized arteries in man (Reinhold et al. 1990). The accumulation and perivascular infiltration of leukocytes was also seen in the microcirculation of the spinal cord in the same histological selections prior to the onset of white matter necrosis, the lesion characteristic of late radiation-induced damage to the central nervous system (CNS) (Hopewell

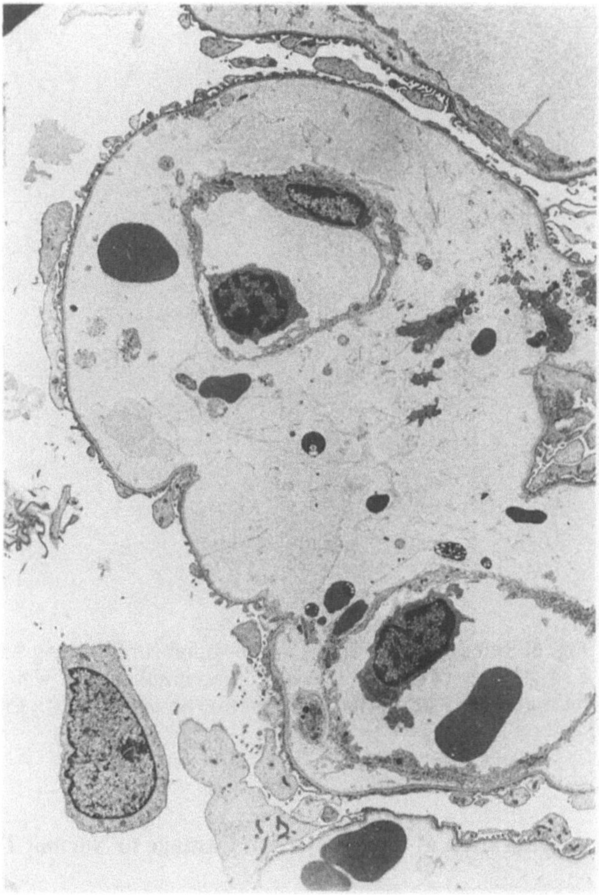

Fig. 4. A pronounced reduction in the size of the glomerular capillary lumen due to the presence of a subendothelial transudate lifting the endothelium away from the glomerular capillary basement membrane. Leukocytes are present within the lumen of both capillaries. Electron micrograph from a renal biopsy obtained 12 weeks after radiation with a single dose of 9.8 Gy of γ-rays. ($\times$2000)

1979). This may also account for the progressive increase in cells, that were termed microglia, in the rat brain after irradiation (Mildenberger et al. 1990). Microglia, the mononuclear-phagocyte system in the CNS (Hickey and Kimura 1988), would appear to infiltrate from the blood. It is an open question as to whether microglia actively destroy viable myelin within the irradiated CNS. However, in other conditions, such as the inflammatory demyelinating lesions of experimental encephalomyelitis, a link with blood-borne cells would appear to have been established, as has the initial lymphocyte/endothelial cell interaction (Raine et al. 1990).

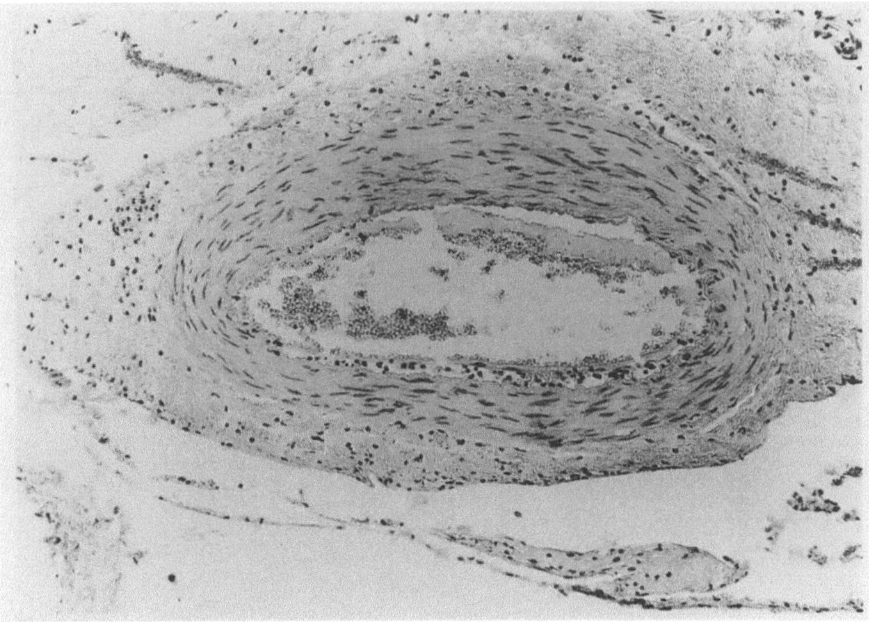

Fig. 5. Inferior spinal artery in the spinal cord of a pig 9 weeks after irradiation with a single dose of 29 Gy. There is on accumulation of white cells, possibly leukocytes, on the endothelial surface. (Hematoxylin and eosin, ×150)

Amelioration of Late Radiation Damage to Normal Tissues

The identification of endothelial cells as a potential primary target cell population, damage to which eventually leads to the expression of late radiation effects, suggests that it may be possible to develop treatment strategies for the modification of the direct and indirect effects of radiation on endothelial cell function. There are no pathognomonic characteristics that can identify the lesions of radiation injury to the vasculature. The changes that have been reported, which include blood vessel wall thickening, vessel dilation, endoarteritis, leukocyte accumulation, the perivascular infiltration of white cells, and thrombosis are not unique to radiation injury but are also, for example, the events consequent on cerebral vascular disease, peripheral vascular disease, and shock. They may all represent secondary effects resulting from endothelial cell loss or modified endothelial cell function. The prevention of these secondary events along lines proposed for other types of vascular-mediated injury would appear to represent a rationale for the amelioration of radiation-induced late effects in normal tissues. Examples of these approaches will be outlined below.

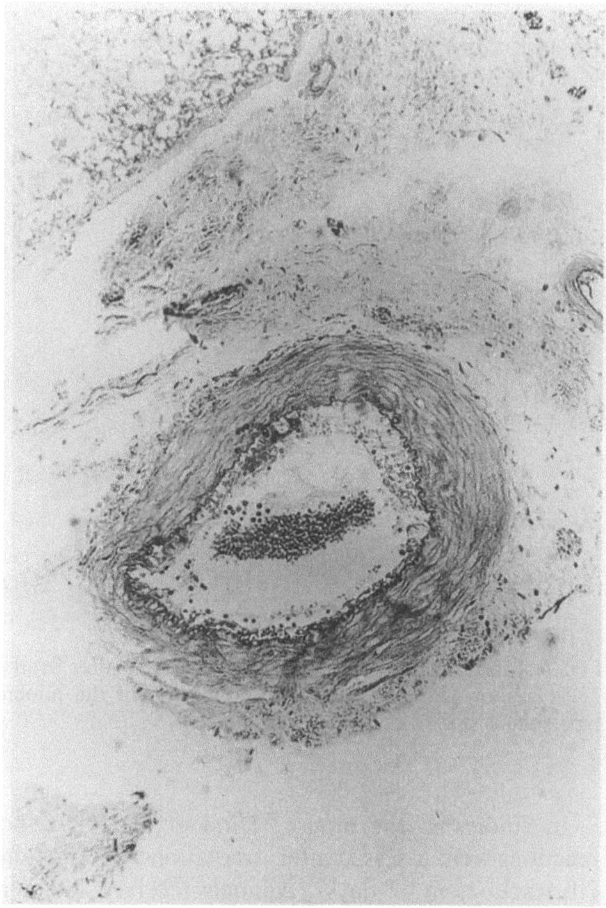

Fig. 6. Inferior spinal artery of a pig 11 weeks after irradiation with a single dose of 29 Gy. There is continued white cell accumulation on the surface of endothelial cells, separation of the endothelium from the internal elastic lamina, and the accumulation of amorphous material in the subendothelial space. (Luxol fast blue, PAS ×150)

Application of Hemorheological Agents

Pentoxifylline is a potent hemorheological agent used in the treatment of several conditions including peripheral and cerebral vascular disease (Aviado and Parker 1984; Muller and Lehrach 1981). Its actions are numerous and include an increased deformability and reduced stickiness of leukocytes, and a reduction in red cell aggregation and platelet aggregation/adhesion, thereby lowering blood viscosity. There is also a reduction in TXA_2 synthesis; PGI_2 levels are increased.

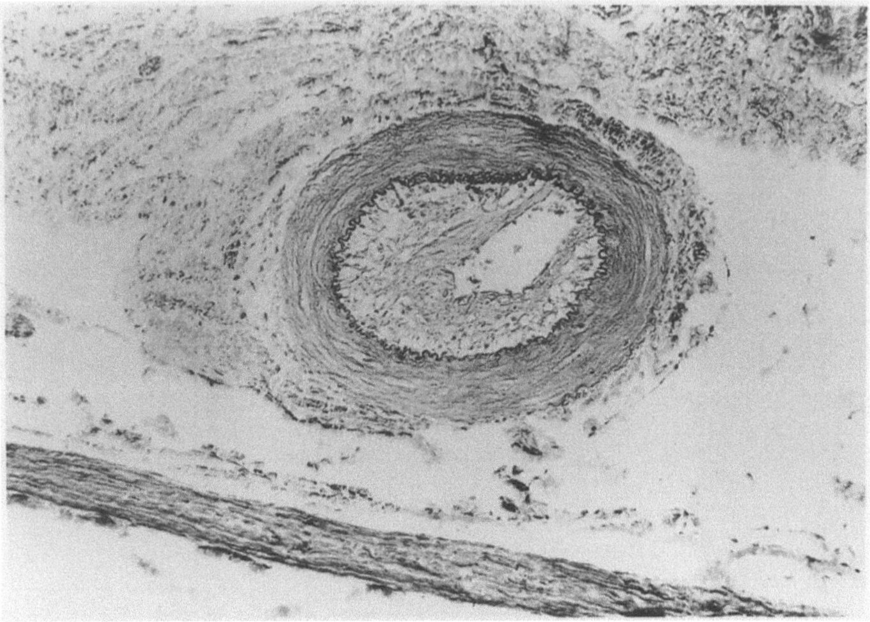

Fig. 7. Inferior spinal artery of a pig 14 weeks after irradiation with a single dose of 27.5 Gy shows almost complete obliteration of the lumen of the vessel by fibrous-type tissue. (Luxol fast blue, PAS ×150)

In studies in the mouse (Dion et al. 1989), both early and late skin reactions were assessed after irradiation with fractionated doses of 40–70 Gy (10 fractions in 12 days). Animals received either pentoxifylline (50 mg/kg daily) or saline subcutaneously from the first day of irradiation for the full observation period of 30 weeks. Treatment with pentoxifylline had no effect on the severity of the acute skin reaction; however, the magnitude of the late response was significantly reduced. Probit analysis of the results given by Dion et al. (1989) for the dose-related incidence of animals showing a late skin score of ⩾3.0 suggested a dose-modification factor (DMF) of approximately 1.4. This calculation assumed that the slopes of the dose–effect curves for treated and control animals were the same (Fig. 8). The applicability of these very significant findings, which have potentially important implications for radiotherapy, have to be confirmed in other late-responding normal tissues.

Oxygen-Derived Free Radicals and Post-ischemic Tissue Injury

Some of the ischemia that develops in tissues after irradiation will be transient, and as reperfusion takes place reperfusion injury could exacerbate

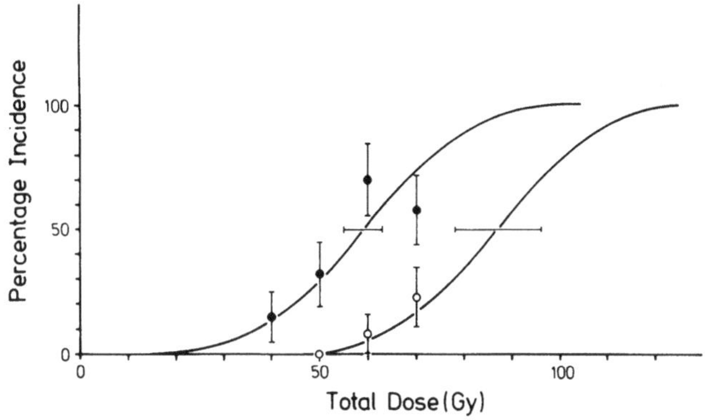

Fig. 8. Dose-related changes in the proportion of mice showing a late radiation response with a score of $\geqslant 3.0$ in the skin of the foot, 18–30 weeks after irradiation with total doses given in 10 fractions over 12 days. Animals were given daily subcutaneous injections of either pentoxifylline (*open circles*) or saline (*filled circles*) from the first day of irradiation. Error bars indicate ±SE. (Dose–effect curves based on data provided in Dion et al. 1988)

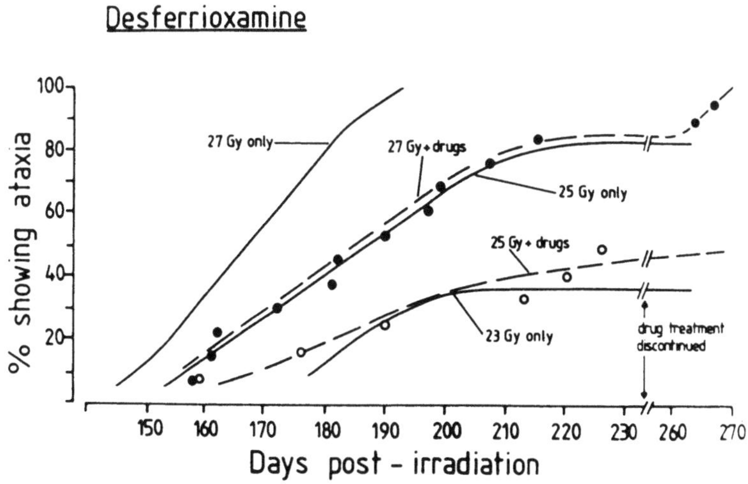

Fig. 9. The time-related incidence of rats developing ataxia after irradiation of the spinal cord with single doses of X-rays. Irradiation was either given alone (*continuous line*) or was given to animals that received desferrioxamine (*broken line*) from 17 to 34 weeks after irradiation. (From Hornsey et al. 1990, with permission)

the initial radiation-induced damage. Reperfusion injury occurs because superoxide radicals or H_2O_2 are converted to damaging hydroxyl radicals (Weisfeldt 1987). This reaction requires iron as a catalyst. In studies in the rat (Hornsey et al. 1990) animals were fed a low-iron diet from 12 weeks after local irradiation of the spinal cord and received disferrioxamine mesylate, an iron chelating agent, from 17 weeks after irradiation (30 mg in 0.3 ml subcutaneously, three times weekly). These animals showed a later time of development and a lower incidence of ataxia, related to white matter necrosis, than those receiving radiation alone (Fig. 9). This change in response represents a small but significant DMF of approximately 1.1.

Modification of Eicosanoid Metabolism

It has been shown that the administration of the essential fatty acid, precursors of prostaglandins, can modify eicosanoid pathways. Gammalinolenic acid (GLA) will preferentially increase exogenous levels of prostaglandin E_1 (PGE_1), which has a range of desirable actions (Horrobin 1988) including the blocking of PGE_2 and TXA_2 production (Fig. 10). TXA_1 has few of the potentially damaging effects of TXA_2. To examine the potential advantages of modifying prostaglandin pathways on late radiation damage to skin, pigs were given GLA for approximately 4 weeks prior to irradiation to allow for a new equilibrium to be reached, and for 16 weeks after irradiation of small, 22.5 mm diameter areas of skin with single doses of 20–40 Gy of $^{90}Sr/^{90}Y$ β-rays. GLA was given orally in the form of an oil (So-1100 8%–10% by volume; Scotia Pharmaceuticals), 3 ml/day. The results were compared with

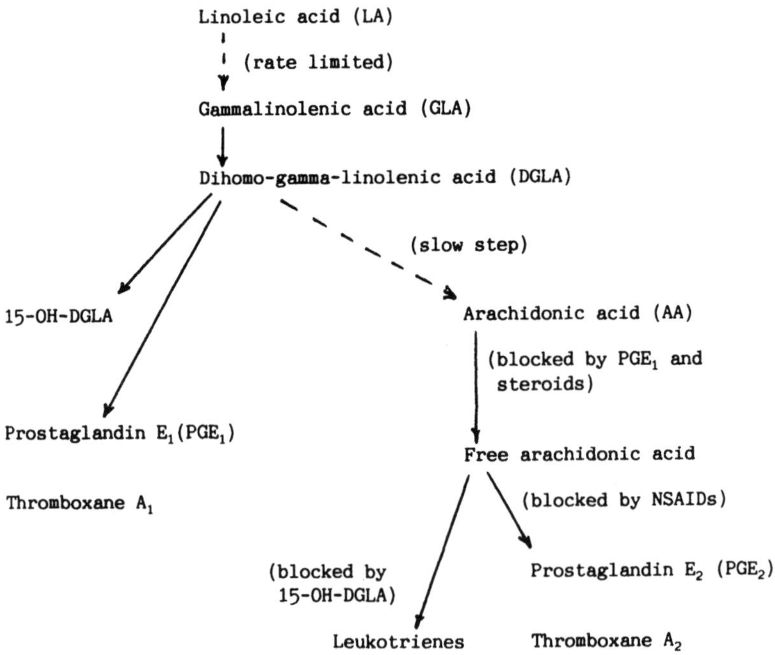

Fig. 10. The proposed pathways for the derivation of prostaglandins of the E_1 and E_2 series from essential fatty acids

Table 1. Variation in the ED_{50} values (±SE) for the late reactions in pig skin of necrosis (N) and dusky/mauve erythema (D/E) following different pre- and post-irradiation treatments

Treatment time (wk)	Reaction	ED_{50} ± SE (Gy)		DMF
		GLA	Placebo	
−4	D/E	26.5 ± 1.3	27.5 ± 1.1	0.96 ± 0.06
	N	34.8 ± 1.4	35.0 ± 1.5	0.99 ± 0.06
−4/+16	D/E	35.9 ± 1.9	24.8 ± 1.5	1.45 ± 0.12[a]
	N	40.6 ± 1.3	35.7 ± 1.6	1.14 ± 0.06[a]

[a] Significant DMF (⩽0.02)

the response seen in irradiated animals receiving a placebo (sunflower oil) and in animals receiving GLA or the placebo for only 4 weeks prior to irradiation. It has been proposed that prostaglandins may protect against damage from ionizing radiation (Steel and Catravas 1988).

For the late skin reactions of dusky/mauve erythema (an indicator of dermal ischemia) and dermal necrosis, significant modification of the response was seen in animals that received GLA over the time course for the development of these late reactions (Table 1). No modification of the responses was seen when GLA was only given prior to irradiation, indicating no direct radioprotection from raised exogenous levels of PGE_1.

The greater DMF for the dusky/mauve erythema reaction (DMF 1.45 ± 0.12), as compared with dermal necrosis (DMF 1.14 ± 0.06), may reflect the presence of inflammation that is usually associated with this response. Leukotrienes, specifically leukotriene B_4 (LTB_4), have a major role to play in inflammation (Smith 1982) and their production is blocked by another product of GLA administration, 15-OH-dihomo-gamma-linolenic acid (15-OH-DGLA), (Horrobin and Manku 1990). This could explain, at least in part, why GLA also produced a marked reduction in the severity of the acute erythematous reaction in pig skin (Hopewell et al. 1992).

Conclusions

Endothelial cells are lost from the walls of blood vessels within a few weeks of irradiation with equivalent therapeutic doses; the half time was of the order of 8 weeks. Comparison of the dose–effect relationships for the reduction in endothelial cell number or of that for direct or indirect changes in endothelial cell function suggests that subclonogenic proliferation may be sufficient to help to preserve vascular integrity after irradiation.

The changes in endothelial cell function and changes in the vessels after irradiation are not pathognomonic and would suggest that therapies effective in the amelioration of other vascular-mediated lesions may also be effective in reducing the consequences of the vascular component in late radiation-induced damage. Hemorheological agents, compounds that modify the consequences of reperfusion injury, and the modulation of eicosanoid metabolism have all been shown to be effective in reducing the severity of late radiation-induced damage, by a degree that is associated with dose modification factors of between 1.1 and 1.4. The prospects of the safe delivery of a 10%–40% higher radiation dose to normal tissues would be of significant therapeutic advantage in many treatment sites. The successful amelioration of radiation damage by interventional therapies that are targeted to the vasculature provides indirect evidence as to the importance of vascular damage in the pathogenesis of late radiation-induced effects in normal tissues.

References

Archambeau JO, Ines A, Fajardo LF (1984) Response of swine skin microvasculature to acute single exposures of x-rays: quantification of endothelial changes. Radiat Res 98:37–51

Allen JB, Sagerman RH, Stuart MJ (1981) Irradiation decreases vascular prostacyclin formation with no concomitant effects on platelet thromboxane production. Lancet 2:1193–1196

Aviado DM, Porter JM (1984) Pentoxifylline: a new drug for the treatment of intermittent claudication. Pharmacotherapy 6:297–307

Boisseau MR (1991) Microcirculation and microrheology. In: Vanhoutte PM, Douste-Blazy Ph (eds) Fish oil and blood–vessel wall interactions. Libbey Eurotext, Paris, pp 17–36

Calvo W, Hopewell JW, Reinhold HS, van den Berg AP, Yeung TK (1987) Dose-dependent and time-dependent changes in the choroid plexus of the irradiated rat brain. Br J Radiol 60:1109–1117

Dinerman JL, Mehta JL (1990) Endothelial, platelet and leukocyte interactions in ischemic heart disease: insight into potential mechanisms and their clinical relevance. J Am Coll Cardiol 16:207–222

Dion MW, Hussey DH, Osborne JW (1989) The effect of pentoxifylline on early and late radiation injury following fractionated irradiation in C_3H mice. Int J Radiat Oncol Biol Phys 17:101–107

Dunn MM, Drab EA, Rubin DB (1986) Effects of irradiation on endothelial cell polymorphonuclear leukocyte interactions. J Appl Physiol 60:1932–1937

Fajardo LF (1989) The unique physiology of endothelial cells and its implications in radiobiology. Front Radiat Ther Oncol 23:96–112

Fike JR, Gillette EL (1978) ^{60}Co gamma and negative Pi meson irradiation of microvasculature. Int J Radiat Oncol Biol Phys 4:825–828

Gassmann A (1899) Zur Histologie der Roentgenulcera. Fortschr Rontgenstr 2:199–207

Hickey WF, Kimura H (1988) Perivascular microglial cells of the CNS are bone-marrow derived and present antigen in vivo. Science 239:290–292

Hirst DG, Denekamp J, Hobson B (1980) Proliferation studies of the endothelial and smooth muscle cells of the mouse mesentery after irradiation. Cell Tissue Kinet 13:91–104

Hopewell JW (1979) Late radiation damage to the central nervous system: a radiobiological interpretation. Neuropathol Appl Neurobiol 5:329–343

Hopewell JW (1983) Radiation effects on vascular tissue. In: Potten CS, Hendry JH (eds) Cytotoxic insult to tissue. Churchill Livingstone, Edinburgh, pp 228–257

Hopewell JW, Patterson TJS (1972) The effect of previous x-irradiation on the revascularization of free skin grafts in the pig. Biorheology 9:45

Hopewell JW, Calvo W, Reinhold HS (1989) Radiation effects on blood vessels: role in normal tissue damage. In: Steel GG, Adams GE, Horwich A (eds) The biological basis of radiotherapy, 2nd edn. Elsevier, Amsterdam, pp 101–113

Hopewell JW, Robbins MEC, Scott C (1992) The effects of So-1100 in reducing the severity of radiation-induced damage to pig skin. In: Nigam S, Honn KV, Mornott LJ, Walden T (eds) Eicosanoids and other bioactive lipids in cancer, inflammation and radiation injury. Kluwer Acad Pub (Boston), pp 345–348

Hornsey S, Myers R, Jenkinson T (1990) The reduction of radiation damage to the spinal cord by post-irradiation administration of vasoactive drugs. Int J Radiat Oncol Biol Phys 18:1437–1442

Horrobin DF (1988) Prostaglandin E_1: physiological significance and clinical use. Wien Klin Wochenschr 10:471–477

Horrobin DF, Manku MS (1990) Clinical biochemistry of essential fatty acids. In: Horrobin DF (ed) Omega-6 essential fatty acids: pathophysiology and roles in clinical medicine. Liss, New York, pp 21–53

Jaffe EA (1987) Cell biology of endothelial cells. Hum Pathol 18:234–239

Lipowsky HH, House SD, Firnell JC (1988) Leukocyte endothelial adhesion and microvascular hemodynamics. Adv Exp Med Biol 242:85–93

Matzner Y, Cohn M, Hyfim E, Razin E, Futs Z, Buchanan MR, Haas TA, Vlodarsky I, Eldar A (1988) Generation of lipid neutrophil chemoattractant by irradiated bovine aortic endothelial cells. J Immunol 140: 2681–2685

Mildenberger M, Beah TG, McGear EG, Ludgate CM (1990) An animal model of prophylatic cranial irradiation: histological effects at acute, early and delayed stages. Int J Radiat Oncol Biol Phys 18: 1051–1060

Mühsam R (1904) Über Dermatitis der Hand nach Roentgenbestrahlung (Fingeramputation). Arch Klin Chir 74(2):434–453

Muller R, Lehrach F (1981) Haemorheology and cerebrovascular disease: multifunctional approach with pentoxifylline. Curr Med Res Opin 7:253–263

Pearson JD (1991) Endothelial cell biology. Radiology 179:9–14

Pober JS, Cotran RS (1991) What can be learned from the expression of endothelial adhesion molecules in tissues? Lab Invest 64:301–305

Raine CS, Cannella B, Duijvestijn AM, Cross AH (1990) Homing to central nervous system vasculature by antigen-specific lymphocytes. II. Lymphocyte/endothelial cell adhesion during the initial stages of autoimmune demyelination. Lab Invest 63:476–489

Reinhold HS (1972) Radiation and the microcirculation. Front Radiat Ther Oncol 6:44–51

Reinhold HS (1974) Cell viability in the vessel wall. Curr Top Radiat Res Q 10:9–28

Reinhold HS, Buisman GH (1973) Radiosensitivity of capillary endothelium. Br J Radiol 46:54–57

Reinhold HS, Hopewell JW, Buisman GH (1985) Colony regeneration techniques in vascular endothelium. In: Potten CS, Hendry JH (eds) Cell clones. Churchill Livingstone, Edinburgh, pp 160–169

Reinhold HS, Fajardo LF, Hopewell JW (1990) The vascular system. Adv Radiat Biol 14:177–226

Reinhold HS, Hopewell JW, Calvo W, Keyeux A, Reyners H (1991) Vasculo-connective tissue. In: Scherer E, Streffer C, Trott K-R (eds) Radiopathology of organs and tissues. Springer, Berlin Heidelbery New York, pp 243–268

Rubin P, Casarett GW (1968) Clinical radiation pathology, vols I and II. Saunders, Philadelphia

Sinzinger H, Cromwell M, Firbas W (1984) Long-lasting depression of rabbit aorta prostacyclin formation by single-dose irradiation. Radiat Res 97:533–536

Smith MJH (1982) Biological activities of leukotriene B_4 (isomer III). In: Samuelsson B, Paoletti R (eds) Advances in prostoglandin, thromboxane and leukotriene research, vol 9. Raven, New York, pp 282–292

Steel LK, Catravas GN (1988) Protection against ionizing radiation with eicosanoids. In: Polgar (ed) Eicosanoids in radiation. Kluwer, Boston, pp 79–87

Ward WF, Molteni A, Solliday NH, Jones GE (1985) The relationship between endothelial dysfunction and collagen accumulation in irradiated rat lung. Int J Radiat Oncol Biol Phys 11:1985–1990

Ward WF, Molteni A, Ts'ao CH, Solliday NH (1987) Pulmonary endothelial cell dysfunction induced by unilateral as compared to bilateral thoracic irradiation in rats. Radiat Res 111:101–106

Ward WF, Solliday NH, Molteni A, Port CD (1983) Radiation injury in rat lung II: angiotensin-converting enzyme activity. Radiat Res 96:294–300

Weisfeldt ML (1987) Reperfusion and reperfusion injury. Clin Res 35:13–20

Withers HR, Peters LJ, Kogelnik HS (1980) The pathobiology of late effects of irradiation. In: Meyn RE, Withers HR (eds) Radiation biology in cancer research. Raven, New York, pp 439–448

The Time Factor for Late Reactions in Radiotherapy: Repopulation or Intracellular Repair?

J.H. Hendry and Y.-M. Jen

Department of Experimental Radiation Oncology, Paterson Institute for Cancer Research, Christie Hospital (NHS) Trust, Manchester M20 9BX, UK

Introduction

When doses in radiotherapy are protracted over increasing periods of time, it is generally considered that very little extra dose is required (the time factor) to reach tolerance for late reactions. This is in contrast to repopulation in early-reacting tissues and in tumors (e.g., Withers et al. 1988). Nevertheless, time factors have been reported for late-reacting tissues, and even small values could sometimes be more important than in the cases of early-reacting normal tissues and tumors because of the greater steepness of dose–incidence curves for injury in late-reacting organs (e.g., Thames et al. 1989; Hendry 1989).

Time factors are often expressed as the extra dose per day, using 2-Gy fractions, required to be isoeffective or to reach tolerance. Higher doses per day would be required using lower doses per fraction, and vice versa. This can be expressed mathematically using the linear quadratic model, with the time factor expressed as $\gamma/(\alpha + \beta d)$ in Gy/day (Tucker and Travis 1990). The maximum value of (γ/α) applies when $d = 0$ i.e., using very low doses per fraction or low-dose-rate exposures. The value of the time factor (Gy/day) using any particular dose per fraction, d, is:

$$\frac{(\text{Gy/day})_{\text{max}}}{1 + \dfrac{d}{\alpha/\beta}}$$

where α/β is the fractionation sensitivity chracteristic of a particular tissue. Also, doses can be normalized to the common dose per fraction of 2 Gy:

$$\text{Normalized dose} = D\frac{(\alpha/\beta + d)}{(\alpha/\beta + 2)}$$

where D is the dose given in fractions of dose d.

Recent Results in Cancer Research, Vol. 130

Some unexpected time factors have been reported for late-reacting tissues. For example, a value of 0.29 Gy/day was reported for telangiectasia in skin, in contrast to 0 Gy/day for early desquamation (Turesson and Notter 1984; Thames et al. 1990). This is the opposite of what might be expected for slowly -renewing vasculature versus more rapidly renewing epidermis. Also, a significant time factor between 18 and 39 days overall treatment was reported for the pig kidney using X-rays but not using neutrons (Robbins et al. 1991a). If repopulation was the cause of the effect for X-rays, it is difficult to see why this should not also happen after irradiation with neutrons (see below).

This chapter summarizes the evidence for the presence of time factors in late-reacting tissues in man and in experimental systems, and addresses the question of whether long-term intracellular repair contributes to these effects.

Human Data

The human evidence is summarized in Table 1. Clearly seen is the expected high dose per day found in oral mucosa, and the unexpected lack of it in skin. Also, the lack of an effect of a 3-week interval between two courses of radiotherapy of the larynx contrasts with the time factor observed for late reactions in skin, oral cavity, and lung. Interestingly, the opinions of 170 radiotherapists in the United Kingdom support the notion of a time factor for tissue tolerance. In the survey by the Royal College of Radiologists (Priestman et al. 1989) 6 cases were described, and opinions on treatment protocols were obtained. These data were assumed by Hendry and Roberts (1991) to be either isoeffective or at least at isotolerance levels, which is likely to be true for the 2 radical cases anyway. Although the values of Gy/day will have quite large errors attached, it is interesting that the two values for breast are of the same order, as are the two values for bronchus. Noteworthy also is the fact that the values of Gy/day for the radical treatment were equivalent to time exponents of 0.16 and 0.14 respectively in the Ellis formula (Ellis 1967), with the other exponents being 0.22, 0.11, 0.15 and 0.50 (Hendry and Roberts 1991). These are of the same order or higher than the original value of 0.11, which was based on early skin reactions.

Experimental Data

The experimental evidence is summarized in Table 2. Seen here is the slow-repair phenomenon reported in the lung, its possible effect in callus inhibition, and the lack of it in spinal cord. With increasing overall times, a time factor becomes important for the spinal cord, the tumour bed, and the

Table 1. Estimated values of the extra dose per day tolerated by human tissues when treatment is prolonged (Thames et al. 1990; Hendry and Roberts 1991)

Tissues	Time range	Dose per day (Gy)	Reference
Early reactions			
Oral mucosa	Toward end of 6-week treatment	1.8	Thames et al. (1990)
Acute responses head and neck	11–49 days	0.6	Fowler (1991)
Skin (desquamation)	to 6 weeks	0	Turesson and Notter (1984)
Late reactions			
Skin (telangiectasia)	11–40 days	0.29	Turesson and Thames (1989)
	3 weeks split	0	
Oral cavity	15–80 days	0.29	Maciejewski et al. (1990)
Larynx	3 weeks split	0	Overgaard et al. (1988)
Lung (pneumonitis)	12–60 days	0.45	van Dyk et al. (1989)
RCR survey			Hendry and Roberts (1991)
Radical			
Breast	15–59 days	0.56	
Vocal cord	18–52 days	0.43	
Palliation			
Bronchus	1–40 days	0.98	
Breast	1–26 days	0.79	
Uncertain value			
Bronchus	1–40 days	0.76	
Rectum	12–52 days	0.92	

kidney (in the pig). In the last case, interestingly, the values appear to depend on the level of injury (i.e., 0.21 to 0.42, etc.) and the fraction size (i.e., 0.21 to 0.36, etc.).

Recovery occurs also *after* irradiation, at least in endothelium and in parenchymal colony-forming cells in liver and in kidney (Table 3). Thus in the kidney, the repair that occurs *during* a course of fractionation continues to occur *after* it is completed.

A summary of the data for recovery in vivo using cellular endpoints (colony formation and chromosome damage) is shown in Fig. 1. For simplicity the data are presented in the form of dose reduction factors (DRF), for equivalent effect when the assay time after irradiation is delayed. The origin of all the lines is at DRF = 1.0, t = 1 day. This shows the substantial early or late recovery in various types of cells which can be detected either in the small subpopulation of cells capable of forming colonies or in the larger complement of cells capable of at least one division to express chromosome aberrations or micronuclei. Interestingly, a line

Table 2. Values of the time factor in experimental tissues expressed as the extra dose per day required to reach the endpoint when the treatment time is increased, normalized to 2 Gy per fraction. Values calculated from data reported in the literature, using α/β ratios quoted in the original articles or assumed to be 3 Gy

Tissue endpoint	Time range (days)	Dose/day (Gy)	Reference
During fractionation			
Lumbar cord,	1–16	0	White and Hornsey (1978)
paralysis	16–32	1.6	
Cervical cord,	1–15	0	White and Hornsey (1980)
paralysis	15–60	0.50	
	60–120	0.37	
Lung, pneumonitis	1–9	0.83–1.12	Field and Hornsey (1974);
	9–28	0.31	Field et al. (1976)
Lung, pneumonitis	1–7	0.56–3.14	Travis and Down (1981)
and breathing rate	7–28	0.08–0.26	
Tumor bed	1–42	0	Terry et al. (1988)
	42–84	0.18	
Callus inhibition	1–7	0.43–0.66	Hayashi and Suit (1971)
	7–28	0.04–0.07	
Kidney function	4–40	0.23–0.47	Williams and Denekamp (1984);
	20–40	0.16–0.69	Williams et al. (1985)
Kidney function	5–39	−0.05	Hopewell and Wiernik (1977)
(pig)	18–39	0.43	
Kidney function	18–39	0.21–0.36	Robbins et al. (1991a)
(pig)		0.31–0.44	
		0.42–0.50	
After fractionation			
Endothelium,	0–16	1.04	Reinhold and Buisman (1975)
fluorescence index	16–32	0.79	
Tumor bed	1–180	0.003–0.04	Hill et al. (1989)
Liver, hepatocyte	14–42	0.37	Fisher et al. (1988)
colonies	42–330	0.60	
Kidney, epithelial colonies	1–42	0.18	Jen and Hendry (1993)

describing a time exponent of 0.11 would cross the right upper line at about the label (4, 8), indicating the quite substantial amount of this type of recovery.

Repopulation or Repair?

It is difficult to separate the components of repopulation and intracellular repair in the recovery phenomena without having a way of affecting one but

Table 3. Values of the time factor for kidney clonogens X-irradiated in situ and assayed in vitro

Time range (days)	Dose per day (Gy)
During irradiation	
2–4	0.20
4–8	0.55
16–40	0.077
2–40[a]	*0.12*
After irradiation	
1–42[a]	0.18
42–180	−0.03
180–365	0.050
1–365	0.034

Values of dose per day are shown for fractionated irradiations with increasing interfraction intervals followed by assay after one further interval, or a constant interfraction interval (12 h) followed by increasing delay periods before subsequent assay. The values were calculated from dose – response curves, using an isosurvival level of 0.1 which corresponded to about 8 Gy single dose or 17 Gy in the 8 fractions used in these experiments (Jen and Hendry 1993)
[a]Note data for same time range

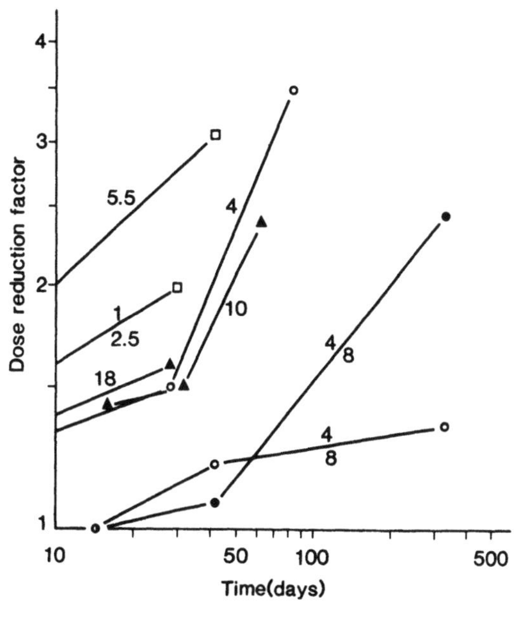

Fig. 1. Dose reduction factors (DRF) as a function of time delay after irradiation and before assay for colony formation or chromosome damage. The DRF was calculated as the factorial increase in dose required to produce the same effect as at 1 day after irradiation. *Filled symbols* refer to colony formation, and *open symbols* to chromosome damage, for parenchymal cells in liver (*circles*) and thyroid (*squares*), and endothelium (*triangles*). The single doses (Gy) used in these studies are stated on the lines, which all have an origin at DRF = 1 at day 1 (log scales)

not the other. One of the best ways of achieving this is to use high linear energy transfer (LET) radiation where the repair component is markedly less, and then to see if the recovery phenomenon is the same (which would imply repopulation as a mechanism) or reduced (implying repair as the important parameter).

There are several examples of a slower recovery after neutrons than after X-rays. The first was reported by Curtis (reviewed in 1967) who measured chromosome aberrations in rat hepatocytes. With reference to control levels, there was a decline in aberration yield up to 1 year after 4 Gy X-rays but not after 2 Gy fission neutrons. Repeated injections of carbon tetrachloride accentuated the decline in the number of aberrations to control levels and beyond because of cell death followed by compensatory cell proliferation and selection against the chromosomally aberrant cells. The long-term differential (unstimulated) decline in aberration frequencies after neutrons or X-rays was confirmed in liver by Tates et al. (1982), scoring micronuclei, and in another organ, the thyroid, by Scott et al. (1984). In a third organ, the kidney, a similar effect was seen, namely a differential recovery of colony-forming efficiency after neutrons or X-rays (Jen and Hendry 1993). The differential was also found for the time factor (during fractionation) for functional injury in the pig kidney (Robbins et al. 1991a). Hence three organ systems show a similar pattern of differential recovery after X-rays or neutrons using various endpoints.

Regarding repopulation and LET, no significant differences have been noted in the rate of appearance and disappearance of skin reactions in rodents or in humans, or in survival times of rodents irradiated with $LD_{50/30}$ doses of X-rays or neutrons (data reviewed by Hendry 1972). However, longer survival times for mice injected with neutron-irradiated than with X-irradiated lymphoma cells were reported, at the same incidence of deaths (Berry 1971). Also a longer doubling time for regenerating hemopoietic stem cells was reported after neutrons than after X-rays, using doses giving the same initial level of cell survival (Hendry 1972). This difference was ascribed to differential host influences on repopulation rates, because following transplantation into similarly treated recipient animals there was no difference in the new repopulation rate.

Any true differences in repopulation rates should be reflected in the clone size distribution. However, in studies with both 14 MeV neutrons (Nias 1968) and 3.2 MeV α-particles (Westra and Barendsen 1966), no differences were noted. This implies the same distribution among cells of the lesions responsible for small colony formation and slow growth for both radiation types. Hence it is unlikely that differential repopulation rates are the reason for the differential recovery phenomena.

Considerations of cell turnover rates are rather speculative and inconclusive. In the kidney, for example, the average duration of S phase is 8 h and the labelling index is 0.2% (Soranson 1990). This indicates an average cell cycle time of around $0.33/0.002 = 165$ days. The D_0 which applies for mitotic death of a cell at its first division in vivo is unknown but it could easily range between 5 and 20 Gy (Hendry 1983; Hopewell 1983). Hence the dose equivalent for the successful division of a cell is $D_0\ln2$. This gives 0.01 and 0.04 Gy/day if the above D_0 values are chosen, showing that such estimated time factors are of the same order as those measured late after irradiation for kidney clonogens (Table 3), but smaller than those estimated at earlier times either after or during irradiation for the clonogens and for the functional injury (Table 2). Accelerated cell turnover has been reported in bladder, lung, spinal cord, and kidney (reviewed by Thames and Hendry 1987; Soranson 1990), which may increase somewhat these speculative calculated values of Gy/day.

Regarding repair, there is indeed evidence for less and slower repair of high-LET lesions within single cells. The method of premature chromosome condensation (PCC) has been used to reveal chromosome lesions in the interphase nucleus (Goodwin et al. 1989; Bedford and Goodhead 1989). For the same initial number of chromatin breaks, 90% rejoined by 7 h after X-rays compared with only 50% after neon ions, with far fewer ring PCC aberrations being formed (Goodwin et al. 1989). Also the relative biological effectiveness (RBE) of 2.6 for chromosome breaks, for 3.2 MeV α-particles with respect to X-rays (Bedford and Goodhead 1989), was in contrast to the much higher RBE of about 10 for the subsequent production of chromosome-type exchange aberrations observed at mitosis. With respect to double-strand breaks in DNA, the lesions responsible for subsequent chromosome exchanges and fragments, a slower rate of rejoining, and a greater proportion of breaks unrepaired (by the last sampling time) have been reported after α-radiation than after low-LET irradiation (Blocher 1988; Frankenberg-Schwager et al. 1990). All these observations indicate that repair differentials are likely to be responsible for recovery differentials observed in vivo, and hence that long-term recovery is likely to include a component of repair as well as presumably some repopulation.

Further Implications

It should not be assumed that if there is a long half-time for repair during fractionation, then recovery will necessarily continue after the fractionation course is completed. Spinal cord is an example where a long half-time of about 6 h has been detected (Feng et al. 1991), but there is no postirradiation recovery until very long times afterwards, which implicates repopulation occurring late (reviewed by van der Kogel 1991).

Another point is that although *cellular* repair may continue, this may not be reflected in *tissue* recovery. An example here is the kidney, showing long-term cellular repair during and after irradiation (see above). But recovery is not seen in terms of the re-irradiation response of the kidney, using long recovery intervals and functional assessments of injury (Stewart et al. 1989;

Stewart and Oussoren 1990; Robbins et al. 1991b). Possible reasons for this are that injury from the first treatment continues to be expressed at the time of the second, so that recovery is masked, or that the cell population recovery somehow is not translated properly into functional tissue recovery.

Notwithstanding these differences between endpoints and between tissues, it is fairly clear that intracellular repair is not solely a short-term phenomenon. Hence it may be important for some tissues, for example (1) in re-treatment situations when such recovery is curtailed, and (2) in carcinogenesis when high RBE values are observed (Scott et al. 1984; Hendry 1991).

Acknowledgments. J.H. Hendry is supported by the Cancer Research Campaign (UK). He thanks Ann Kaye for help in the preparation and typing of the manuscript.

References

Bedford JS, Goodhead DT (1989) Breakage of human interphase chromosomes by alpha particles and X-rays. Int J Radiat Biol 55:635–643

Berry RJ (1971) LET dependence of lethal and non-lethal radiation damage in mammalian cells. Int J Radiat Biol 20:184

Blocher D (1988) DNA double-strand break repair determines the RBE of α particles. Int J Radiat Biol 54:761–771

Curtis HJ (1967) Biological mechanisms of delayed radiation damage in mammals. In: Ebert M, Howard A (eds) Current topics in radiation research, vol 3. North-Holland, Amsterdam, pp 139–174

Ellis F (1967) Fractionation in radiotherapy. In: Deeley TJ, Wood CAP (eds) Modern trends in radiotherapy, vol 1. Butterworths, London, pp 34–51

Feng Y, Guttenberger R, Thames HD, Stephens LC, Ang KK (1991) Repair kinetics in rat cervical spinal cord: significance for multiple fractions per day treatment. In: Chapman JD, Dewey WC, Whitmore GF (eds) Radiation research, vol 1. Academic, San Diego, p 185 (Congress abstracts)

Field SB, Hornsey S (1974) Damage to mouse lung with neutrons and X-rays. Eur J Cancer 10:621–627

Field SB, Hornsey S, Kutsutani Y (1976) Effect of fractionated irradiation on mouse lung and a phenomenon of slow repair. Br J Radiol 49:700–707

Fisher DR, Hendry JH, Scott D (1988) Long-term repair in vivo of colony-forming ability and chromosomal injury in X-irradiated mouse hepatocytes. Radiat Res 113:40–50

Frankenberg-Schwager M, Frankenberg D, Harbich R, Adamczyk C (1990) A comparative study of rejoining of DNA double-strand breaks in yeast irradiated with 3.5 MeV α-particles or with 30 MeV electrons. Int J Radiat Biol 57:1151–1168

Goodwin E, Blakely E, Ivery G, Tobias C (1989) Repair and misrepair of heavy-ion-induced chromosomal damage. Adv Space Res 9(10):83–89

Hayashi S, Suit HD (1971) Effect of fractionation of radiation dose on callus formation at site of fracture. Radiology 101:181–186

Hendry JH (1972) A difference in haemopoietic stem cell repopulation after D-T neutrons or X-irradiation. Int J Radiat Biol 22:279–283

Hendry JH (1983) Mathematical aspects of colony growth, transplantation kinetics, and cell survival. In: Potten CS, Hendry JH (eds) Cell clones; manual of mammalian cell techniques. Churchill Livingstone, Edinburgh, pp 1–12

Hendry JH (1989) Response of human organs to single (or fractionated equivalent) doses of irradiation. Int J Radiat Biol 56:691–700

Hendry JH (1991) The slower cellular recovery after higher-LET irradiations including neutrons, focusses on the quality of DNA breaks. Radiat Res 128[Suppl 1]:111–113

Hendry JH, Roberts SA (1991) The sensitivity of human tissues to changes in dose fractionation: deductions from the RCR survey among UK radiotherapists. Clin Oncol 3:22–27

Hill SA, Smith KA, Williams KB, Denekamp J (1989) The fractionated response of mouse stroma after X-rays and neutrons: influence of early vs late expression of damage. Radiat Oncol 16:129–137

Hopewell JW (1983) Radiation effects on vascular tissue. In: Potten CS, Hendry JH (eds) Cytotoxic insult to tissue: effects on cell lineages. Churchill Livingstone, Edinburgh, pp 228–257

Hopewell JW, Wiernik G (1977) Tolerance of the pig kidney to fractionated X-irradiation. In: IAEA (eds) Radiobiological research and radiotherapy. IAEA, Vienna, pp 65–73

Jen YM, Hendry JH (1993) Dose-fractionation sensitivity of mouse kidney clonogens measured using different interfraction intervals and postirradiation assay times. Radiother Oncol (to be published)

Maciejewski B, Withers HR, Taylor JMG, Hliniak A (1990) Dose fractionation and regeneration in radiotherapy for cancer of the oral cavity and oropharynx: part 2. Normal tissue responses: acute and late effects. Int J Radiat Oncol Biol Phys 18:101–111

Nias NHS (1968) Clone size analysis: a parameter in the study of cell population kinetics. Cell Tissue Kinet 1:153–165

Overgaard J, Hjelm-Hansen M, Vendelbo Johansen L, Anderson AP (1988) Comparison of conventional and split-course radiotherapy as primary treatment in carcinoma of the larynx. Acta Oncol 27:147–152

Priestman TJ, Bullimore JA, Godden TP, Deutsch GP (1989) The Royal College of Radiologists' Fractionation Survey. Clin Oncol 1:39–46

Reinhold HS, Buisman GH (1975) Repair of radiation damage to capillary endothelium. Br J Radiol 48:727–731

Robbins MEC, Barnes DWH, Campling D, Hopewell JW, Knowles JF, Sansom JM, Simmonds RH (1991a) The relative biological effectiveness of fractionated doses of fast neutrons ($42\,MeV_{d\rightarrow Be}$) for normal tissues in the pig. Br J Radiol 64:823–830

Robbins MEC, Bywaters T, Rezvani M, Golding SJ, Hopewell JW (1991b) Residual radiation-induced damage to the kidney of the pig as assayed by retreatment. Int J Radiat Biol 60:917–928

Scott D, Gellard PA, Hendry JH (1984) Differential rates of loss of chromosomal aberrations in rat thyroids after x-rays or neutrons. Radiat Res 97:64–70

Soranson A (1990) Proliferation and function in normal and perturbed mouse kidney following irradiation. PhD thesis, CNAA, UK

Stewart FA, Oussoren Y (1990) Re-irradiation of mouse kidneys: a comparison of retreatment tolerance after single and fractionated partial tolerance doses. Int J Radiat Biol 58:531–544

Stewart FA, Luts A, Lebesque JV (1989) The lack of long term recovery and reirradiation tolerance in the mouse kidney. Int J Radiat Biol 56:449–462

Tates AD, Broerse JJ, Neuteboom I, deVogel N (1982) Differential persistence of chromosomal damage induced in resting rat-liver cells by X-rays and 4.2 MeV neutrons. Mutat Res 92:275–290

Terry NHA, Ang KK, Hunter NR, Milas L (1988) Tissue repair and repopulation in the tumour bed effect. Radiat Res 114:621–626

Thames HD, Hendry JH (1987) Fractionation in radiotherapy. Taylor and Francis, London

Thames HD, Hendry JH, Moore JV, Ang KK, Travis EL (1989) The high steepness of dose–response curves for late-responding normal tissues. Radiother Oncol 15:49–53

Thames HD, Bentzen SM, Turesson I, Overgaard M, van den Bogaert W (1990) Time-dose factors in radiotherapy: a review of the human data. Radiother Oncol 19:219–235

Travis EL, Down JD (1981) Repair to mouse lung after split doses of X-rays. Radiat Res 89:166–174

Tucker SL, Travis EL (1990) Comments on a time-dependent version of the linear-quadratic model. Radiother Oncol 18:155–163

Turesson I, Notter G (1984) The influence of the overall treatment time in radiotherapy on the acute reaction: comparison of the effects of daily and twice-a-week fractionation on human skin. Int J Radiat Oncol Biol Phys 10:607–619

Turesson I, Thames HD (1989) Repair capacity and kinetics of human skin during fractionated radiotherapy: erythema, desquamation, and telangiectasia after 3 and 5 year's follow-up. Radiother Oncol 15:169–188

Van der Kogel AJ (1991) The nervous system: radiobiology and experimental pathology. In: Schere E, Streffer C, Trott K-R (eds) Radiopathology of organs and tissues. Springer, Berlin Heidelberg New York, pp 191–212

Van Dyk J, Mah K, Keane TJ (1989) Radiation-induced lung damage: dose-time-fractionation considerations. Radiother Oncol 14:55–69

Westra A, Barendsen GW (1966) Proliferation characteristics of cultured mammalian cells after irradiation with sparsely and densely ionizing radiations. Int J Radiat Biol 11:477–485

White A, Hornsey S (1978) Radiation damage to the rat spinal cord: the effect of single and fractionated doses of X-rays. Br J Radiol 51:515–523

White A, Hornsey A (1980) Time dependent repair of radiation damage in the rat spinal cord after x-rays and neutrons. Eur J Cancer 16:957–962

Williams MV, Denekamp J (1984) Radiation-induced renal damage in mice: influence of fraction size. Int J Radiat Oncol Biol Phys 10:885–893

Williams MV, Stewart FA, Soranson JA, Denekamp J (1985) The influence of overall treatment time on renal injury after multifraction irradiation. Radiat Oncol 4:87–92

Withers HR, Taylor JMG, Maciejewski B (1988) The hazard of accelerated tumor clonogen repopulation during radiotherapy. Acta Oncol 27:131–146

The Response of Tissues to Very Low Doses per Fraction: A Reflection of Induced Repair?

M.C. Joiner, B. Marples, and H. Johns

CRC Gray Laboratory, Mount Vernon Hospital, Northwood, Middlesex HA6 2JR, UK

Introduction

The linear-quadratic (LQ) equation is now used widely to model and predict the increase in total dose with decreasing dose per fraction needed for an isoeffective response to radiotherapy in normal tissues and tumors (Joiner 1989). This relationship reflects the gradual decrease in radiation effectiveness with lowered doses due to these doses being further and further back "on the shoulder" of the underlying survival curve for the cells at risk. Although there has been some indication in experimental studies in vivo that the LQ model can underpredict radiation response to doses per fraction in the range 1–2 Gy relative to higher doses per fraction, this appears to be due to incomplete repair between successive doses (Thames et al. 1988). Alternatively, studies on pig skin have suggested that the LQ model can overpredict radiation effect in the range 2–6 Gy, but this has been attributed to a combination of cellular repopulation and cell cycle redistribution affecting *net* tissue response (Hopewell and van den Aardweg 1991). Thus for doses greater than 1 Gy per fraction, the LQ model describes the radiation response of normal tissues reasonably well.

As part of our program for testing the ability of the LQ model to describe a range of normal tissue and tumor responses, we have evaluated the effect of very low doses per fraction, less than 2 Gy and typically down to 0.1 Gy, on skin and kidney (Joiner et al. 1986; Joiner and Johns 1988). Lung has also been tested down to 0.15 Gy per fraction by Gray Laboratory workers (Parkins and Fowler 1986). These studies have been made possible by utilizing an experimental design in which only a part of the underlying damage equivalent to full tissue tolerance is produced by the X-ray fractions of interest, and the balance is supplied by a "top-up" dose of low-energy (high-LET) neutrons (Joiner 1987; Joiner *et al.* 1989, 1992). These neutrons are used for the top-up because the effect they produce is little influenced by factors which otherwise modulate X-ray sensitivity, such as position in the

Recent Results in Cancer Research, Vol. 130

cell cycle and oxygen. Additionally, there is little or no fractionation effect for neutrons of this energy and to a first approximation the amount of underlying damage contributed by the top-up is directly proportional to the neutron dose, enabling the effect of the X-ray treatment of interest to be easily deduced from the top-up dose needed to produce measurable tissue reactions: the smaller the top-up dose needed, the larger is the effect of the X-ray treatment.

The project has now been extended and we have been able to compare these data obtained in vivo with direct measurements of survival made on V79 cells in vitro exposed to very low *single* doses of X-rays. These measurements have been made possible by using a computerized microscope (DMIPS, dynamic microscopic image processing scanner) for locating and identifying cells (Palcic and Jaggi 1986).

Experimental Methods

Irradiation

For the studies in vivo, fractionated treatments were delivered with 240 kVp X-rays (half value layer = 1.3 mm Cu) at high dose rate: 2.3 Gy/min for skin irradiation and 2.5 Gy/min for kidney irradiation. For the lung studies quoted from the literature, dose rate was 1.8 Gy/min. Top-up doses were d(4)-Be neutrons produced by the reaction of 4 MeV deuterons with a thick beryllium target; mean energy was 2.3 MeV (Folkard 1986). Cells in vitro were irradiated with single doses of 250 kVp X-rays (half value layer = 1.46 mm Cu) at dose rates of 0.016 Gy/min (0.01–0.5 Gy), 0.44 Gy/min (0.2–5 Gy) or 1.7 Gy/min (1–10 Gy). The dose rate was selected according to the dose delivered, so that exposure times were always greater than 35 s in order to maintain dosimetric accuracy.

Normal Tissue Studies

Acute skin reactions were scored during the period 10–32 days after irradiation, and an average value calculated (Denekamp 1973; Douglas and Fowler 1976; Joiner 1989). The skin scoring scale ranges from 0 to 3, with a single X-ray dose of ~23 Gy required for an average skin reaction of 1.5, which corresponds to transient moist desquamation at about day 20 postirradiation. Late renal damage was assessed from typically 25–40 weeks postirradiation, using decreased clearance of EDTA from the plasma, reduction in hematocrit, and increased urine output as endpoints (Joiner and Johns 1988). At 29 weeks postirradiation, equivalent mid-range responses are typically 3% residual EDTA per milliliter plasma, 40% hematocrit, and 15 urination events per day for an X-ray dose of ~21.5 Gy delivered in 2 fractions (Joiner and Johns 1988), compared with values of ~0.4% residual

EDTA, ~50% hematocrit, and ~6.3 urination events per day in unirradiated age-matched animals (Stevens et al. 1991). The studies on lung by Parkins and Fowler (1986), cited in Fig. 4, used breathing frequency to assess an acute phase of lung damage at about 28 weeks postirradiation and mortality as an endpoint for a late phase of damage by about 48 weeks postirradiation. Typically in this system, for single-dose schedules ED_{50} (dose at which 50% of animals exhibited breathing frequency >1.2 times that in unirradiated animals) at 28 weeks and $LD_{50/48\,weeks}$ are both ~11 Gy. These values of *functional* damage have been used as the specification of "full tissue tolerance" in these experimental systems.

Analysis of these top-up experiments has been carried out using the methods described in detail by Joiner et al. (1986), Joiner and Johns (1988), Joiner et al. (1989), and Johns and Joiner (1991). In particular, extrapolated total X-ray doses were calculated which would be needed to reach full tissue tolerance if the treatment had all been given with X-ray fractions alone instead of partially with X-ray fractions plus a subsequent top-up; this calculation has been described by Joiner and Denekamp (1986).

In Vitro Studies

Samples of Chinese hamster V79-379A cells, maintained routinely in suspension culture in the logarithmic phase of growth (Watts et al. 1986), were allowed to attach to the bottom surface of tissue culture flasks which were then filled completely with culture medium, sealed, and irradiated with either X-rays or neutrons at room temperature (21°–25° C). Following irradiation, a DMIPS cell analyser (Palcic and Jaggi 1986; Spadinger and Palcic 1991) was used to locate and record the positions of ~300 cells in each flask, which was then incubated at 37° C for 3.5 days to allow six or seven divisions producing colonies of greater than 50 cells from a single surviving cell. At this time, the location of each recorded cell was revisited automatically to determine whether a colony was present and, if it was, to measure its size. The fraction of surviving cells at each dose level was determined in the conventional way as the plating efficiency of the irradiated cells divided by the plating efficiency of the unirradiated cells. The full protocol for these experiments has been described by Marples and Joiner (1992).

Normal Tissue Studies

Skin

Figure 1 shows the relationship between extrapolated total dose needed to achieve an isoeffect and dose per fraction, for an experiment using 20 initial

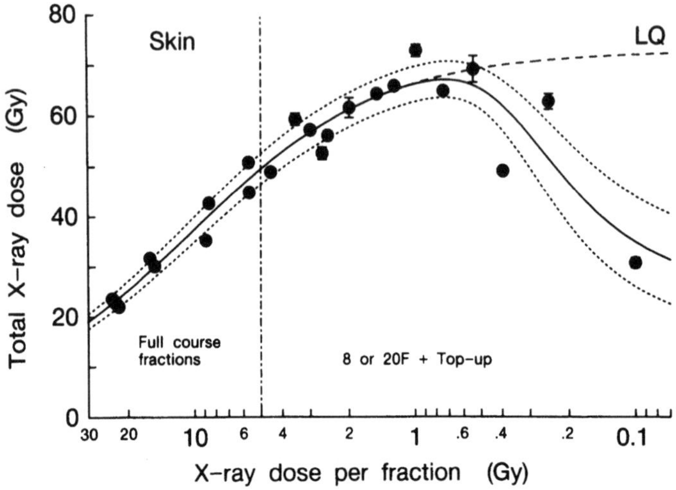

Fig. 1. Total dose required to achieve full acute skin tolerance (see text) in mice feet as a function of dose per fraction in the range 0.1–20 Gy. Experiments used either a full course of fractions (no top-up) or 8 or 20 X-ray fractions followed by a neutron top-up dose. Errors are SEM, within the data points if not shown. The data are well-fitted by the LQ model (*dashed line*) in the dose per fraction range above 1 Gy. Below 0.6 Gy per fraction, the LQ model underpredicts the effect of X-rays and total dose decreases with decreasing dose per fraction. Total dose is better predicted over the complete range of dose per fraction by a modified LQ model which includes induced repair, shown by the *continuous line*; 95% confidence limits on the mean (expected) values of the fit are shown *dotted*. (Data from Joiner et al. 1986)

fractions of X-rays as low as 0.1 Gy, followed by a single neutron top-up (Joiner et al. 1986). Additionally, Fig. 1 includes data from experiments using 8 higher-dose X-ray fractions plus top-up and full courses of X-ray fractions (no top-up) for comparison. The isoeffect level chosen for the analysis in Fig. 1 was an average skin reaction of 1.5 (see above). The linear-quadratic (LQ) model has been used successfully in previous studies (Douglas and Fowler 1976) to describe this relationship. Thus the survival of the underlying target-cell population is given by

$$E' = -\log(\mathrm{SF}) = n(\alpha d + \beta d^2) \qquad (1)$$

where SF is the surviving fraction, d is the dose per fraction given in n fractions, and α and β are constants in the model which together describe the shape of the survival curve: a higher ratio of α/β indicates a more "linear" survival curve and correspondingly less effect of fractionation. This may be seen by rearranging Eq. 1 to give the relationship between total dose $D = nd$ and dose per fraction, for a fixed level of damage E. Thus,

$$D = \frac{E/\alpha}{1 + d/(\alpha/\beta)} \qquad (2)$$

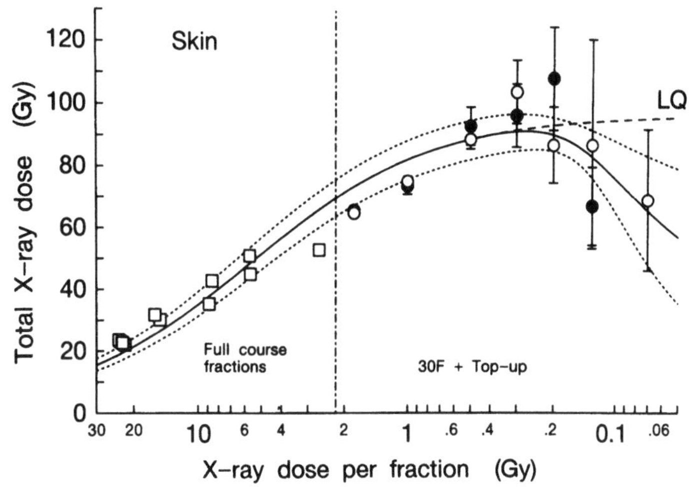

Fig. 2. Experiments similar to those summarized in Fig. 1, but using 30 X-ray fractions plus neutron top-up given either before (●) or after (○) the X-ray schedule. There is no significant difference between these two protocols, and at low doses per fraction the LQ model again underpredicts the effect of X-ray treatment. However, in this 30-fraction study the phenomenon is not as pronounced as shown in Fig. 1, and the maximum value of total dose occurs at a lower dose per fraction. Errors are SEM, within the data points if not shown. *Continuous line*, fit of the induced repair model; *dotted lines*, 95% confidence limits on mean (expected) values of the fit

This equation is shown in Fig. 1 as a continuous/dashed line (labelled LQ). Down to doses per fraction of 0.6 Gy the data fit the LQ model very well, but below this dose there is a significantly reduced total dose compared with the LQ prediction: the LQ model *underestimates* the true effect of these low doses per fraction.

Figure 2 summarizes a further experiment on mouse skin, using 30 initial fractions of X-rays as low as 0.07 Gy, plus a single neutron top-up. In this study we also tested the influence of giving the neutron top-up dose either before or after X rays (filled and open symbols respectively); clearly there was no significant difference in the effect of X-rays measured using these two protocols. However, again there is evidence of an increased effect of low X-ray doses per fraction (<0.2 Gy) compared with the simple LQ model, as indicated by a reduction in total dose needed for an isoeffect (skin reaction = 1.5). In these 30-fraction X-ray experiments, low dose per fraction sensitivity is not as marked as in the 20-fraction study shown in Fig. 1; additionally deviation from the LQ model occurs at a lower dose per fraction so that the maximum total dose measured is higher – about 100 Gy in Fig. 2 compared with about 70 Gy in Fig. 1. The reason for this difference between these two studies is not yet understood.

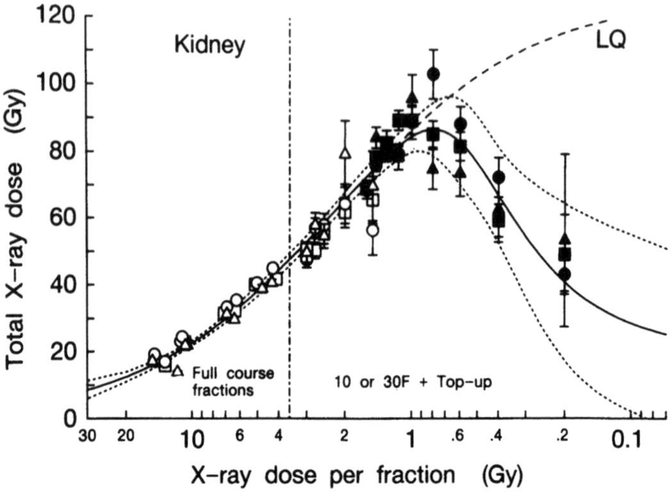

Fig. 3. Relationship between total dose and dose per fraction for late renal damage in the mouse assayed at 29 weeks postirradiation by EDTA clearance (■, □), hematocrit (●, ○), and urination frequency (▲, △). Irradiation was with 10 (*open symbols*) or 30 (*filled symbols*) X-ray fractions followed by a neutron top-up treatment, and is compared with the response to a full course of X-ray fractions (no top-up). The LQ model underpredicts the effect of X-ray treatment with doses per fraction less than 0.8 Gy; however, the induced repair model (*continuous line*; *dotted lines*, 95% confidence limits) fits all the data well. Errors are SEM, within the data points if not shown

Kidney

In the late-reacting tissue of kidney we have tested the effect of X-ray doses per fraction down to 0.2 Gy in an experiment using 30 X-ray fractions followed by a neutron top-up treatment given in two fractions (Joiner and Johns 1988). Figure 3 summarizes the data; data from three assays of renal damage (see above) are included. Additionally included for comparison are data from experiments using 10 higher-dose X-ray fractions (1.5–3.5 Gy per fraction) plus top-up and full courses of X-ray fractions (no top-up). All these data are in close agreement and show clearly an increased effect of small X-ray dose fractions, with total dose reaching a maximum average of about 92 Gy at 1 Gy per fraction, decreasing by a factor of 1.9 to about 49 Gy at 0.2 Gy per fraction.

Lung

We examined further the data published previously on the dose-fractionation response of mouse lung (Parkins et al. 1985; Parkins and

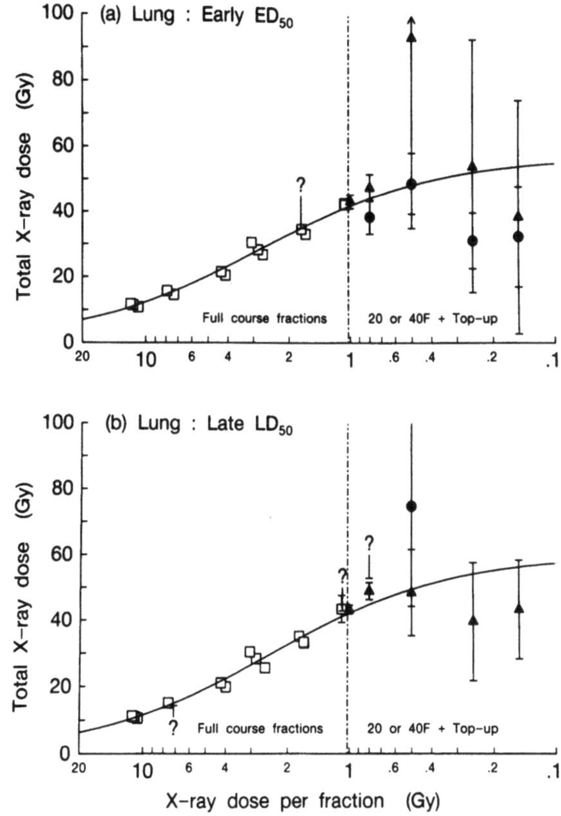

Fig. 4a,b. Total dose to the mouse lung needed for an increase in breathing rate by 20% compared with controls in half the subjects measured at 28 weeks (ED_{50}, **a**) or total dose needed for mortality in half the subjects (LD_{50}, **b**) at 44–48 weeks. Irradiations were full course X-ray fractionation (□), 20 X-ray fractions with a neutron top-up (●), and 40 X-ray fractions with a neutron top-up (▲). Errors are SEM, within the data points if not shown. Although not significant in these studies, there is a trend towards a greater effect of low-dose X-ray fractionation compared with the LQ model. (Data from Parkins et al. 1985; Parkins and Fowler 1985, 1986; and Dr. C.S. Parkins, personal communication)

Fowler 1985, 1986). These experiments used 1 to 40 fractions in a full course of treatment (no top-up), and 20 low-dose fractions plus a neutron top-up. These data are shown in Fig. 4 in the same format as Figs. 1–3. Also shown on Fig. 4 are unpublished data from an experiment using 40 low-dose X-ray fractions plus neutron top-up. These data were kindly supplied by Dr. C.S. Parkins at the Gray Laboratory. The lines drawn in Fig. 4 show the fit of the LQ model to only the full-course fractionation data (open symbols, dose per fraction >1 Gy). The ratio of α/β from this fit was 2.8 Gy, similar to the values quoted previously (Parkins et al. 1985; Parkins and Fowler 1985). In these experiments the data from both the early and late phases of response indicate a trend that X-rays become more effective as the dose per fraction is reduced below 0.8 Gy. Unfortunately, however, the errors on the total dose estimates below 1 Gy per fraction do not permit a firm conclusion to be made and it would be useful to repeat these experiments.

Studies of Cells In Vitro

Beck-Bornholdt et al. (1989) have measured the total X-ray dose needed to control the R1H rhabdomyosarcoma in the rat, using from 6 up to 126 dose fractions. No top-ups were used in their study. It was found that curative doses were lower, and net growth delay per gray higher, for the 126-fraction schedule (dose per fraction <0.5 Gy) compared with the schedules using 6–42 fractions (dose per fraction >1 Gy). The cellular basis for tumor response to radiotherapy is well understood and these results seem to underline the possibility that increased sensitivity of tissues to low-dose fractions is caused by an increased killing of stem cells per unit radiation dose.

To investigate this phenomenon further, we carried out a large series of 56 experiments in which we measured the survival of V79 hamster cells after exposure to *single* doses of 250 kVp X-rays or d(4)-Be neutrons. These experiments comprised a total of 412 separate assessments of cell survival after X-ray doses in the range 0–10 Gy, with 86% of the measurements made at doses less than 1 Gy, 78% made at less than 0.5 Gy, and 60% made at less than 0.25 Gy. Figure 5 shows the results from a typical experiment. In this example the response to X-ray doses above 0.5 Gy is well described by a conventional downward-bending survival curve; in Fig. 5 the continuous line shows the LQ model (Eq. 1 with $n = 1$) fitted to the X-ray data at doses of $\geq$0.6 Gy. For neutrons, V79 cell survival was always reduced exponentially with dose; the straight dashed line indicates this in Fig. 5. The X-ray data below 0.5 Gy deviate from the expected response extrapolated from higher doses. Just as in the systems in vivo described above, low X-ray doses are more effective than predicted. Indeed, in this example, X-ray doses <0.2 Gy were almost as effective as neutrons.

Each of the 56 experiments (for example Fig. 5) included neutron as well as X-ray responses. This strategy was implemented so that as well as measuring X-ray survival directly, a comparison could be made between neutron and X-ray survival: it is less likely that the apparent increase in X-ray sensitivity at low doses shown in Fig. 5 could be an artifact of the specialized procedure (with the DMIPS) used to measure cell survival, since dose-related changes were not seen in the neutron response. Therefore, at the same high level of cell survival, X-ray and neutron *doses* were similar. By taking advantage of the exponential neutron survival curve in each experiment, this comparison was expressed as a relative biological effectiveness (RBE) by relating each X-ray survival point to the neutron survival line, and calculating the ratio of X-ray to neutron dose required to achieve

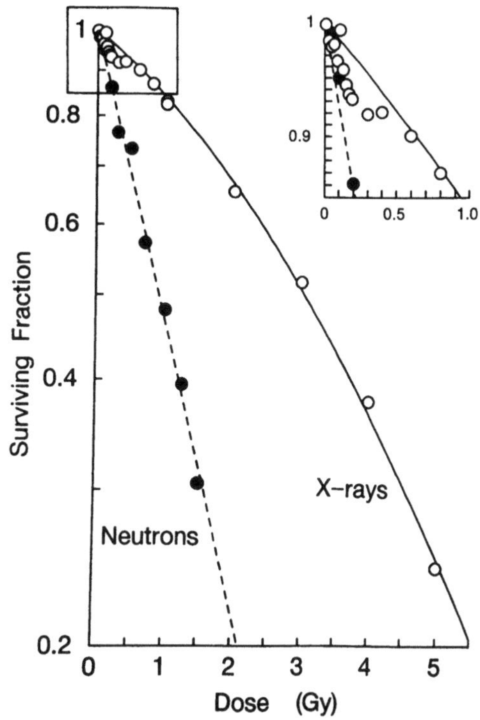

Fig. 5. Typical experiment using V79 hamster cells in vitro irradiated with single doses of X-rays or neutrons. At X-ray doses >0.6 Gy, the dose–survival relationship conforms to a conventional LQ model. At X-ray doses <0.6 Gy, the LQ model substantially underpredicts the effect of X-rays. The response to neutrons is described by a simple exponential survival curve and there is no indication of increased sensitivity to low-dose neutrons. At X-ray doses <0.2 Gy, the response to X-rays and neutrons is similar

this level of survival. We have found that an advantage of this technique is that interexperimental variations in the X-ray survival response are reduced in the RBE data, presumably because slight changes in radiosensitivity from time to time affect both the X-ray and neutron responses similarly. Figure 6 summarizes the 412 RBE values from all the experiments. Since the response to neutrons was exponential, increasing RBE corresponds directly to increasing X-ray resistance. Thus a low RBE at low X-ray doses indicates high X-ray sensitivity; the RBE is well below the prediction made with the LQ model extrapolated from doses above 2 Gy, shown by the dashed line. As the X-ray dose increases, RBE increases, which reflects increasing X-ray resistance. RBE reaches a peak at about 1–1.5 Gy after which it decreases with increasing dose, which is the conventional picture due to the downward bending of the X-ray survival curve. For example, at an X-ray dose of 0.1 Gy, RBE was 2.1 corresponding to an effective X-ray D_0 of 2.7 Gy (neutron D_0 = 1.3 Gy); for 1 Gy X-rays, RBE was 3.9 corresponding to an

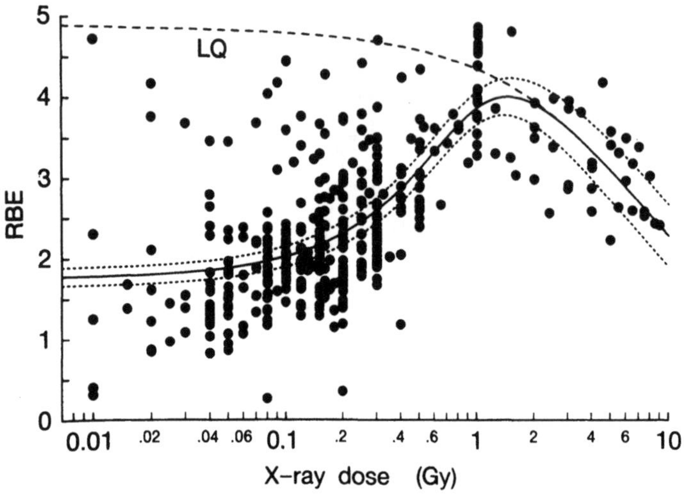

Fig. 6. Data from 56 experiments (e.g., Fig. 5) where each estimate of cell survival after a single X-ray dose is expressed as an RBE value relative to the line fitted to survival after neutrons, measured in the same experiment (see text). These data show clearly the increased effect of low-dose X-rays as mirrored by a decreasing RBE with decreasing dose; the LQ model (*dashed line*) substantially underpredicts low-dose X-ray sensitivity

effective X-ray D_0 of 5.2 Gy. Thus X-ray radioresistance increased by a factor of 1.9 as X-ray dose increased from 0.1 to 1 Gy.

The data obtained in vitro seem to leave no doubt that low (<1 Gy) X-ray doses (or doses per fraction in vivo) are much more effective than expected, or predicted from any reasonable extrapolation (e.g., with the LQ model) from high-dose data.

A Model to Describe the Data

How can both the in vivo and in vitro data be explained? One possibility is that the sensitive response at low doses is a consequence of a small subpopulation of cells (for example in a particular position within the cell cycle) with exquisite radiosensitivity. When this model was fitted to the in vitro data, it predicted that this population would comprise about 3% of the total cells, but would have an increased sensitivity to X-rays by a factor of about 50 compared with the rest of the cell population. This seems unlikely. Additionally, further experiments in vitro (Marples and Joiner 1992) rule out the existence of a stable genetic subpopulation and also indicate that low-dose sensitivity and the relationship shown in Fig. 6 occur regardless of the phase of the cell cycle at the time of irradiation. It is also hard to reconcile a mechanism based on cell cycle progression with the data on mouse kidney, where estimates of labelling index are generally less than 0.5% (Wilson et al. 1987).

An alternative explanation is that low-dose sensitivity represents a "resting" response to radiation, and that higher doses become less effective at killing cells per unit dose because they produce increased amounts of DNA damage which stimulate or induce repair systems or other stress proteins or protective mechanisms. Such radiation-induced systems that protect against chromosomal damage have been documented in human lymphocytes (Tuschl et al. 1980; Shadley and Wolff 1987; Shadley and Wiencke 1989) and in hamster cells (Ikushima 1987, 1989), and induced repair has been proposed to explain the shapes of highly radioresistant lepidopteran cell survival curves (Koval 1984, 1986, 1988). It is now documented that ionizing radiation can induce expression of certain genes, for example the *gadd45* system (Papathanasiou et al. 1991). We propose, therefore, that the data presented here could reflect repair induction as the X-ray dose is increased. Since this is essentially an effect on survival restricted to the first gray of X-radiation, such a mechanism would have to affect predominantly the α term in the linear-quadratic equation (Eq. 1). A simple modification of the LQ model is to make α in Eq. 1 decrease with dose, thus

$$\alpha = \alpha_{\mathrm{RES}}[1 + g\,\exp(-d/d_{\mathrm{c}})] \tag{3}$$

where two new parameters are defined: d_{c} represents the dose at which 63% $(1 - e^{-1})$ of induction has occurred and g is the amount by which α at very low doses (α_{SENS}) is larger that α at high doses (α_{RES}). Thus $\alpha_{\mathrm{SENS}} = \alpha_{\mathrm{RES}}(1 + g)$. Equation 2 therefore becomes

$$D = \frac{E/\alpha_{\mathrm{RES}}}{1 + g\,\exp(-d/d_{\mathrm{c}}) + d/(\alpha_{\mathrm{RES}}/\beta)} \tag{4}$$

The continuous lines in Figs. 1, 2 and 3 represent this equation fitted to the data for skin and kidney, using nonlinear least squares regression. In all these cases, the fit of this simple model is very good. To fit the data in Fig. 6, Eqs. 1 and 3 are expressed as the RBE compared with an exponential response to neutrons given by $E' = n(\alpha_{\mathrm{N}} d_{\mathrm{N}})$ in analogy with Eq. 1. Thus

$$\mathrm{RBE} = \frac{\alpha_{\mathrm{N}}/\alpha_{\mathrm{RES}}}{1 + g\,\exp(-d/d_{\mathrm{c}}) + d/(\alpha_{\mathrm{RES}}/\beta)} \tag{5}$$

The continuous line in Fig. 6 shows the excellent fit of this equation to the data. It appears, therefore, that a concept of induced repair, as implemented simply in Eq. 3, can adequately account for the phenomenon of unexpected radiosensitivity to low X-ray doses, which we have seen both in vivo and in vitro. Interestingly, low-dose sensitivity does not appear to be a feature of the response to neutrons either in vitro (Fig. 5) or in vivo (data not shown). Since the spectrum of initial DNA lesions is very different for high- and low-LET radiations, this possibly suggests that repair induction, if

Table 1. Parameters g and d_c in the simple induced repair model

Parameter	Lower 95% confidence limit	Value	Upper 95% confidence limit
Skin in vivo[a]			
g	0.62	2.02	3.42
d_c	0.07	0.16	0.26
Skin in vivo[b]			
g	−0.07	1.88	3.83
d_c	0.01	0.07	0.12
Kidney in vivo[c]			
g	−2.92	5.66	14.2
d_c	0.04	0.19	0.34
V79 cells in vitro[d]			
g	1.27	1.78	2.30
d_c	0.26	0.39	0.52

Data from [a] Joiner et al. (1986) (Fig. 1); [b] Joiner et al. (unpublished) (Fig. 2); [c] Joiner and Johns (1988) (Fig. 3); [d] Marples and Joiner (1992) (Fig. 6)

this is the explanation for this phenomenon, is triggered by specific types of DNA lesion which dominate at low LET – for example single- and double-strand breaks.

Table 1 summarizes the values of g and d_c obtained from the fits of Eqs. 4 and 5 to the data from the different systems. Interestingly, g is highest in the kidney; this tissue is late-reacting with the lowest value of α/β of these systems. Values of d_c, the dose needed to cause significant "induction", are all less than 0.4 Gy but do vary between systems and even, in the skin, between experiments. At usual values of dose per fraction used clinically, therefore, tissues are all "fully induced" and the radiation response appears conventional and is reasonably described by the LQ model. However, these data suggest that the effect of much smaller doses in penumbrae or in multiple field treatments, outside the target volume, may need to be reassessed in critical cases, for example where the target volume is adjacent to spinal cord.

Conclusions

1. Low X-ray doses per fraction (<0.6 Gy) are *more* effective per unit dose compared with higher doses per fraction. This has been confirmed in skin and kidney, and is suggested in lung.
2. V79 cells also demonstrate the same pattern of sensitivity to low *single* X-ray doses in vitro.
3. An explanation is that this phenomenon reflects increasing radioresistance as X-ray dose is increased from zero to about 1 Gy, due to the induction of repair systems or other radioprotective mechanisms.

Acknowledgments. This work was supported entirely by the Cancer Research Campaign of the UK. We are grateful to Dr. C.S. Parkins for supplying us with the data on which Fig. 4 is based.

References

Beck-Bornholdt HP, Maurer T, Becker S, Omniczynski M, Vogler H, Wurschmidt F (1989) Radiotherapy of the rhabdomyosarcoma R1H of the rat: hyperfractionation - 126 fractions applied within 6 weeks. Int J Radiat Oncol Biol Phys 16:701–705

Denekamp J (1973) Changes in the rate of repopulation during multifraction irradiation of mouse skin. Br J Radiol 46:381–387

Douglas BG, Fowler JF (1976) The effect of multiple small doses of X-rays on skin reactions in the mouse and a basic interpretation. Radiat Res 66:401–426

Folkard M (1986) Determination of d(3)-Be and d(4)-Be neutron spectra using a recoil proton spectrometer. Phys Med Biol 31:135–144

Hopewell JW, van den Aardweg GJMJ (1991) Studies of dose-fractionation on early and late responses in pig skin: a reappraisal of the importance of the overall treatment time and its effects on radiosensitization and incomplete repair. Int J Radiat Oncol Biol Phys 21:1441–1450

Ikushima T (1987) Chromosomal responses to ionizing radiation reminiscent of an adaptive response in cultured Chinese hamster cells. Mutat Res 180:215–221

Ikushima T (1989) Radio-adaptive response: characterization of a cytogenetic repair induced by low-level ionizing radiation in cultured Chinese hamster cells. Mutat Res 227:241–246

Johns H, Joiner MC (1991) A simple method for fitting curves to dose–effect data for functional damage. Int J Radiat Biol 60:533–541

Joiner MC (1987) The design and interpretation of top-up experiments to investigate the effects of low radiation doses. Int J Radiat Biol 51:115–130

Joiner MC (1989) The dependence of radiation response on the dose per fraction. In: McNally NJ (ed) The scientific basis for modern radiotherapy. British Institute of Radiology, London, pp 20–26 (BIR Report 19)

Joiner MC, Denekamp J (1986) Evidence for a constant repair capacity over 20 fractions of X-rays. Int J Radiat Biol 49:143–150

Joiner MC, Johns H (1988) Renal damage in the mouse: the response to very small doses per fraction. Radiat Res 114:385–398

Joiner MC, Denekamp J, Maughan RL (1986) The use of top-up experiments to investigate the effect of very small doses per fraction in mouse skin. Int J Radiat Biol 49:565–580

Joiner MC, Rojas A, Johns H (1989) Does the repair capacity of skin change with repeated exposure to X-rays? Int J Radiat Biol 55:993–1005

Joiner MC, Rojas A, Johns H (1992) A test of equal effect per fraction in the kidney of the mouse. Radiat Res 130:227–235

Koval TM (1984) Multiphasic survival response of a radioresistant lepidopteran insect cell line. Radiat Res 98:642–648

Koval TM (1986) Inducible repair of ionizing radiation damage in higher eukaryotic cells. Mutat Res 173:291–293

Koval TM (1988) Enhanced recovery from ionizing radiation damage in a lepidopteran insect cell line. Radiat Res 115:413–420

Marples B, Joiner MC (1992) The response of V79 cells to low radiation doses: evidence of enhanced sensitivity of the whole cell population. Radiat Res (in press)

Palcic B, Jaggi B (1986) The use of solid state sensor technology to detect and characterise live mammalian cells growing in tissue culture. Int J Radiat Biol 50:345–352

Papathanasiou MA, Kerr NCK, Robbins JH, McBride OW, Alamo I, Barrett SF, Hickson ID, Fornace AJ (1991) Induction by ionizing radiation of the *gadd45* gene in cultured human cells: lack of mediation by protein kinase C. Mol Cell Biol 11:1009–1016

Parkins CS, Fowler JF (1985) Repair in mouse lung of multifraction X-rays and neutrons: extension to 40 fractions. Br J Radiol 58:225–241

Parkins CS, Fowler JF (1986) The linear quadratic fit for lung function after irradiation with X-rays at smaller doses per fraction than 2 Gy. Br J Cancer 53 [Suppl VII]:320–323

Parkins CS, Fowler JF, Maughan RL, Roper MJ (1985) Repair in mouse lung for up to 20 fractions of X-rays or neutrons. Br J Radiol 58:225–241

Shadley JD, Wiencke JK (1989) Induction of the adaptive response by X-rays is dependent on radiation intensity. Int J Radiat Biol 56:107–118

Shadley JD, Wolff S (1987) Very low doses of X-rays can cause human lymphocytes to become less susceptible to ionizing radiation. Mutagenesis 2:95–96

Spadinger I, Palcic B (1992) The relative biological effectiveness of ^{60}Co γ-rays, 55 kVp X-rays, 250 kVp X-rays and 11 MeV electrons at low doses. Int J Radiat Biol 61:345–353

Stevens G, Joiner MC, Joiner B, Johns H, Denekamp J (1991) Early detection of damage following bilateral renal irradiation in the mouse. Radiother Oncol 20:124–131

Thames HD, Ang KK, Stewart FA, van der Schueren E (1988) Does incomplete repair explain the apparent failure of the basic LQ model to predict spinal cord and kidney responses to low doses per fraction? Int J Radiat Biol 54:13–19

Tuschl H, Altmann H, Kovac R, Topaloglou A, Egg D, Gunther R (1980) Effects of low-dose radiation on repair processes in human lymphocytes. Radiat Res 81:1–9

Watts ME, Hodgkiss RJ, Jones NR, Fowler JF (1986) Radiosensitisation of Chinese hamster cells by oxygen and misonidazole at low X-ray doses. Int J Radiat Biol 50:1009–1021

Wilson GD, Soranson JA, Lewis AA (1987) Cell kinetics of mouse kidney using bromodeoxyuridine incorporation and flow cytometry: preparation and staining. Cell Tissue Kinet 20:125–133

Clinically Important Factors Modifying the Response of Tumors and Normal Tissue to Radiation Therapy

K.-H. Hübener, M. Baumann, A. Krüll, and R. Schwarz

Department of Radiation Therapy, University Hospital-Eppendorf, W-2000 Hamburg 20, Fed. Rep. of Germany

Introduction

The aim of curative radiation oncology is to destroy all tumor cells without producing major damage in normal tissues. As early as 1936 the radiologist Hermann Holthusen related such uncomplicated local tumor control to tumor response on the one hand and normal tissue tolerance on the other (Fig. 1). Holthusen showed that both the probability of eradicating carcinoma of the skin and the probability of developing telangiectasia as a late normal tissue reaction increase as a sigmoid function of radiation dose. At each dose level the probability of uncomplicated local tumor control can be calculated as the product of the probability of achieving local tumor control and the probability of preventing normal tissue damage (Holthusen 1936; Busch 1987).

Several predictors of the position of tumor control curves relative to normal tissue damage curves are currently available to the radiooncologist (Peters et al. 1982; Suit and Walker 1988). These allow treatment strategies to be tailored to individual patients to some degree. Among the most widely used predictors are tumor histology, grade, stage, and localization, as well as the patient's sex, age, and performance status. However, uncomplicated local tumor control rates are not only dependent on these parameters and the skills of the radiooncologist; they can also be significantly modified by noxious factors that affect the patient before, during, or after treatment. Such confounding factors can either increase the radioresistance of the tumor, or increase the acute or late toxicity of radiation.

Anemia as an Example of a Noxious Factor that Increases the Radioresistance of Tumors

A variety of animal and human tumors have been shown to contain hypoxic cells. Since these are more radioresistant than well-oxygenated cells, tumor

Recent Results in Cancer Research, Vol. 130

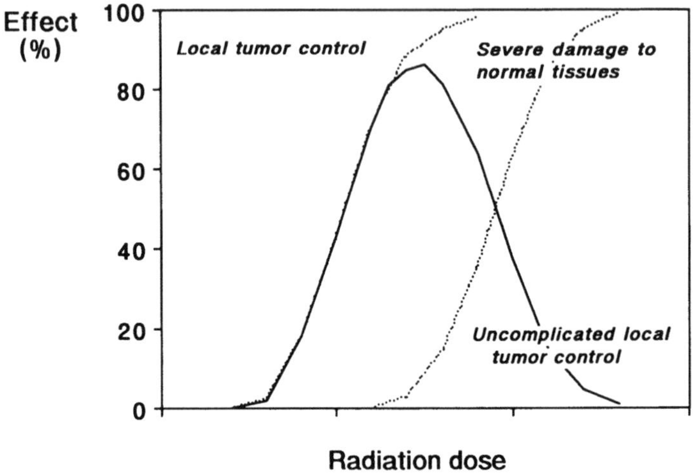

Fig. 1. Relationship of uncomplicated local tumor control by radiation to tumor control probability and the rate of severe normal tissue damage (Holthusen 1936)

hypoxia is an important factor that can limit the success of radiation treatment (Gray et al. 1953; Moulder and Rockwell 1984; Hirst 1986; Vaupel et al. 1989). Several reports indicate that this problem may be aggravated in the presence of anemia.

In a prospective clinical trial, Bush and collegues (Bush 1986; Bush et al. 1978) randomized 132 patients suffering from stage IIB or III carcinoma of the cervix into a group that received transfusion for maintenance of a hemoglobin level ≥12.5 g/100 ml during radiotherapy and a group that did not (Table 1). The results show that in the control patients, local failures occurred significantly more often at hemoglobin levels <12.5 g/100 ml than at higher hemoglobin concentrations. Transfusion to hemoglobin levels

Table 1. Results of a randomized trial on the effect of maintenance of a hemoglobin (Hb) level ≥12.5 g/100 ml by transfusion on the incidence of local failure after radiation therapy (RT) of stage IIB and III carcinoma of the cervix (Bush et al. 1978; Bush 1986)

Treatment arm	Hb prior to RT (g/100 ml)	Hb during RT (g/100 ml)	Incidence of local failure (%)
Control	<12.5	10–12.5[a]	44[b]
	≥12.5	≥12.5	21
Transfusion	<12.5	≥12.5	15[b]
	≥12.5[c]	≥12.5	23

[a] Transfused prior to RT to a Hb level of 10 g/100 ml
[b] The difference between these subgroups is significant ($p < 0.01$)
[c] Randomized to the transfusion arm but not transfused since the Hb level prior to treatment was already ≥12.5 g/100 ml

$\geqslant$12.5 g/100 ml could significantly decrease this rate of local failures to the same incidence that was observed in non-anemic patients in the control and the transfusion arm of the trial.

Similar results were reported by Overgaard et al. (1986) who retrospectively evaluated the records of about 1000 patients treated for squamous cell carcinoma of the head and neck. Local tumor control was highly dependent on the hemoglobin level. The threshold hemoglobin level for improved local tumor control was found to be $\geqslant$13 g/100 ml in female patients, and $\geqslant$14.5 g/100 ml in male patients. This sex-related dependence of local tumor control by radiation therapy on the hemoglobin level was confirmed in a comprehensive statistical analysis of patients with squamous cell carcinoma of the oropharynx (Bentzen et al. 1991).

In a recent review Dische (1991) compiled data from 25 different retrospective trials. Twenty-three of these studies report an adverse prognosis for anemic patients treated by radiation therapy when compared with similar patients who were not anemic. Some of this difference may be explained by more advanced disease in patients with low hemoglobin levels; however, evidence suggests that an increased fraction of hypoxic tumor cells in anemic patients is also a major factor in their poorer prognosis.

At our institution we currently attempt to transfuse anemic patients prior to curative radiation therapy so as to achieve at least the lowest reference values given by our hematology laboratory for male or female patients. That this is not a small task is illustrated by the cumulative frequency of the hemoglobin levels of 100 consecutive patients referred to our department (Fig. 2): approximately one third of our patients would need transfusions

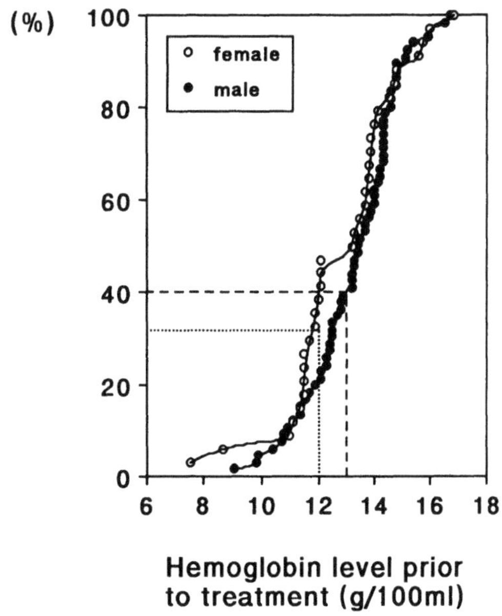

Fig. 2. Cumulative frequency of hemoglobin levels prior to treatment of 100 consecutive patients referred to the Department of Radiation Therapy, University Hosptial Hamburg-Eppendorf

before the start of treatment by the standards outlined above. Since such a program is expensive and extremely difficult to organize, it appears highly desirable to obtain more detailed data on optimal hemoglobin levels for patients undergoing radiation treatment for tumors of different histologies and stages.

Smoking and Preexisting Disease in Tumor-Surrounding Organs as Examples of Noxious Factors that Increase the Acute and Late Normal Tissue Toxicity of Radiation Therapy

It is well documented that the majority of patients undergoing radiation treatment for head and neck cancers and lung tumors have been heavy smokers for many years. In our experience it is difficult for many of these patients to quit smoking and, despite the warnings of their physicians, a considerable proportion continue to smoke during radiation therapy.

Rugg and collegues (1990) showed for patients with head and neck cancers that the time to resolution of mucositis increased from about 12 weeks for patients who never smoked or quit smoking before therapy to more than 20 weeks for patients who continued to smoke during treatment (Table 2).

The usual consequence of unexpected severe acute reactions during radiation therapy is the interruption of treatment. The reasoning for this is to allow acutely reacting normal tissues such as skin, mucosa, and bone marrow to regenerate. However, clonogenic tumor cells may repopulate the tumor during such treatment gaps, thereby increasing the dose necessary to achieve local tumor control.

This was demonstrated by Overgaard et al. (1988) who retrospectively evaluated local tumor control rates after treatment of larynx carcinoma with either continuous fractionated irradiation (5 fractions of 1.8–2.0 Gy per week) or "split-course" radiotherapy, that is an interruption of the treatment for 3 weeks after the first 20 fractions had been applied. Table 3 shows that the dose necessary to obtain 65% local tumor control increased

Table 2. Effect of smoking during radiation therapy (RT) on acute mucositis (Rugg et al. 1990)

Patient group	Number of patients	Weeks after start of RT to resolution of mucositis
Never smoked	8	12[a]
Stopped smoking prior to RT	18	14
Temporary abstinence	7	18
Continued to smoke during RT	8	23

[a] Mean values

Table 3. Effect of an interruption of fractionated radiation therapy on tumor control doses

Tumor	Endpoint	Continuous treatment	Interrupted treatment	Duration of interruption (weeks)	Reference
Larynxcarcinoma (human)	TCD_{65}[a]	57.4 Gy (55.8 to 59.0)[b]	69.4 Gy (65.8 to 73.3)	3	Overgaard et al. (1988)
Rhabdomyosarcoma (rat)	TCD_{37}	76.3 Gy (74.5 to 78.0)	78.2 Gy (75.3 to 81.1)	1	Würschmidt et al. (1991)
			87.2 Gy (78.4 to 94.9)	2	

[a] TCD_x, radiation dose necessary to control x % of the tumors locally
[b] 95% confidence limits given in parentheses

from 57.4 Gy for continuous radiation treatment to 69.4 Gy for the split-course regimen.

Similar findings are reported by Würschmidt and colleagues (1991) who investigated the effect of a treatment gap during radiation therapy with 30 fractions (5 fractions per week) on the local control rate of the rat rhabdomyosarcoma R1H. In this experiment the treatment was interrupted for 1 or 2 weeks after the first 20 fractions had been applied. Table 3 shows that the dose necessary to control 37% of the tumors locally increases from 76 Gy for a continuous course of treatment to 87 Gy for a treatment gap of 2 weeks.

These studies illustrate that if the acute toxicity of radiation therapy is increased to such a degree that interruptions of the treatment become necessary, a reduced probability of local tumor control is expected for affected patients. If noxious factors are the cause of these increased acute reactions, abstinence from such factors is expected to be effective in further improving the results of radiation treatment.

Unfortunately this situation is much more complex in the case of increased late normal tissue damage, for example after irradiation of organs which were already damaged before treatment. Since late normal tissue damage occurs several months or even years after completion of radiation therapy, correction of the treatment is not possible for an individual patient. Therefore clinical treatment strategies are based on so-called tolerance doses. These are doses at which for a given fractionation schedule and a given treatment volume late normal tissue damage is expected in a certain percentage, say 5% (TD_5), of patients (Rubin and Casarett 1968). As a general rule the accepted incidence of damage decreases with the severity of the side effect, and in a variety of clinical situations only doses well below TD_1 will be accepted. Since it is often impossible to evaluate retrospectively the impact of preexisting disease or other noxious factors on late morbidity after irradiation, small subsets of patients with increased radiosensitivity caused by such factors may easily affect clinically accepted tolerance doses. Therefore, in contrast to increased acute normal tissue damage caused by noxious factors which preferentially reduce the tumor control probability for affected patients, increased late normal tissue damage caused by confounding factors may, via tolerance doses, reduce the chance of local tumor control for all patients undergoing radiotherapy. Apart from the development of predictive assays for late radiation injury, the most promising way to minimize this problem is to evaluate thoroughly all known risk factors in patients undergoing radiation treatment and to report those factors in clinical studies.

Consequences for Clinical Radiation Oncology

Anemia, smoking, and preexisting disease in irradiated organs are only three examples of a host of different factors that modify the response of tumors and normal tissues to radiation therapy. At present only scant data are available on the prevalence of those factors in cancer patients; however, the three examples listed above clearly illustrate that a considerable proportion of all patients undergoing curative radiation treatment are at risk. To minimize the influence of those confounding factors on the results of clinical radiation therapy, the following approaches appear to be useful:

1. Possible risk factors should be identified in clinical and radiobiological studies, and screening assays for such risk factors should be developed.
2. Clinical-epidemiological studies should evaluate the proportion of patients undergoing radiotherapy who are at risk for known risk factors.
3. Every patient referred to radiation therapy should be screened for important risk factors, and efforts should be made to instruct patients how to avoid such influences.
4. Clinical studies should be stratified according to risk factors. Individualized treatment strategies can then be developed for patients according to whether or not they are influenced by confounding factors.

References

Bentzen SM, Johansen LV, Overgaard J, Thames HD (1991) Clinical radiobiology of squamous cell carcinoma of the oropharynx. Int J Radiat Oncol Biol Phys 20:1197–1206

Busch M (1987) Risiken und Heilungschancen bei der Tumortherapie. In: Scherer E (ed) Strahlentherapie, 3rd edn. Springer, Berlin Heidelberg New York, pp 299–317

Bush RS (1986) The significance of anaemia in clinical radiotherapy. Int J Radiat Oncol Biol Phys 12:2047–2050

Bush RS, Jenkin RDT, Allt WEC, Beale FA, Bean H, Dembo AJ, Pringle JF (1978) Definitive evidence for hypoxic cells influencing cure in cancer patients. Br J Cancer 37 [Suppl III]:302–306
Dische S (1991) Radiotherapy and anaemia: the clinical experience. Radiother Oncol 20 [Suppl]:35–40
Gray LH, Conger AD, Ebert M, Hornsey S, Scott OCA (1953) The concentration of oxygen dissolved in tissues at the time of irradiation as a factor in radiotherapy. Br J Radiol 26:638–648
Hirst DG (1986) Anemia: a problem or an opportunity in radiotherapy? Int J Radiat Oncol Biol Phys 12:2009–2017
Holthusen H (1936) Erfahrungen über die Verträglichkeitsgrenze für Röntgenstrahlen und deren Nutzanwendung zur Verhütung von Schäden. Strahlentherapie 57:254–269
Moulder JE, Rockwell S (1984) Hypoxic fractions of solid tumors: experimental techniques, methods of analysis, and a survey of existing data. Int J Radiat Oncol Biol Phys 10:695–712
Overgaard J, Sand-Hansen H, Jorgensen K, Hjelm-Hansen M (1986) Primary radiotherapy of larynx and pharynx carcinoma: an analysis of some factors influencing local control and survival. Int J Radiat Oncol Biol Phys 12:515–521
Overgaard J, Hjelm-Hansen M, Vendelbo-Johansen L, Andersen AP (1988) Comparison of conventional and split-course radiotherapy as primary treatment in carcinoma of the larynx. Acta Oncol 27:147–152
Peters LJ, Withers HR, Thames HD, Fletcher GH (1982) Keynote address. The problem: tumor radioresistance in clinical radiotherapy. Int J Radiat Oncol Biol Phys 8:101–108
Rubin P, Casarett GW (1968) Clinical radiation pathology. Saunders, Philadelphia
Rugg T, Saunders M, Dische S (1990) Smoking and mucosal reactions to radiotherapy. Br J Radiol 63:554–556
Suit HD, Walker AM (1988) Predictors of radiation response in use today: criteria for new assays and methods of verification. In: Chapman JD, Peters LJ, Withers HR (eds) Prediction of tumor treatment response. Pergamon, New York, pp 3–19
Vaupel P, Kallinowski F, Okunieff P (1989) Blood flow, oxygen and nutrient supply, and metabolic microenvironment of human tumors: a review. Cancer Res 49:6449–6465
Würschmidt F, Beck-Bornholdt HP, Vogler H, Jung H (1991) Radiotherapy of the rhabdomyosarcoma R1H of the rat: split course versus continuous fractionation. Strahlenther Onkol 167:26–30

II. Radiation Response of Mucosa and Skin, Muscle and Bladder

Dose–Response Relationships for Late Effects on Skin and Mucosa

I. Turesson

Department of Oncology, Sahlgrenska Hospital, 413 45 Gothenburg, Sweden

Introduction

The dose–response relationship is a very fundamental concept in radiotherapy for treatment of malignant diseases. The Poisson statistics, the number and types of target cells or functional tissue units, and their radiosensitivity determine the location and steepness of the dose–response curve in an individual patient. However, the dose–response curve estimated from a group of patients is always flatter than the individual one due to heterogeneity concerning the number and radiosensitivity of the target units and variation in the absorbed dose (Gilbert 1974; Thames and Hendry 1987).

In this chapter the dose–response characteristics for late effects derived from various fractionation schedules are described. The data were collected prospectively for skin and mucosa from patients treated for breast carcinoma and head and neck tumors.

The dose–response curve using probit analysis is characterized by:

1. The dose at 50% incidence of effect, ED_{50}, which is used for determination of isoeffect doses.
2. The absolute steepness, the probit width, K, which is the dose increment that would alter the incidence from 16% to 50% or from 50% to 84%.
3. The relative steepness, γ_{50}, which is the increase in incidence per 1% increase in dose on the steep part of the curve; γ_{50} is dimensionless (Brahme 1984).
4. The inverse radiosensitivity, D_0, of the target units for the tissue effect, which is related to the slope. D_0 can be derived from $dP/dD = -(P \ln P)/D_0$ using the LQ-Poisson model for tissue injury (P) (Thames and Hendry 1987).

Assays

Dose–response data were collected for skin telangiectasia up to 10 years after postoperative radiotherapy of the internal mammary nodes of breast cancer patients. The data include 1, 2, and 5 fractions per week with 3 or 4 dose levels per schedule. Altogether 286 fields were used. Details were published previously (Turesson 1991). However, it is worth noting that these data were collected from a well-defined, uniform, and simple radiotherapy material, and the unique feature of this study is the careful dosimetric control performed at each treatment session using thermoluminescence dosimetry (TLD).

Dose–response characteristics were also analyzed for the clinically important mucosa morbidity, such as necrosis and death from complications, 5 years after radiotherapy of advanced head and neck tumors. The details were presented previously (Turesson 1991).

Characteristics of Skin Telangiectasia

Skin telangiectasia was scored on an arbitrary 6-point scale, which covers the whole range of detectable changes: no, minimal, distinct, very marked, partially confluent, and totally confluent (score 0, 1, 2, 3, 4, and 5). The fractionation sensitivity measured by α/β was determined to 2.8 (1.7, 3.8) Gy using the linear-quadratic (LQ) model. However, a significant effect of the overall treatment time was found, and in using the LQ + time model α/β was estimated to be 4.2 (3.4, 4.8) Gy, γ/β to be 1.9 Gy^2/day and γ/α to be 0.46 Gy/day (Turesson and Thames 1989).

As is typical for late-responding tissues, skin telangiectasia progressed continuously with time, and the progression rate was strongly dose dependent (Turesson 1989). There was also a significant individual variation in progression rate for the same treatment (Turesson 1990; Tucker et al. 1992).

Results

An important consequence of the continuous progression of late effects is that the location and slope of the dose–response curve change with follow-up time. This is illustrated in Fig. 1 for skin telangiectasia and 5 × 1.8 Gy/week at 3, 5, and 10 years' follow-up. For score $\geqslant$3 (Fig. 1a) the dose–response curve is flat between 35 and 70 Gy at 3 years, but significantly steeper over the same dose range at 5 and 10 years. For score $\geqslant$4 (Fig. 1b) no dose–response relationship can be distinguished in this dose range at 3 years and only a weak dose response is seen at 5 years, in contrast to the steep curve at 10 years. The isoeffect dose, ED_{50}, is dramatically reduced between 3 and 10 years. Thus, for a progressive endpoint it is evident by comparison of the dose response for score $\geqslant$3 and score $\geqslant$4 that

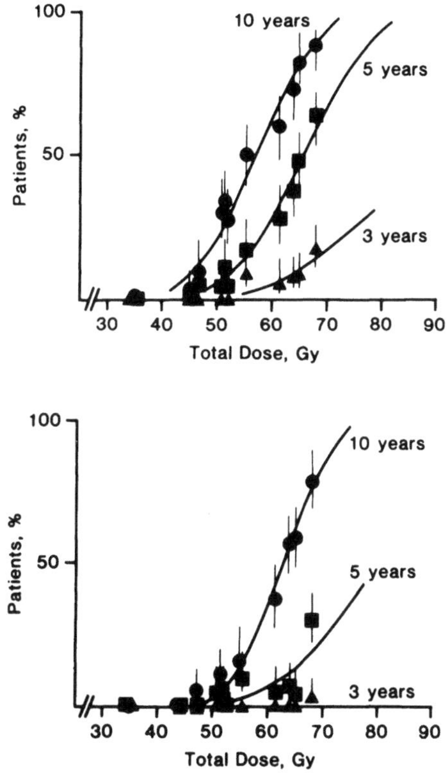

a

b

Fig. 1. **a** Dose–response relationship for telangiectasia score ⩾3 at 3(▲), 5(■), and 10(●) years' follow-up for 5 × 1.8 Gy/week. Error bars represent ± SE. **b** Dose–response relationship for telangiectasia score ⩾4 at 3(▲), 5(■), and 10(●) years' follow-up. Error bars represent ±SE. (From Turesson 1990, by permission of Pergamon Press)

the location and steepness vary not only with the length of follow-up but also with the degree of damage used as the endpoint.

The latter phenomenon is outlined in more detail from the data presented in Fig. 2, showing dose–incidence curves for various degrees of telangiectasia and 3 fractionation schedules at 10 years' follow-up time. It is evident that the ED_{50} increases when a higher degree of damage is used as the endpoint. The steepness of the curve is also higher the higher the score. All three dose schedules show the same pattern. For the sake of simplicity, only the figures of the dose–response parameters for distinct telangiectasia (score ⩾2) and partially confluent telangiectasia (score ⩾4) and 5 × 1.8 Gy/week will be shown here (Table 1). A complete analysis is presented elsewhere (Turesson 1991).

The isoeffect doses, ED_{50}, are 52.6 and 62.0 Gy for 1.8 Gy per fraction for score ⩾2 and score ⩾4 respectively. ED_{50} decreases with increasing

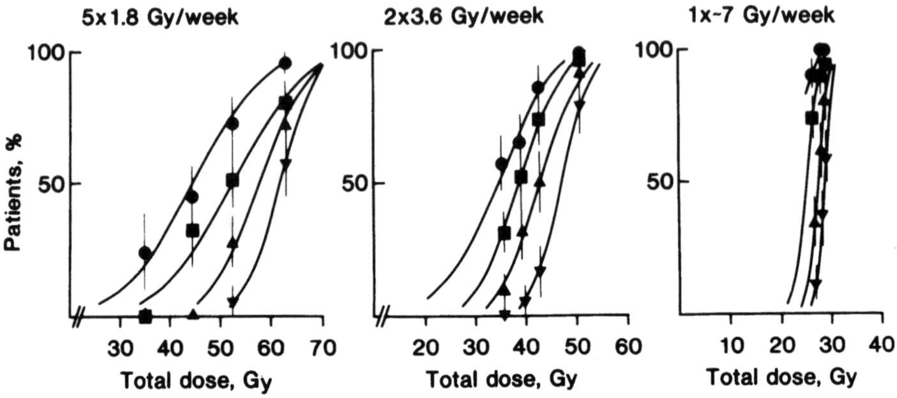

Fig. 2. Dose–response curves for various degrees of telangiectasia (⩾1, ●; ⩾2, ■; ⩾3, ▲; ⩾4, ▼) 10 years after radiotherapy, for three fractionation schedules. Error bars represent ±SE. (From Turesson 1991, by permission of Elsevier)

Table 1. Dose–response characteristics for skin telangiectasia at 5 × 1.8 Gy/week

Degree 10 years	ED_{50} (Gy)	*K* (Gy)	γ_{50}	D_{0eff} (Gy)
Score ⩾ 2	52.6	11.2	1.9	9.9
Score ⩾ 4	62.0	5.7	4.3	5.0

fraction size. The fractionation sensitivity, α/β, derived by direct analysis (Thames et al. 1986), does not differ significantly between different degrees of damage: 2.0 (1.0, 2.9) Gy for score ⩾2 and 2.7 (2.1, 3.5) Gy for score ⩾4.

The absolute steepness, measured as the probit width *K* of the dose–response curve, for 1.8 Gy per fraction is 11.2 and 5.7 Gy for score ⩾2 and score ⩾4 respectively, i.e., the steepness increases by almost a factor of 2 for the higher degree of damage. $K = 5.7$ Gy means that this dose increment will increase the incidence by 34%.

The relative steepness, measured as γ_{50}, is 1.9 and 4.3 for score ⩾2 and score ⩾4, respectively, for 5 × 1.8 Gy/week. As does the absolute steepness, the relative steepness also increases significantly with higher degree of damage. A γ_{50} value of 4.3 means that the incidence increases by 4.3 for a 1% increase in dose on the steep part of the curve.

From the LQ-Poisson model, γ_{50} is expected to be independent of fraction size. Very similar γ_{50} values were also found for 1.8 and 3.6 Gy per fraction. However, γ_{50} is also predicted to be higher when the dose–response curve is generated with a fixed fraction number (here $N = 4$) compared with a fixed fraction size (here 1.8 and 3.6 Gy). This was verified by the significantly

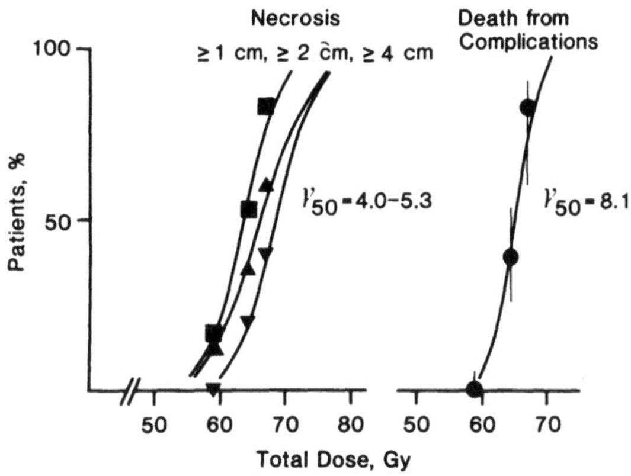

Fig. 3. Dose–response curves for various degrees of necrosis and fatal complications 5 years after radiotherapy of advanced head and neck tumors (2 fractions/day × 4/week; $\Delta t = 4\,h$; d = 2.1, 2.3, 2.4 Gy; N = 28)

higher γ_{50} (4.6 and 6.4 for score ≥2 and score ≥4, respectively) determined for the four-fraction schedule.

The inverse radiosensitivity, D_{0eff}, is 9.9 and 5.0 Gy for score ≥2 and score ≥4, respectively, for 1.8 Gy per fraction. The decrease with higher score is predictable from the higher steepness with higher score. D_{0eff} decreases with increasing dose per fraction and is therefore only relevant as a measure of radiosensitivity if it is related to fraction size.

An analogous analysis was done for late complications after radiotherapy of advanced head and neck tumors. Figure 3 shows the dose–response data for 50 patients treated twice a day, with a 4 h interval, with 2.1, 2.3 and 2.4 Gy per fraction and 28 fractions in 5.5 weeks. The treatment technique was very similar for all patients. The morbidity was scored regularly at least up to 5 years. The dose response for necrosis and death from complications was determined from the actuarial risk at 5 years.

The dose–response characteristics are given in Table 2. There is no difference in steepness for necrosis ≥1 cm, ≥2 cm, and ≥4 cm (Fig. 3), but for death from complications (rupture of the carotid artery, bleeding from necrosis, and severe edema and fibrosis) the steepness is higher by a factor of about 2 with $K = 3.2$ Gy and $\gamma_{50} = 8.1$.

Table 2. Dose–response characteristics for late morbidity in the head and neck region at 2 × ~2.2 Gy/day

Degree 5 years	ED_{50} (Gy)	K (Gy)	γ_{50}	D_{0eff} (Gy)
Necrosis ≥ 2 cm	66.5	6.5	4.0	5.8
Death from complications	64.9	3.2	8.1	2.8

Table 3. Dose–response characteristics for skin telangiectasia, single doses

Degree 10 years	ED_{50} (Gy)	K (Gy)	γ_{50}	D_{0eff} (Gy)
Score ≥ 2	14.1	1.3	4.1	1.2
Score ≥ 4	15.6	0.8	7.3	0.7

Table 4. Dose–response characteristics for late morbidity in the head and neck region, single doses

Degree 5 years	ED_{50} (Gy)	K (Gy)	γ_{50}	D_{0eff} (Gy)
Necrosis ≥ 2 cm	18.7	1.5	4.8	1.4
Death from complications	18.3	0.8	7.6	0.8

Single dose response allows the most proper comparison of dose–response characteristics for various endpoints. Therefore, the equivalent single dose–response curves with K, γ_{50}, and D_0 were calculated for all dose–response curves in Figs. 2 and 3 using the LQ model ($\alpha/\beta = 2.8$ Gy, $T_{\frac{1}{2}} = 3.0$ h). The figures for skin telangiectasia score ≥2 and score ≥4 are given in Table 3 and for mucosa morbidity in Table 4.

The dose–response characteristics found for late skin telangiectasia score ≥2 and score ≥4 are consistent with those derived for necrosis and fatal complications after radiotherapy of the head and neck tumors. The highest steepness determined corresponds to $K = 0.8$ Gy, $\gamma_{50} = 7$, and $D_0 = 0.7$ Gy.

Discussion

Skin telangiectasia in patients showed a continuous progression after radiotherapy, and the rate of progression was found to be strongly dose dependent. These findings have implications for dose–response analysis: the steepness of the dose–response curve increases and the isoeffect dose decreases with the follow-up time (Turesson 1989, 1990). In studying progressive late effects, one has to be cautious in using endpoints that result in a low incidence as these could be misleading concerning the dose–response relationship. This was illustrated for telangiectasia score 3 at 3 years and score 4 at 3 and 5 years (Fig. 1), which showed no or a very weak dose–response relationship. However, due to the dose-dependent progression rate, these endpoints showed a steep dose response at longer follow-up times. In contrast, lower degrees of telangiectasia (scores 1 and 2) are proper endpoints before 5 years' follow-up, showing a steep dose response

(Turesson 1989; Turesson and Thames 1989) even though the damage is very mild and of no clinical importance.

An important finding in the present analysis using skin telangiectasia is that the steepness of the dose-incidence curve at a certain follow-up time depends on the degree of damage. One explanation is related to the number of different types of target cells involved in the tissue response. Possible target cells for telangiectasia are endothelial cells and smooth muscle cells or both(Hopewell, this volume). If two types of target cells are responsible for the measured damage, this will give rise to a steeper dose-response curve than if only one target cell population is engaged. It might be the case that a mild degree of telangiectasia involves only one target cell population but that the higher degree engages both endothelial and smooth muscle cells and possibly also other cell populations such as fibroblasts. This may contribute to the higher steepness of the dose-incidence curve found with increasing degree of skin telangiectasia.

For late effects in the mucosa after radiotherapy of head and neck tumors, there was no difference in steepness between different degrees of necrosis, probably due to the lack of resolution in this small study. However, there was a clear difference between necrosis and fatal complications. It is reasonable to assume that there are more types of target cell populations involved and responsible for complications leading to death than for development of necrosis. This might explain the higher steepness for death compared with necrosis.

A distinction concerning the way the dose-response curve is generated is of importance for the criticality of the prescribed dose and dose distribution in radiotherapy. The steepness is higher when the dose-response curve is generated by a fixed fraction number compared with a fixed dose per fraction (Turesson 1991). Of practical importance is that the relative steepness is independent of the fraction number (Turesson, unpublished data) and the same as for single dose response. In this case, γ_{50} is about 7 for severe late effects (Fig. 4a). The relative steepness is also independent of the dose per fraction. In this case, γ_{50} is about 4 for severe late effects (Fig. 4b). In agreement with these findings for skin telangiectasia, the LQ-Poisson model predicts a higher steepness for curves generated by a fixed fraction number than for curves generated by a fixed fraction size (Thames and Hendry 1987).

The situation with a fixed fraction number is applicable to the dose distribution of the irradiated volume. If there is a volume of significant size with 110%, the risk for severe damage increases by 70% within that volume. The situation with a fixed dose per fraction is applicable to the prescribed dose and modification of the total dose. If we want to change the total dose we usually modify the number of fractions. An increase of 10% in this case will increase the risk for severe damage by 40%.

The inverse radiosensitivity, D_0, derived for skin telangiectasia and mucosa morbidity was surprisingly small, 0.7-0.8 Gy, for severe late effects

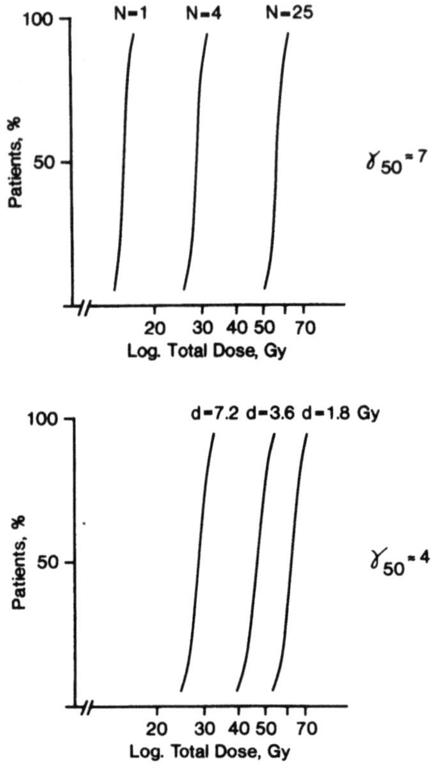

Fig. 4. a Dose–response steepness for severe late effects generated by a fixed fraction number: N = 1, N = 4 and N = 25. **b** Dose–response steepness for severe late effects generated by a fixed dose per fraction: d = 1.8 Gy, d = 3.6 Gy, and d = 7.2 Gy

(Tables 3 and 4). However, the values agree extremely well with those derived from experimental data for various functional injuries to kidney, lung, and spinal cord, which all varied between 0.6 and 0.8 Gy (Thames et al. 1989). This finding suggests that the heterogeneity is not much greater between individual patients than between inbred animals.

It is essential to relate the dose–response characteristics of late effects to acute reactions and tumor control. The parameters for mucositis at ED_{50} = 31.5 Gy were K = 3.8 Gy, γ_{50} = 3.3, and $D_{0\mathrm{eff}}$ = 3.3 Gy for a fraction size of 2.0 Gy at ED_{50}. The parameters for tumor control were ED_{50} = 58.9 Gy, K = 9.3 Gy, γ_{50} = 2.5, and $D_{0\mathrm{eff}}$ = 8.2 Gy for a fraction size of 2.1 Gy at ED_{50}. Thus, it is clear that the steepness of the dose–response curve is significantly less for both acute reactions and tumor control than for late effects. The implication for radiotherapy is that the criticality of the prescribed dose and dose distribution should be determined by the late tissue effects.

Conclusions

Skin telangiectasia in patients has been extensively studied as a model for late radiation effects. The fractionation sensitivity is in agreement with that for various late functional injuries determined experimentally with α/β close to 3 Gy. Also, as typical for late effects, telangiectasia progresses continuously and the progression rate is strongly dose dependent. Consequently, the location and steepness of the dose–response curve vary with the length of follow-up and the degree of damage used as the endpoint. At a certain follow-up time, the steepness increases with higher degree of telangiectasia. The highest steepness determined for telangiectasia score $\geqslant 4$ (partially confluent or more) at 10 years corresponded to $K = 0.8$ Gy, $\gamma_{50} = 7$, and $D_0 = 0.7$ Gy. The dose–response characteristics found for skin telangiectasia were consistent with those determined for necrosis and fatal complications 5 years after radiotherapy of head and neck tumors in our department.

References

Brahme A (1984) Dosimetric precision requirements in radiation therapy. Acta Radiol Oncol 23:379–391

Gilbert CW (1974) A double minus log transformation of mortality probabilities. Int J Radiat Biol 25:633–663

Thames HD, Hendry JH (1987) Fractionation in radiotherapy. Taylor and Francis, London

Thames HD, Rozell ME, Tucker SL, Ang KK, Fischer DR, Travis EL (1986) Direct analysis of quantal radiation response data. Int J Radiat Biol 49:999–1009

Thames HD, Hendry JH, Moore JV, Ang KK, Travis EL (1989) The high steepness of dose–response curves for late-responding normal tissues. Radiother Oncol 15:49–53

Tucker SL, Turesson I, Thames HD (1992) Evidence for individual differences in the radiosensitivity of human skin. Eur J Cancer 28A:1783–1791

Turesson I (1989) The progression rate of late radiation effects in normal tissue and its impact on dose–response relationships. Radiother Oncol 15:217–226

Turesson I (1990) Individual variation and dose dependency in the progression rate of skin telangiectasia. Int J Radiat Oncol Biol Phys 19:1569–1574

Turesson I, Thames HD (1989) Repair capacity and kinetics of human skin during fractionated radiotherapy: erythema, desquamation and telangiectasia after 3 and 5 years' follow-up. Radiother Oncol 15:169–188

Turesson I (1991) Characteristics of dose-response relationship for late radiation effects: an analysis of skin telangiectasia and of head and neck morbidity. Radiother Oncol 20:149–158

Early and Late Normal Tissue Injury after Postmastectomy Radiotherapy

S.M. Bentzen and M. Overgaard

Danish Cancer Society, Department of Experimental Clinical Oncology, and Department of Oncology, University Hospital of Aarhus, 8000 Aarhus C, Denmark

Introduction

Postmastectomy radiotherapy has played – and continues to play – a leading role in the clinical radiobiology of normal tissues. There are several reasons for this:

1. The loco-regional control rate is relatively high in these patients: in the Danish Breast Cancer Cooperative Group (DBCG) high-risk pre- and postmenopausal patients had an actuarial 10-year loco-regional control rate ranging between 83% and 94% (Overgaard et al. 1988). (High-risk patients according to the DBCG 1977 criteria are those in whom histologically positive lymph nodes were found, or the diameter of the primary tumor exceeded 5 cm, or there was microscopic evidence of invasion of the skin or the deep fascia.) Thus observation of normal tissue reactions in the treated region is possible without the confounding effect of progressive loco-regional disease.
2. The life expectancy of these patients is sufficient to allow long-term follow-up in a large proportion of them, which is necessary for studying the radiobiology of late-responding normal tissues in humans where the typical latent periods are several years. Even in high-risk patients the crude survival rate at 5 years is about 50% or better. Patients with incomplete follow-up, either because they are alive without having reached a specific endpoint at the time of the analysis, or have died from any cause, give rise to time-censored observations. Statistical methods are available to analyze such data in a multivariate setting, for example by means of the mixture model (Farewell 1977; Bentzen et al. 1989d,e) or the Cox proportional hazards model (Cox 1972; Taylor et al. 1987).
3. A number of tissues are included in the irradiated area which means that several endpoints are evaluable in each patient. Late endpoints that have been analyzed include subcutaneous fibrosis, telangiectasia,

Recent Results in Cancer Research, Vol. 130

pulmonary fibrosis, spontaneous rib fractures, impaired shoulder movement, brachial plexopathy, and persistent arm edema. Acute endpoints include erythema, moist desquamation, and radiation-induced pneumonitis. Among these, the most extensive quantitative studies have been on endpoints in the skin and the subcutis; however, impaired shoulder movement, a functional endpoint, has also been thoroughly analyzed.

4. Postmastectomy radiotherapy often involves different doses to a specific reference point and/or different radiation qualities. Examples are the application of a wax bolus to increase the surface dose around the surgical scar, or the use of an abutted electron field to treat the chest wall while minimizing the dose to the lung.
5. Finally, breast cancer is unfortunately the most common cancer in women in western countries, which means that relatively large series of patients treated with a consistent policy may be collected in a short time period even within a single institution.

Radiobiological topics of interest have been fractionation sensitivity, latent periods, interactions between treatment modalities, and the steepness of dose–response relationships. It is the aim of this article to review what has been learned from clinical radiobiological studies in postmastectomy radiotherapy during the last decade. One of the current hopes for reducing the level of treatment sequelae is to use predictive assays to identify patients with a high risk of developing severe complications and, ideally, to suggest a therapeutic alternative in such cases. Here we look at the hypothesis of a host factor, as for example a common intrinsic radiosensitivity in various tissues, by testing whether patients with a stronger-than-expected response for one endpoint also tend to have an increased probability of reaching another normal tissue endpoint. First, a brief summary is presented of the radiotherapy technique and the patient material in the Aarhus study of postmastectomy radiotherapy.

Radiotherapy Technique and Dosimetry

The target area in postmastectomy radiotherapy includes the chest wall, the surgical scar, the internal mammary chain nodes, the supra- and infraclavicular nodes, and the parasternal and axillary lymph nodes. A variety of field techniques have been devised to treat these regions. In the following a brief description is given of the radiotherapy technique used in the Danish Breast Cancer Cooperative Group (Overgaard et al. 1987, 1988). All patients were treated by an anterior 8 MV photon field covering the axillary and the infra- and supraclavicular areas. Individually shaped shielding blocks, positioned by means of skin marks drawn during fluoroscopy, protected the humerus from the level of the caput humeri, the larynx, and the lung below the level of the second rib. The shielded part of the chest wall was treated by an abutted electron field. The energy of the electron beam was chosen after ultrasound measurement of the thickness of the chest wall in the intercostal spaces. The surgical scar was covered by a 5 mm wax bolus with a margin of 3 cm. The area underneath the wax bolus (referred to as the axillary field), the open photon field (the supraclavicular field), and the electron field provided three independent scores of early and late radiation reactions.

The treatment technique remained essentially unchanged during the period from 1978 to 1982. However, beginning in 1981 the fractionation schedule was changed from 2 to 5 fractions per week. In the group given 2 fractions per week, 88 patients received a maximum absorbed dose of 51.36 Gy and 75 patients received a minimum target dose, specified at the level of the mid-axilla, of 36.6 Gy. In both cases the dose was delivered in 12 fractions over a period of 37–46 days. In the group given 5 fractions per week, 66 patients received a minimum target dose of 40.92 Gy in 22 fractions in an overall time of 29–35 days. In addition to these 229 patients another 90 patients received postmastectomy radiotherapy and adjuvant chemotherapy (see below). Inter-patient variations in the absorbed dose resulted in part from the two different dose prescriptions in the 12-fraction group, and partly from the patient-to-patient variation in the depth of the mid-axilla. For reference points close to the surface, corrections for field-size-dependent scatter from the block-supporting Plexiglas tray contributed additional variability (Bentzen et al. 1988).

Evaluation of Normal Tissue Injury

Early reactions (erythema and moist desquamation) were evaluated routinely by members of the staff or junior staff on the last day of treatment. The clinical description was used for retrospective scoring of the grade of reaction using an ordinal 4-point scale (Table 1). All late endpoints were scored by the same physician after a follow-up time of between 16 and 71 months using the scoring system summarized in Table 1. Time progression of late radiation injury was allowed for by means of a mixture model (Bentzen et al. 1989d).

Dosimetric Reference Points

A key problem in clinical radiobiology is to establish biologically relevant dosimetric reference points for the various endpoints. Standard practices of dose specification, such as using the maximum absorbed dose or the central dose, are of virtually no use for injury to superficially located tissues. Establishing a more relevant reference dose may be based on anatomical considerations, as in the case of telangiectasia where the reference depth of

Table 1. Scoring of normal tissue endpoints discussed here (Overgaard et al. 1987)

Endpoint	Grade 0	Grade 1	Grade 2	Grade 3
Moist desquamation	None	<10% of field	10%–49% of field	⩾50% of field
Erythema	None	Mild	Moderate	Severe with dry desquamation
Telangiectasia	None	$<1/cm^2$	$1-4/cm^2$	$>4/cm^2$
Subcutaneous fibrosis	None	Mild (just palpably increased firmness)	Moderate (definitely increased firmness)	Severe (very marked firmness, retraction and fixation)
Impaired shoulder movement	None	Slight reduction	Significant reduction	Severe reduction
Late arm edema	None	More than 2 cm difference in circumference		

0.1 mm was chosen to be immediately beneath the epidermis. For impaired shoulder movement, the so-called frozen shoulder, the dosimetric reference point was selected at 18 mm depth. This is a representative depth for calculating the dose received by the pectoralis major muscle at the level of the anterior axillary fold. Another approach was taken for subcutaneous fibrosis in the Aarhus study. A dosimetric reference depth of 4.1 mm was used for subcutaneous fibrosis. This depth was established by comparing isoeffective doses estimated from the axillary and supraclavicular fields as a function of the assumed (effective) depth of the target cell population. A reference depth of about 4 mm must be assigned in order to obtain consistent isoeffect estimates from these two areas (Bentzen et al. 1988).

Relative Biological Effectiveness of High-Energy Electrons

The relative biological effectiveness (RBE) of high-energy electrons relative to megavoltage photons is generally assumed to be close to unity (ICRU 1984). However, at small tissue depths, relative to the depth of the maximum absorbed dose point, electronic equilibrium has not yet been established and a difference in RBE might be expected. Although such a difference in most situations would not influence dose prescriptions in clinical radiotherapy, it should be taken into consideration for normal tissue endpoints in superficially located tissues. Because of differences in the depth–dose distributions for electrons and photons the ratio between isoeffective doses for these two radiation qualities is not an RBE in a rigorous sense but rather an equivalent effect ratio (ICRP-ICRU 1963). In any case, the doses in the relevant reference point for a specific endpoint must be corrected by the apparent RBE if electron and photon data are to be analyzed jointly. The RBE for telangiectasia in the Aarhus material was 0.89 (95% confidence limits 0.85, 0.93) for telangiectasia and 0.88 (0.86, 0.91) for subcutaneous fibrosis (Bentzen and Overgaard 1991).

Latency

Radiation reactions in human tissues are expressed after a characteristic time period: the latent time. The clinically and biologically important distinction between early and late responses is based on their latent periods, which in humans are typically measured in weeks and years, respectively.

There are two main motives for studying latency in clinical radiobiology. First, latency is a biological characteristic of the expression of radiation-induced tissue injury. The time progression of late radiation injury is a fundamental biological phenomenon that needs no further justification to be the subject of study. In principle latent-time distributions may carry important information on tissue structure and kinetics (Wheldon et al. 1982), an aspect that has been quantitatively investigated only to a limited extent.

The second motive is crucial: in order to obtain valid estimates of incidence and radiobiological parameters time-censored observations must be allowed for. A censored observation is the technical term for a subject with incomplete follow-up, in this case a patient who had not reached the endpoint at the time of the last examination. Such a patient carries the positive information that she has been alive without having developed the radiation reaction in question at a given time after the end of treatment. Statistical methods, often termed actuarial methods, are available for obtaining incidence estimates (Berkson and Gage 1952; Kaplan and Meier 1958) or for multivariate analysis of this type of data (Cox 1972; Farewell 1977). The application of multivariate methods to time-censored radiobiological data has been discussed previously (Bentzen et al. 1989d, e; Taylor et al. 1987). Failing to use appropriate statistical methods may, depending on the frequency of censoring, lead to considerable underestimates of the incidence of a given complication (e.g., Schultheiss et al. 1986; Bentzen et al. 1989d; Turesson and Notter 1986; Turesson 1989).

Extensive studies of latency have been conducted, especially for telangiectasia (Turesson and Notter 1986; Turesson 1989; Bentzen et al. 1990b) but also for subcutaneous fibrosis (Bentzen et al. 1989d) and impaired shoulder movement (Bentzen et al. 1989b). The results of these studies may be summarized briefly as follows. Late endpoints in humans progress in severity with time, at least within the first 3 years or more after the end of treatment. This means that the proportion of patients expressing a specific grade of radiation injury will also increase with time. Although a plateau is reached in the incidence of the endpoint, the effects in some patients will continuously progress in severity. The latent time depends on the grade of reaction being considered, with higher grades being expressed at progressively longer follow-up times. The estimated time at which 90% of the ultimately expected incidence has been reached is shown in Table 2 for the three endpoints. Furthermore, the latent period is strongly dependent on the biological effectiveness of the treatment: grade 3 reactions in the Gothenburg series had an estimated median latent time ranging from 11 years to 4.8 years as the total dose was increased from 40 to 70 Gy with 2 Gy per fraction (Bentzen et al. 1990b). This is of concern in the design of follow-up patterns in clinical radiobiology: assessing the incidence of a given reaction at a fixed point in time may underestimate the incidence in some dose-fractionation schedules. One more caveat: it remains to be settled whether combined modality treatment precipitates the late injury.

Fractionation Sensitivity

Since the early 1980s the linear-quadratic (LQ) model has come into widespread use as a means of quantifying the response of normal tissue to changes in dose per fraction. Several biophysical models of cellular radiation injury predict approximately linear-quadratic dose–effect relationships (Goodhead 1987). Yet these models have, as yet, not played any significant role in the justification of the LQ model. At present the LQ model is not regarded as mechanistic at the cellular level. Conceptually, the LQ model and its application have been justified by its assumed validity for an underlying population of target cells responsible for the expression of damage (Thames et al. 1982), and this has been a fruitful point of view. However, it is possible to apply the model operationally without this assumption (Fowler 1983).

The main reason for the influence of the LQ model in the field of fractionation studies is the discovery that fractionation sensitivity may be characterized by the ratio between the two parameters of the model, α/β, and that this ratio is significantly different in early- and late-responding tissues (Thames et al. 1982). High fractionation sensitivities, that is low α/β values, are seen in late-responding normal tissues, and relatively low fractionation sensitivities (α/β around 10 Gy) are seen in early-responding tissues. The validity of this observation, originally made from experimental animal studies, has been tested in clinical radiobiology (Thames et al. 1990). Again, most quantitative studies have been conducted in postmastectomy radiotherapy and, as summarized in Table 2, the pattern seen in experimental studies does actually correspond to what is seen in clinical studies.

A famous presentation of the LQ model is the plot of isoeffective doses for various endpoints in experimental animals, which has been nicknamed the spaghetti plot. With our current knowledge on fractionation sensitivities of human tissues it is possible to construct a clinical "spaghetti plot" (Fig.

Table 2. α/β ratios and latency for late radiation injury after postoperative radiotherapy

Tissue	Endpoint	α/β (Gy)	LT_{90} (years)	Reference
Subcutis	Fibrosis	1.9 (0.8, 3.0)	3.2 (2.3, 3.9)	Bentzen et al (1989d)
Vasculature	Telangiectasia	2.8 (−0.1, 8.1)	4.7 (2.8, 6.5)	Bentzen and Overgaard (1991)
		2.8 (1.7, 3.8)	?	Turesson and Thames (1989)
		3.9 (2.7, 4.8)[a]	?	Turesson and Thames (1989)
		2.6 (2.2, 3.3)[b]	2–15[c]	Bentzen et al. (1990b)
Lung	Fibrosis	3.6 (?)	?	Overgaard (1985)
Bone	Necrosis	≈2. (–, –)	<3 (?)	Overgaard (1988)
Muscle/vasculature/cartilage	Impaired shoulder movement	3.5 (0.7, 6.2)	3.9 (3.1, 4.6)	Bentzen et al. (1989b)
Subcutis/muscle	Nipple retraction	2.5 (?)	?	Van Limbergen et al. (1989)
Lymphatic system	Late arm edema	6. (–, –)[d]	?	Bentzen et al. (1989b)
Nerve	Brachial plexopathy	≈2. (?)	?	Powell et al. (1990)

?, not available; (?), 95% confidence limits not available; (–, –), 95% confidence limits too large to be estimated by standard methods
[a] With correction for overall treatment time (see Turesson and Thames 1989)
[b] Reanalysis of graded response data from Turesson and Thames (1989) with latent-time correction
[c] Depends on grade of reaction and toxicity of treatment (Bentzen et al. 1990b)
[d] Confounded by extent of axillary dissection

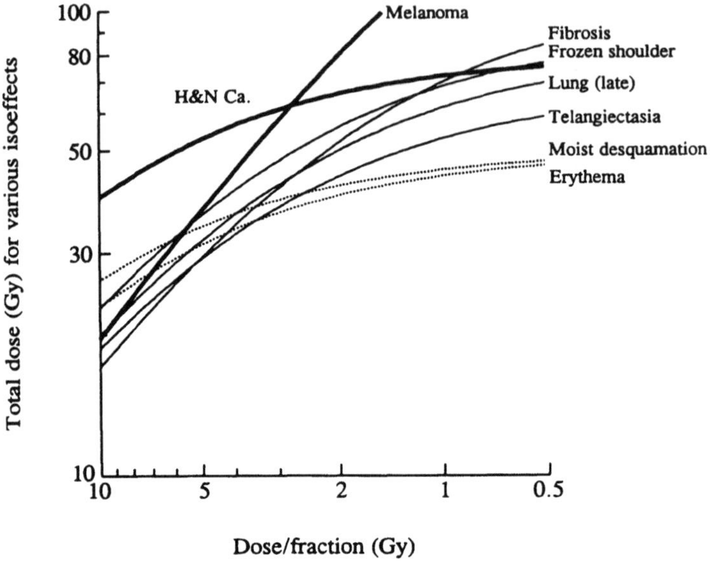

Fig. 1. Change in isoeffective dose for various isoeffects for clinical endpoints. *Dashed curves* are for early reactions, *continuous curves* for late reactions. All normal tissue endpoints are from postmastectomy radiotherapy studies (data in Table 2, where references may be found). Data for two tumors are plotted: squamous cell carcinoma of the tonsil, $\alpha/\beta = 7.2\,Gy$ (Maciejewski et al. 1989), and malignant melanoma, $\alpha/\beta = 0.6\,Gy$ (Bentzen et al. 1989a). No α/β estimate is available for adenocarcinoma of the breast

1). The general observation for the late-responding normal tissues is that change in isoeffective dose with fraction size is more rapid than that seen for the early-responding tissues. One consequence of this is that fractionation schedules which are isoeffective with respect to early reactions will not be so with respect to late reactions.

Fractionation Sensitivity of Tumors

By analogy with experimental animal data, human tumors have been supposed to be characterized by a low fractionation sensitivity, similar to that of early-responding tissues. This proposition seems to hold true for squamous cell carcinoma, but even though melanoma may be the exception that proves the rule, it seems likely that the biological diversity among human tumors is larger than among human normal tissues.

There are only very limited data on the effect of changed fractionation on tumor control in breast cancer. Patients treated with postmastectomy radiotherapy may be free of disease or have only microscopic disease at the time of radiotherapy. In the Aarhus study, comparing the 4-year loco-regional control rates revealed no significant difference between the two fractionation schedules, suggesting that the two arms, which were roughly equivalent with respect to the incidence of early reactions, were isoeffective in controlling subclinical disease. However, this does not allow a more rigorous estimation of the α/β ratio. Regarding repopulation of tumor cells during therapy, there are some indications (see Thames et al. (1990) for a summary) that this effect is less important in breast cancer than it is in squamous cell carcinoma of the head and neck.

Repair Kinetics

Few clinical data exist on the kinetics of sublethal damage repair. The only quantitative study, to our knowledge, is the analysis by Turesson and Thames (1989) of telangiectasia after postmastectomy radiotherapy with intervals between fractions varying from 15 min to several days. The repair half-time was estimated at 3.4 (2.8, 4.2) h. A remarkable finding in the Gothenburg study was that overall treatment time appeared to influence the level of telangiectasia. Repopulation is not a likely explanation for this, as the introduction of a 3-week pause in the treatment course did not significantly reduce the incidence of telangiectasia. Likewise an influence of overall treatment time on the incidence of late complications has been sought in the Aarhus study, but without any demonstrable effect. Admittedly, the variation in overall treatment time is limited in this study. The more likely explanation for the finding in the Gothenburg study seems to be a slow repair component, apparently incomplete even with a 24 h interval between fractions. It remains to be clarified to what extent slow repair, a phenomenon of obvious importance in the design of schedules with multiple fractions per day, is also a problem with other late endpoints. At the time of writing, studies in the rat spinal cord indicate that this may be so (K.K. Ang, personal communication 1991).

Dose–Response Relationships

Dose–response curves for late injury after postmastectomy radiotherapy are remarkably steep. The steepness may be quantified by means of the normalized dose–response gradient, γ, that is the percentage increase in complication rate for a 1% increase in dose. More formally γ is defined as (Brahme 1984):

$$\gamma = D\frac{\Delta P}{\Delta D}$$

where ΔP and ΔD are increases in the probability of reaching the endpoint and in the total dose, respectively. In the limit where $\Delta D \longrightarrow 0$ the quotient on the right-hand side approaches the derivative of the complication-probability function for dose D. Because of the sigmoid shape of the dose–response curve, γ depends on the incidence level at which it is estimated. Here, the 50% level is chosen. Also, from the mixture model formulation of the LQ model, the steepness is expected to increase with increasing observation time and with increasing grade of the endpoint in question. This has indeed been shown empirically to hold for telangiectasia (Turesson 1990). Furthermore, the steepness depends on whether the dose–response relationship is estimated for a constant number of fractions, $\gamma_{N,50}$, or for a constant dose per fraction, $\gamma_{d,50}$. In the first case, an increase (or decrease) in dose is accompanied by an increase (decrease) in fraction size as well, which leads to an increased (decreased) biological effective dose. As a consequence, the dose–response curve is steeper in that case, or formally $\gamma_{N,50} > \gamma_{d,50}$. The steepness of relevance for hot or cold spots and for patients being systematically over- or under-dosed is $\gamma_{N,50}$, as the number of fractions will be equal to a prescribed number in such cases. If, on the other hand, the total dose to a group of patients is deliberately changed, such a change will most commonly be made with a fixed dose per fraction in which case $\gamma_{d,50}$ is the relevant steepness measure.

Table 3 shows the γ factors derived for three late endpoints after post-mastectomy radiotherapy. Thames and colleagues (1989) reanalyzed dose–response data for three late-responding tissues in experimental animal models: kidney, lung, and spinal cord. These authors noted that the dose–response curves for late responses in these three tissues are steeper than those for acute responses in skin and gut, but suggested that the steepness for human late responses would be decreased by inter-patient heterogeneity. However, converting the steepnesses estimated in that study into values of γ yields values between 3.2 and 5.6, i.e., in the same range as the steepness of the clinical dose–response curves analyzed here. Turesson (1990) found a $\gamma_{d,50}$ of 2.5 for her grade $\geq$3 telangiectasia at 10 years of follow-up that

Table 3. Steepness of the dose–response curve: the Aarhus experience

Endpoint	Grade	$\gamma_{N,50}$[a]	$\gamma_{d,50}$[b]
Fibrosis	≥2	5.7	3.3
Impaired shoulder movement	≥2	6.6	4.8
Telangiectasia	3	3.2	2.2
	≥2	1.4	1.0

[a] Normalized dose–response gradient with a fixed number of fractions (22)

[b] Normalized dose–response gradient with a fixed dose per fraction (2.0 Gy)

was in good agreement with the value for grade 3 telangiectasia in the Aarhus series. For grade ≥4 Turesson estimated the value to be 3.5 at 10 years. These values are in good agreement with those derived from the Aarhus series in which grade ≥2 telangiectasia appears to be roughly equivalent to grade ≥1 telangiectasia on the Gothenburg scale (Bentzen et al. 1990b). The increase in steepness with increasing grade of reaction is also seen here, where the dose–response curve for grade 3 telangiectasia is steeper than that for grade ≥2 telangiectasia.

Precision Requirements in Isoeffective Dose Calculations

The high steepness of the dose–response curve for late radiation injury in humans has obvious implications for radiotherapy. The incidence and severity of late complications depend critically on the exact absorbed dose. Likewise, if the dose prescription is changed, for example to exploit a possible benefit from altered fractionation, the α/β ratio has to be determined quite accurately to ensure a high probability of the level of normal tissue complications being within a clinically acceptable range. This is illustrated in Fig. 2 where the uncertainty in the isoeffective dose estimate for subcutaneous fibrosis is plotted as a function of dose per fraction. The reference schedule is assumed to employ 2 Gy per fraction. The uncertainties

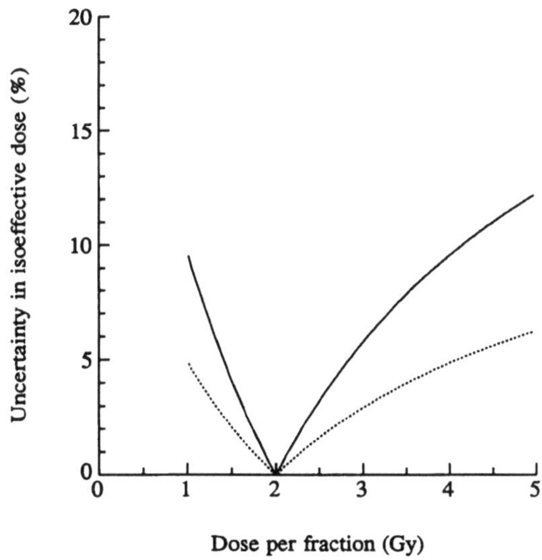

Fig. 2. Uncertainty in the isoeffective dose for grade ≥2 subcutaneous fibrosis calculated by means of the LQ model for a change in dose per fraction. The reference fraction size was 2 Gy, α/β = 1.9 (0.8, 3.0) Gy. *Dashed curves* and *continuous curves* indicate the approximate standard error and 95% confidence limits (both expressed as a percentage of the estimated total dose), respectively

in the figure are calculated using the propagation-of-error technique and should be regarded as approximate values. Nevertheless, they provide a useful impression of the precision requirement when using the LQ formula for practical isoeffect calculations. As an example, assume that a fractionation schedule is changed from 60 Gy with 2 Gy per fraction to a schedule employing 5 Gy per fraction. The biologically equivalent dose for subcutaneous fibrosis is easily calculated using the isoeffect formula derived from the LQ model (Withers et al. 1983) with $\alpha/\beta = 1.9$ Gy (Table 2). It is about 33.9 Gy. But because of the uncertainty in the α/β ratio there will be an uncertainty in the estimated isoeffective dose with 5 Gy per fraction. From the continuous curve in Fig. 2 it is seen that the 95% confidence limits for the estimated total dose will be ±12%, or in this case ±4.1 Gy. Another example is the estimation of the range of doses per fraction for which the 95% confidence interval of the estimated isoeffective dose is within ±5% of that dose. This interval is approximately 1.4–2.8 Gy. Because of the very steep dose–response curves for late reactions even an uncertainty in isoeffective dose within ±5% may yield a clinically unacceptable uncertainty in the predicted incidence of late sequelae. The uncertainties depicted in Fig. 2 become especially large in the case of low α/β ratios and when extrapolating to low doses per fraction.

Interaction Between Radiotherapy and Other Treatment Modalities

Several treatment modalities have a place in the treatment of breast cancer: surgery, radiotherapy, chemotherapy, endocrine therapy and, in advanced cases, hyperthermia. Following Steel and Peckham (1979) a therapeutic gain from combined modality treatment might result from four mechanisms: spatial cooperation, independent toxicities, normal tissue protection, or enhanced tumor response. As an example, the classical rationale behind the use of modified radical mastectomy and postoperative radiotherapy for breast cancer is to reduce the overall toxicity by combining two less-than-radical modalities without compromising the long-term loco-regional control rate. Nevertheless, the incidence of late arm edema, defined here as a more than 2 cm difference in the circumference of the ipsilateral and contralateral arms, was significantly dependent not only on radiation dose and dose per fraction but also on the extent of the axillary dissection (Bentzen et al. 1989b). Thus if surgical procedures are intensified a dose reduction may be needed to maintain an acceptable level of late arm edema.

Despite the increasing use of combined adjuvant systemic therapy and postoperative radiotherapy in breast cancer, surprisingly few data have been published quantifying the effect of adding the two modalities. In the Aarhus study, adjuvant CMF (cyclophosphamide, methotrexate, and 5-fluorouracil) and postoperative radiotherapy have been found significantly to increase the risk of developing marked subcutaneous fibrosis (Bentzen et al. 1989c). Late and acute complications were scored in 90 patients who received adjuvant chemotherapy in combination with radiotherapy according to the DBCG 77 protocols (Andersen et al. 1981; Overgaard et al. 1987). Radiotherapy and the first cycles of chemotherapy were given concomitantly. One cycle of

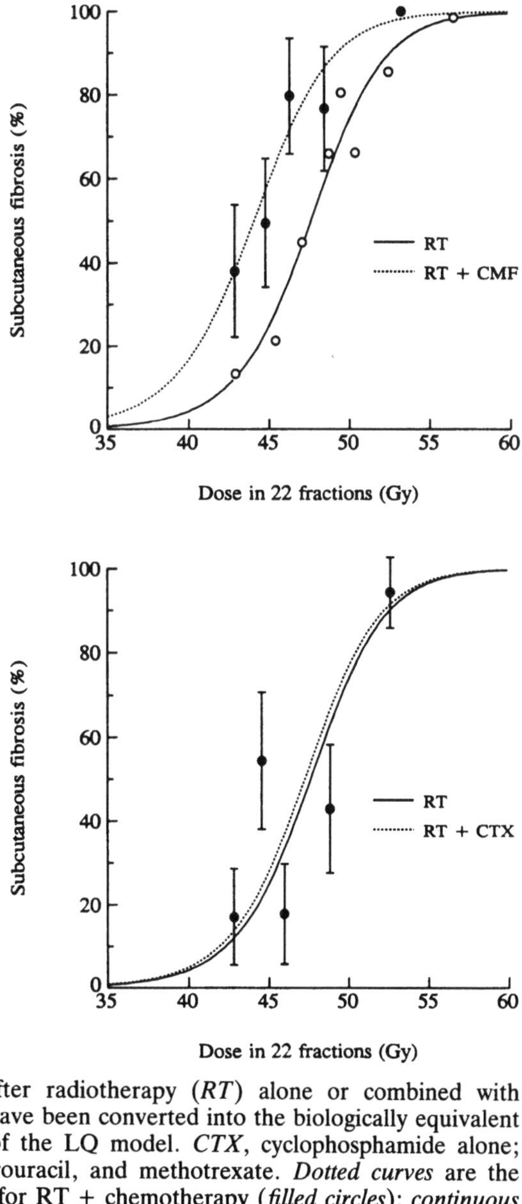

Fig. 3. Subcutaneous fibrosis after radiotherapy (*RT*) alone or combined with chemotherapy. Radiation doses have been converted into the biologically equivalent dose in 22 fractions by means of the LQ model. *CTX*, cyclophosphamide alone; *CMF*, cyclophosphamide, 5-fluorouracil, and methotrexate. *Dotted curves* are the best fitting dose-response curve for RT + chemotherapy (*filled circles*); *continuous curves* are for RT alone (*open circles*). Data in the *upper panel* are redrawn from Bentzen et al. (1989c)

cyclophosphamide (CTX) consisted of 130 mg/m^2 administered perorally (p.o.) daily from days 1 to 14. This schedule was given to 45 patients. One cycle of CMF consisted of 80 mg/m^2 CTX p.o. daily from days 1 to 14, 30 mg/m^2 methotrexate intravenously (i.v.) on days 1 and 8, and 500 mg/m^2 5-fluorouracil i.v. on days 1 and 8. CMF was given to 45 patients. In both schedules, cycles of chemotherapy were given every 4 weeks for a total of 12 cycles. The radiotherapy technique was identical to that of patients treated with radiotherapy alone. Five fractions per week were given to 28 and 27 patients in the CTX and CMF groups, respectively.

Both CTX and CMF significantly increased the level of acute reactions relative to radiotherapy alone (Bentzen et al. 1989c). For the late reactions the findings are summarized in Fig. 3. Patients receiving CMF and radiotherapy had a statistically significantly increased risk of developing marked (grade $\geqslant 2$) fibrosis. The estimated risk of ultimately developing this late reaction after 44 Gy in 22 fractions increased from 19% to 50% for the combined therapy group. When CTX was given alone no significant increase in the incidence of fibrosis was found (Fig. 3). The importance of the timing of the two modalities is not known. In the analysis, the effect of CMF or CTX was assumed to be to reduce the target cell content of the irradiated tissue, but it was not possible to discriminate between this and other biological explanations for the increased toxicity of the combined treatment.

Predisposing Factors

Individualization of treatment regimens is of great potential value in cancer therapy. While much attention has been paid to predictive assays of tumor response to radiotherapy (Peters et al. 1988b), the real problem for the clinician is to optimize the therapeutic differential between normal tissue injury and tumor response, preferably in the individual patient. Thus predictors of normal tissue response are *a priori* of equal importance (Peters 1990). Such predictors can be divided roughly into two categories: clinical predisposing factors and predictive assays (that is laboratory tests assessing the probability of normal tissue injury after a specific treatment schedule). New developments in data analysis have enhanced the capability for identifying predisposing factors in a multivariate setting (Thames et al. 1986; Bentzen et al. 1990a).

Factors influencing the development of late radiation reactions have been sought in the Aarhus study (Bentzen et al. 1989b) in patients treated with radiotherapy alone, and the results are summarized in Table 4. For subcutaneous fibrosis only total dose and dose per fraction had a significant influence. These two factors were significant for all late endpoints investigated. For impaired shoulder movement, age above 60 years was a predisposing factor in developing reduced mobility of the ipsilateral relative to the contralateral shoulder. However, participation in a physical rehabilita-

Table 4. Factors of importance for late sequelae after postmastectomy radiotherapy

Endpoints	Factors influencing incidence
Telangiectasia	Total dose
	Dose per fraction
	Previous moist desquamation
Fibrosis	Total dose
	Dose per fraction
Arm edema	Total dose
	Dose per fraction
	Extent of axillary dissection
Frozen shoulder	Total dose
	Dose per fraction
	Patient's age
	Physical exercise
	Subcutaneous fibrosis (?)

tion program had a beneficial effect in reducing the probability of this complication. Finally, subcutaneous fibrosis was tested and was found to predispose to frozen shoulder. The occurrence of this endpoint is a likely indication of the presence of muscular fibrosis as well, and this may explain the observed predisposition. There was no increased risk associated with postoperative complications, lateral tumor location, overall treatment time, late arm edema, or telangiectasia. For the expression of telangiectasia, previous moist desquamation was associated with an increased risk, an observation discussed below.

Consequential Late Reactions

Another problem that has attracted attention is consequential late reactions, that is late reactions seen as sequelae of severe acute reactions (Peracchia and Salti 1981; Peters et al. 1988a). This effect was investigated in the Aarhus study for the acute radiation reactions of erythema and moist desquamation, and the two late endpoints of subcutaneous fibrosis and telangiectasia (Bentzen and Overgaard 1991). A statistically significant predisposition for telangiectasia was found in patients with previous moist desquamation (Table 5). As an example, the incidence of grade 3 telangiectasia following 44 Gy in 22 fractions increased from 27% to 49% in patients having a history of moist desquamation covering more than 10% of the field. This observation may be considered mechanistically as a consequence of the breakdown of the epidermal protection of the endothelial cells. Such a predisposition was not seen for telangiectasia after severe erythema or for subcutaneous fibrosis after either of the two acute radiation reactions.

Table 5. Association between early and late reactions after postmastectomy radiotherapy

	Moist desquamation	Severe erythema
Fibrosis	ns	ns
Telangiectasia	$p = 0.04$	ns

ns, not significant at the 0.05 level

Intrinsic Radiosensitivity

Improved techniques for culturing of human skin fibroblasts open up the possibility of routine clinical use of in vitro assays for cell survival vs dose. Also human epithelial and endothelial cells may be grown in culture with an increasing success rate as laboratory research progresses (Peters et al. 1988b). These developments have stirred an interest in the prospects for in vitro radiosensitivity testing as a guidance for clinical therapy optimization. Loeffler and colleagues (1990) found that the in vitro radiosensitivity of human skin fibroblasts in 5 patients with an unusually strong acute reaction to standard radiotherapy was significantly higher than in fibroblasts from a randomly selected sample of 6 patients with normal acute reactions. Although these results are of considerable interest in themselves they do not allow a direct evaluation of the predictive power of this assay. First, the 5 patients constitute only 0.6% of a population of 811 patients from which they were selected because of their atypical radiation reaction. Thus when applying this method as a predictive assay these patients have to be detected against an (unknown) background of normally responding individuals. Using the criteria defined by Little and Nove (1990) only 3 of these 5 patients would have been classified as being in "the lower range of sensitivity". Secondly, it remains to be established to what extent the in vitro fractionation sensitivity is predictive for the late clinical endpoints that are regarded as the dose-limiting radiation reactions in radiotherapy.

It is possible, however, to throw a little light on the possible existence of a host factor as a major determinant of the response of normal tissues to radiotherapy. At the clinical level, if variability in (genetically determined?) intrinsic radiosensitivity is indeed a major component in the patient-to-patient variability in response to radiotherapy, this should show up as subsets of patients with radiation reactions that are stronger or weaker than expected. An example is the occurrence of subcutaneous fibrosis and telangiectasia in a population of patients treated with a variety of radiotherapy schedules. Patients with a severe grade of fibrosis are more likely also to present with telangiectasia, simply because the incidence and severity of both endpoints increase with increasing dose/dose per fraction. This association due to treatment intensity will almost inevitably influence the clinical impression that some patients tend to present with multiple late radiation sequelae. Bourne and colleagues (1983) showed that patients who had serious early reactions after intracavitary plus external beam radiotherapy for cancer of the uterine cervix had a statistically significantly increased risk of developing late bowel complications. Without discussing that study in detail, it is noteworthy that stratification according to the dose received by the two radiotherapy modalities was not performed, and that patients who had severe complications all had at least one radium insertion. Thus it can not be ruled out that high risk of early and late sequelae was quite simply found in patients who had the highest dose/dose rate.

To overcome this general problem, treatment toxicity must be allowed for before looking for a possible association between two endpoints. One way to do this is to look at the residuals (see Bentzen et al. 1989a for an example of this method), that is the difference between the observed and expected response for a given endpoint, scored in a specific treatment field. This has been done for subcutaneous fibrosis and telangiectasia in the Aarhus series (Bentzen et al. 1992). Highly statistically significant correlations were found between the same endpoint evaluated in two different fields. However, when the two endpoints were mixed, no significant correlation was found. These results weaken the hypothesis about a generally low or high radiosensitivity of all normal tissues in individual patients.

What Next?

The quantitative clinical radiobiology studies that have been conducted in the 1980s have considerably increased our knowledge on the response of human normal tissues to radiotherapy. In the next decade we expect the link between clinical and laboratory research to be further strengthened, and normal tissue radiobiology will increasingly focus on underlying biological mechanisms. The high steepness of dose–response curves for late normal tissue reactions is not only a serious concern to the clinician but also an encouragement to conduct more clinical studies. The attitude that clinical heterogeneities preclude quantitative radiobiological studies has been a self-fulfilling prophecy. In reality, clinical radiobiological studies are not only feasible but much needed.

References

Andersen KW, Mouridsen HT, Castberg T, Fischerman K, Andersen J, Hou-Jensen K, Brincker H, Johansen H, Henriksen E, Rørth M, Rossing N (1981) Organisation of the Danish adjuvant trials in breast cancer. Dan Med Bull 28:102–106

Bentzen SM, Overgaard M (1991) Relationship between early and late normal-tissue injury after postmastectomy radiotherapy. Radiother Oncol 20:159–165

Bentzen SM, Thames HD (1989) Incidence and latency of radiation reactions. Radiother Oncol 14:261–262
Bentzen SM, Christensen JJ, Overgaard J, Overgaard M (1988) Some methodological problems in estimating radiobiological parameters from clinical data: alpha/beta ratios and electron RBE for cutaneous reactions in patients treated with postmastectomy radiotherapy. Acta Oncol 27:105–116
Bentzen SM, Overgaard J, Thames HD, Overgaard M, Hansen PV, von der Maase H, Meder J (1989a) Clinical radiobiology of malignant melanoma. Radiother Oncol 16:169–182
Bentzen SM, Overgaard M, Thames HD (1989b) Fractionation sensitivity of a clinical endpoint: impaired shoulder movement after post-mastectomy radiotherapy. Int J Radiat Oncol Biol Phys 17:531–537
Bentzen SM, Overgaard M, Thames HD, Christensen JJ, Overgaard J (1989c) Early and late normal-tissue injury after postmastectomy radiotherapy alone or combined with chemotherapy. Int J Radiat Biol 56:711–715
Bentzen SM, Thames HD, Overgaard M (1989d) Latent-time estimation for late cutaneous and subcutaneous radiation reactions in a single-follow-up clinical study. Radiother Oncol 15:267–274
Bentzen SM, Thames HD, Travis EL, Ang KK, van der Schueren E, Dewit L, Dixon DO (1989e) Direct estimation of latent time for radiation injury in late-responding normal tissues: gut, lung and spinal cord. Int J Radiat Biol 55: 27–43
Bentzen SM, Thames HD, Tucker SL, Smith C (1990a) New options in direct analysis of dose–response data. Int J Radiat Biol 57:221–225
Bentzen SM, Turesson I, Thames HD (1990b) Fractionation sensitivity and latency of telangiectasia after postmastectomy radiotherapy: a graded response analysis. Radiother Oncol 18:95–106
Bentzen SM, Overgaard M, Overgaard J (1992) Clinical correlations between late normal-tissue endpoints after radiotherapy: implications for predictive assays of radiosensitivity. Eur J Cancer (submitted)
Berkson J, Gage RP (1952) Survival curve for cancer patients following treatment. J Am Stat Assoc 47:501–515
Bourne RG, Kearsley JH, Grove WJ, Roberts SJ (1983) The relationship between early and late gastrointestinal complications of radiation therapy for carcinoma of the cervix. Int J Radiat Oncol Biol Phys 9:1445–1450
Brahme A (1984) Dosimetric precision requirements in radiation therapy. Acta Radiol Oncol 23:379–391
Cox DR (1972) Regression models and life-tables (with discussion). J R Stat Soc [B] 34:178–220
Farewell VT (1977) A model for a binary variable with timecensored observations. Biometrika 64:43–46
Fowler JF (1983) Dose–response curves for organ function or cell survival. Br J Radiol 56:497–500
Goodhead DT (1987) Biophysical models of radiation action; introductory review. In: Fielden EM, Fowler JF, Hendry JH, Scott D (eds) Radiation research, vol 2. Taylor and Francis, London, pp 306–311
ICRP-ICRU (1963) Report of the RBE committee to the International Commissions on Radiological Protection and on Radiological Units and Measurements. Health Phys 9:357–384
ICRU (1984) Radiation dosimetry: electron beams with energies between 1 and 50 MeV. Bethesda, MD, USA: International Commission on Radiation Units and Measurements, Report no 35
Kaplan EL, Meier P (1958) Non-parametric estimation from incomplete observations. J Am Stat Soc [C] 53:457–481

Little JB, Nove J (1990) Sensitivity of human diploid fibroblast cell strains from various genetic disorders to acute and protracted radiation exposure. Radiat Res 123:87–92

Loeffler JS, Harris JR, Dahlberg WK, Little JB (1990) In vitro radiosensitivity of human diploid fibroblasts derived from women with unusually sensitive clinical responses to definitive radiation therapy for breast cancer. Radiat Res 121:227–231

Maciejewski B, Withers HR, Taylor JMG, Hliniak A (1989) Dose fractionation and regeneration in radiotherapy for cancer of the oral cavity and oropharynx: tumor dose–response and repopulation. Int J Radiat Oncol Biol Phys 16:831–843

Overgaard M (1985) The clinical implication of non-standard fractionation. Int J Radiat Oncol Biol Phys 11:1225–1226

Overgaard M (1988) Radiation-induced spontaneous rib fractures in breast cancer patients treated with postmastectomy irradiation: a clinical radiobiological analysis of fraction size and dose response relationships on late bone damage. Acta Oncol 27:117–122

Overgaard M, Bentzen SM, Christensen JJ, Hjøllund Madsen E (1987) The value of the NSD formula in equation of acute and late radiation complications in normal tissue following 2 and 5 fractions per week in breast cancer patients treated with postmastectomy radiotherapy. Radiother Oncol 9:1–12

Overgaard M, Christensen JJ, Johansen H, Nybo-Rasmussen A, Brincker H, van der Kooy P, Frederiksen PL, Laursen F, Panduro J, Sørensen NE, Gadeberg CC, Hjelm-Hansen M, Overgaard J, West Andersen K, Zedeler K (1988) Postmastectomy irradiation in high-risk breast cancer patients: present status of the Danish Breast Cancer Cooperative Group trials. Acta Oncol 27:707–714

Peracchia G, Salti C (1981) Radiotherapy with thrice-a-day fractionation in a short overall time: clinical experiences. Int J Radiat Oncol Biol Phys 7:99–104

Peters LJ (1990) The ESTRO Regaud lecture: Inherent radiosensitivity of tumor and normal tissue cells as a predictor of human tumor response. Radiother Oncol 17:177–190

Peters LJ, Ang KK, Thames HD (1988a) Accelerated fractionation in the radiation treatment of head and neck cancer: a critical comparison of different strategies. Acta Oncol 27:185–194

Peters LJ, Brock WA, Chapman JD, Wilson G (1988b) Predictive assays of tumor radiocurability. Am J Clin Oncol 11:275–287

Powell S, Cooke J, Parsons C (1990) Radiation-induced brachial plexus injury: follow-up of two different fractionation schedules. Radiother Oncol 18:213–220

Schultheiss TE, Thames HD, Peters LJ, Dixon DO (1986) Effect of latency on calculated complication rates. Int J Radiat Oncol Biol Phys 12:1861–1865

Steel GG, Peckham MJ (1979) Exploitable mechanisms in combined radiotherapy–chemotherapy: the concept of additivity. Int J Radiat Oncol Biol Phys 5:85–91

Taylor JMG, Withers HR, Vegesna V, Mason K (1987) Fitting the linear-quadratic model using time of occurrence as the endpoint for quantal response multifraction experiments. Int J Radiat Biol 52:459–468

Thames HD, Withers HR, Peters LJ, Fletcher GH (1982) Changes in early and late radiation responses with altered dose fractionation: implications for dose–survival relationships. Int J Radiat Oncol Biol Phys 8:219–226

Thames HD, Rozell ME, Tucker SL, Ang KK, Fischer DR, Travis EL (1986) Direct analysis of quantal radiation response data. Int J Radiat Biol 49:999–1009

Thames HD, Hendry JH, Moore JV, Ang KK, Travis EL (1989) The high steepness of dose–response curves for late-responding normal tissues. Radiother Oncol 15:49–53

Thames HD, Bentzen SM, Turesson I, Overgaard M, van den Bogaert W (1990) Time–dose factors in radiotherapy. Radiother Oncol 19:219–235

Turesson I (1989) The progression rate of late radiation effects in normal tissues and its impact on dose–response relationships. Radiother Oncol 15:217–226

Turesson I (1990) Individual variation and dose dependency in the progression rate of skin telangiectasia. Int J Radiat Oncol Biol Phys 19:1569–1574

Turesson I, Notter G (1986) The predictive value of skin telangiectasia for late radiation effects in different normal tissues. Int J Radiat Oncol Biol Phys 12:603–609

Turesson I, Thames HD (1989) Repair capacity and kinetics of human skin during fractionated radiotherapy: erythema, desquamation, and telangiectasia after 3 and 5 years' follow-up. Radiother Oncol 15:169–188

Van Limbergen E, Rijnders A, van der Schueren E, Lerut T, Christiaens R (1989) Cosmetic evaluation of breast conserving treatment for mammary cancer. 2. A quantitative analysis of the influence of radiation dose, fractionation schedules and surgical treatment techniques on cosmetic results. Radiother Oncol 16:253–267

Wheldon TE, Michalowski A, Kirk J (1982) The effect of irradiation on function in self-renewing normal tissues with differing proliferative organisation. Br J Radiol 55:759–766

Withers HR, Thames HD, Peters LJ (1983) A new isoeffect curve for change in dose per fraction. Radiother Oncol 1:187–191

Muscle Injury in Experimental Intraoperative Irradiation

E.L. Gillette, B.E. Powers, S. McChesney Gillette, and T.B. Borak

Department of Radiological Health Sciences, Colorado State University, Fort Collins, CO 80523, USA

Introduction

Complications reported for intraoperative radiation therapy (IORT) in humans include fibrosis (Calvo et al. 1989a; Sindelar et al. 1986; Tepper et al. 1984), hemorrhage (Tepper et al. 1984), peripheral neuropathies (Calvo et al. 1989a; Kinsella et al. 1985), bone necrosis (Hoekstra et al. 1988), and pelvic pain (Tepper et al. 1984). Most patients were followed for a relatively short period of time, with few patients observed more than 2 years after irradiation.

Studies of experimental dogs have had relatively short periods of observation or involved few animals at specific doses and time points. Recently, studies were completed of the effect of IORT or IORT combined with external beam radiation therapy (EBRT) 2 or 5 years after irradiation of the paraaortic regions in dogs. Aortic thrombosis and aneurysms, branch artery injury (Gillette et al. 1988, 1989), peripheral neuropathies (LeCouteur et al. 1989), ureteral strictures (McChesney Gillette et al. 1989), bone necrosis, and tumor induction (Powers et al. 1989) were reported.

This report of response of psoas muscles included in the treatment field of dogs at 2 and 5 years after IORT or IORT combined with EBRT also has been reported and is summarized here (Powers et al. 1991).

Materials and Methods

Young adult beagle dogs were randomized to receive variable radiation doses of IORT, IORT combined with 50 Gy EBRT, or EBRT only to the paraaortic area. Dogs observed for 2 years received 15–50 Gy IORT only; 10–42.5 Gy IORT combined with 50 Gy EBRT in 2 Gy fractions; or 50, 60, 70 or 80 Gy EBRT only in 30 fractions. Dogs observed for 5 years after treatment received 17.5–55 Gy IORT only; 10–47.5 Gy combined with

Recent Results in Cancer Research, Vol. 130

50 Gy EBRT in 2 Gy fractions; or 60, 70, or 80 Gy EBRT only in 30 fractions.

Dogs were anesthetized for IORT and placed in dorsal recumbency. A celiotomy was performed as previously described (Gillette et al. 1988). The intestines, kidney, and urinary bladder were retracted from the field and a 5 × 8 cm Plexiglas cone placed over the paraaortic region. The left ureter was retracted for dogs in the 2 year study but was included in the field for the 5 year study. Aorta, vena cava, lumbar nerves, ventral cortex of vertebrae L3–4 through L7, and the left psoas muscle were included in the treatment volume. A 6-MeV electron beam was used with a dose rate of 6.6 Gy/min. The source to surface distance was 125 cm. The D_{max} was 15 mm. Doses were calculated at the 90% isodose line.

A 50 Gy dose was delivered in 2 Gy fractions over a 5 week period immediately prior to IORT for the IORT–EBRT combination. The aorta, vena cava, lumbar nerves, both ureters, a portion of the left kidney, ventral cortex of vertebrae L2 through L7, and the psoas muscle were included in the 5 × 10 cm EBRT field. All EBRT doses were with 6 MV photons delivered through bilateral parallel opposed portals. For dogs receiving EBRT only, 50–80 Gy was given in 30 equal fractions over a 6 week period.

After the dogs were killed, tissues were dissected, labeled and placed in 10% neutral buffered formalin. Transverse sections of the left psoas muscle were embedded in paraffin, sectioned at 5 μm and stained with hematoxylin and eosin and Masson's trichrome. Histomorphometry was done on three sections, spaced 50 μm apart using a 36 point ocular grid in a microscope (Chalkley 1943). The percentages of muscle, connective tissue, capillaries, larger vessels, fat or hemorrhage and fibrin were recorded. Vascular lesions were scored on a scale of 0 to 3. Grade 0 was no lesions, grade 1 was mild fibrosis and/or mild intimal proliferation, grade 2 was marked fibrosis and/or intimal proliferation, and grade 3 was thrombosis, disruption or medial necrosis.

Results

Two Year Study

The psoas muscles were smaller than normal and were firm, pale, and adherent to surrounding tissues and bone. There were focal areas of increased connective tissue associated with loss or shrinkage of muscle fibers. Fibrous connective tissue or masses of hemorrhage and fibrin replaced areas of muscle fiber loss.

Higher doses caused a relative decrease in volume of muscle fibers, an increase in connective tissue, a decrease in the percentage of capillaries, and an increase in the percentage of hemorrhage and fibrin after IORT only. The response was similar for IORT combined with EBRT. The dose causing

Table 1. Isoeffective IORT doses for muscle and vessel injury

	Isoeffective IORT dose (Gy)	
	2 years	5 years
50% decrease in muscle volume		
IORT	21 (–)	34 (28–39)[a]
IORT plus 50 Gy EBRT	23 (15–29)	25 (20–29)
ED_{50} for severe vessel lesions		
IORT	19 (18–21)	26 (24–28)
IORT plus 50 Gy EBRT	16 (13–20)	18 (16–20)

[a] 95% confidence interval

a 50% decrease in the percentage of muscle fibers was 21 Gy IORT only and 23 Gy IORT when combined with 50 Gy EBRT (Table 1). After EBRT only there was minimal increase in percentage of connective tissue with increasing dose but other parameters did not change significantly.

Mild perivascular fibrosis and mild intimal proliferation (grade 1 lesion) were present 2 years after irradiation to lower doses. Severe perivascular fibrosis and severe intimal proliferation (grade 2 lesion) or severe hyalinization, medial necrosis, and disruption of the vessel walls with thrombosis (grade 3 lesion) were present in some arteries and arterioles following higher doses. The ED_{50}s for grade 2 or 3 vessel lesions was 19 Gy IORT only and 16 Gy IORT when combined with 50 Gy EBRT (Table 1). Grade 2 or 3 vessel lesions were not seen in any dogs which received EBRT only.

Perivascular inflammation was present in about 75% of the dogs given IORT doses greater than 15 Gy alone or with EBRT. Inflammation was not present in dogs receiving EBRT only.

Five Year Study

The psoas muscles appeared grossly similar to those in the 2 year study. In 2 dogs which received 47.5 Gy IORT with 50 Gy EBRT the muscle was abscessed. In 3 dogs which received 50 Gy EBRT and 25, 40 or 47.5 Gy IORT, the muscle was replaced by a firm gritty tumor (Powers et al. 1989). Histologically, lesions were similar to that observed at 2 years after irradiation. Connective tissue appeared more dense, remaining muscle fibers appeared larger, and inflammation, hemorrhage and fibrin were less frequent than at 2 years after irradiation. The dogs with tumors had a complete replacement of the muscle by the tumors, which were osteosarcomas (Powers et al. 1989). Those dogs were not included in histomorphometric analysis.

As at 2 years, increasing doses caused a decrease in the percentage of muscle, an increase in the percentage of connective tissue, a decrease in the percentage of capillaries, and an increase in the percentage of hemorrhage and fibrin after IORT only and IORT combined with 50 Gy EBRT (Figs. 1 and 2).

The dose which caused a 50% decrease in the percentage of muscle was 34 Gy IORT only and 25 Gy IORT when combined with 50 Gy EBRT (Table 1). After EBRT only there was a mild decrease of less than 5% in percentage of muscle fibers with increasing dose. There was no significant change in the other parameters.

Vessel lesions were present 5 years after irradiation and were similar in type to those observed 2 years after irradiation. The ED_{50}s for grade 2 or 3 lesions was 26 Gy IORT only and 18 Gy IORT when combined with 50 EBRT (Table 1). One dog receiving 80 Gy EBRT had a grade 2 vessel lesion.

Chronic inflammation was similar to that observed 2 years after irradiation but was less frequent. Inflammation was present mostly at doses of 40 Gy IORT and above, and in dogs receiving IORT with 50 Gy EBRT, mostly at doses of 32.5 Gy IORT and above. Inflammation was not present in dogs receiving EBRT only.

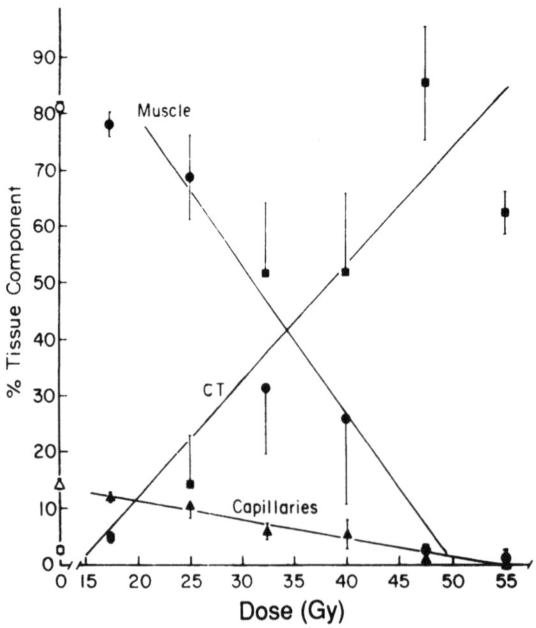

Fig. 1. Dose response of percentage tissue components 5 years after IORT. Mean and SEM are shown. *Open symbols* are control values. *CT*, connective tissue. (After Powers et al. 1991)

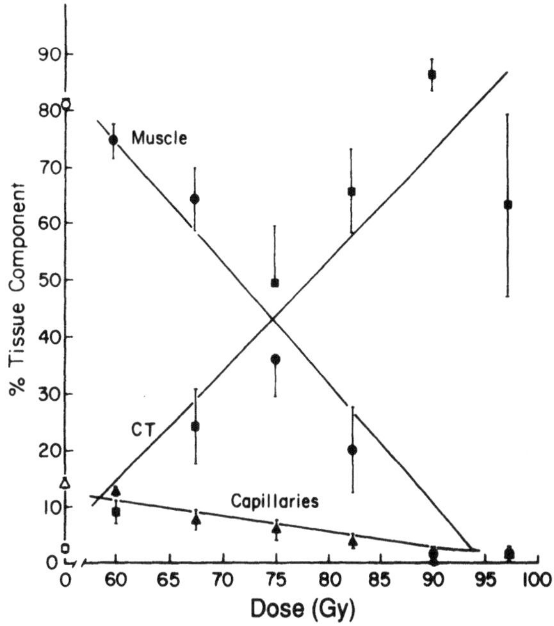

Fig. 2. Dose response of percentage tissue components 5 years after IORT combined with 50 Gy EBRT. Mean and SEM are shown. *Open symbols* are control values. *CT*, connective tissue. (After Powers et al. 1991)

Many dogs had clinical neuropathies due to radiation damage of the lumbar nerves (LeCouteur et al. 1989). The quadriceps muscles, which were outside of the radiation field but supplied by those nerves, were small, firm and pale. Histologically, the muscle fibers were small and angular but there was no significant increase in connective tissue, no vessel lesions nor hemorrhage or fibrin, and no inflammation. This neurogenic muscle atrophy was distinct from the more direct radiation injury to vasculature and muscle in the treatment volume.

Discussion

The left psoas muscle in the IORT field showed injury characterized by loss of muscle fibers, atrophy, and fibrosis. An IORT dose of 21 Gy alone or 23 Gy IORT combined with 50 Gy EBRT caused a 50% decrease in muscle fibers at 2 years. At 5 years those isoeffective doses were 34 Gy IORT only and 25 Gy IORT when combined with 50 Gy EBRT (Table 1). The higher isoeffective doses at 5 years imply some recovery process, possibly muscle regeneration or hypertrophy. Myoblasts have limited potential for regeneration (Cotran et al. 1989). Condensation of the hemorrhage, fibrin and immature loose connective tissue into more mature, dense connective tissue would lead to a relative decrease in those components and an relative increase in muscle volume. Muscle fibers appeared larger at 5 years than at 2 years after irradiation. Muscle fiber hypertrophy would also cause a relative increase in the percentage of muscle counted. The injury to the psoas muscle was not clinically evident. Their lack of function probably would not be detected due to the subtle influence of their action.

Most soft tissue complications in humans are related to abscesses, hemorrhages, fibrosis, and pelvic pain following IORT (Calvo et al. 1989a,b; Sindelar et al. 1982). Two dogs in this study had abscess formation 5 years after 47.5 Gy plus 50 Gy EBRT. The infrequent occurrence of abscesses in humans at IORT doses as low as 10–20 Gy is probably related to tumor or surgical procedures. Pelvic pain could be due to damage to peripheral nerves or due to fibrosis and adhesions caused by the tumor, surgery or irradiation. Pelvic pain was not observed in the dogs of this study. In humans examined 1–18 months after IORT, mild fibrotic changes were observed in the retroperitoneal soft tissues and these increased in severity with increasing time after irradiation (Sindelar et al. 1986). Soft tissue necrosis and fibrosis occurred in young patients treated with IORT for a variety of pediatric tumors (Calvo et al. 1989b). Fibrotic changes also routinely occurred in the retroperitoneal tissues of dogs given IORT at doses of 30 Gy or more in another study (Sindelar et al. 1982). The present study confirms these results as the muscle atrophy and fibrosis seen at doses below 20 Gy, as would be used in humans, were mild. Muscle atrophy and fibrosis were more consistent and severe at doses of 30 Gy and above.

Previous studies of muscle injury following irradiation in rabbits and rats suggest an early effect on myocytes resulting in cell death (Khan 1974; Schwenen et al. 1989; Zeman and Solomon 1971). The later effect which results in further muscle injury is more likely to be due to vascular lesions resulting in ischemia (Khan 1974; Remy et al. 1986; Wegrowski et al. 1988; Zeman and Solomon 1971). The fibrosis which occurs may also be related to vessel damage and ischemia, which may be mediated further by the inflammation that accompanies the vessel damage (Wegrowski et al. 1988).

In this study vascular damage appeared to have a role in causing late muscle atrophy and fibrosis. There was a consistent decrease in the percentage of capillaries with increasing IORT dose at 2 and 5 years after irradiation. Severe vascular injury was seen with an ED_{50} of 16–26 Gy IORT alone or when combined with 50 Gy EBRT at 2 and 5 years after irradiation. Severe vessel injury resulting in vessel rupture probably led to the presence of fibrin and hemorrhage within the muscle. The somewhat lower doses needed to cause vessel lesions and more frequent inflammation at 2 years compared with 5 years after irradiation suggest that a portion of the vascular injury and inflammation had occurred by 2 years. However, in the abdominal aorta and large branch arteries there was a progression of vessel injury between 2 and 5 years (Gillette et al. 1988, 1989). This probably reflects a difference in vessel size, with injury to the smaller arteries, arterioles and capillaries within the psoas muscle occurring earlier than injury to the larger arteries and abdominal aorta. The severe injury that occurred to the aorta and larger branch arteries at 5 years after irradiation could be responsible for the ongoing vessel lesions, hemorrhage and fibrin that were seen in the psoas muscle 5 years after irradiation.

Neurogenic atrophy has been proposed to be a cause of muscle injury after irradiation and may have contributed to the muscle atrophy seen in the dogs in this study. However, the doses required to produce electrophysiological abnormalities and severe histological lesions of nerve fiber loss and fibrosis were lower than that required to cause severe muscle injury (LeCouteur et al. 1989). The ED_{50} for severe vessel lesions in and around nerves (LeCouteur et al. 1989) was very similar to the ED_{50} for vessel lesions in the psoas muscle. This is to be expected as these were similarly sized vessels and are probably different sections of the same vessel. Furthermore, neurogenic atrophy of muscle is characterized by small, angular fibers with relatively little fibrosis (Cotran et al. 1989) and was seen in muscles outside the radiation field. In contrast the irradiated muscle had, in addition to fiber atrophy, abundant fibrosis, vascular lesions, inflammation, hemorrhage and fibrin formation. These latter lesions would not be found if neurogenic atrophy were the sole cause for the muscle injury seen in this study.

The lack of an effect of 50 Gy EBRT in causing some lesions may be because the large single IORT dose obscured the relatively smaller contribution of the 50 Gy EBRT given in 2 Gy fractions. The IORT dose was responsible for producing the majority of the lesions seen in the psoas muscles. At both 2 and 5 years after irradiation, dogs receiving 50–80 Gy EBRT only in 2–2.67 Gy fractions had either no or only minimal lesions.

In summary, muscle was resistant to fractionated irradiation up to 80 Gy. Radiation-induced muscle atrophy was associated with significant fibrosis and vascular lesions, which distinguishes this muscle injury from that caused solely by neurogenic atrophy. The lesions produced were largely a function of the single IORT dose rather than EBRT given in fractions. In general, 20–25 Gy in combination with 50 Gy EBRT was reasonably well tolerated by the sublumbar musculature. Doses above 25 Gy IORT could lead to significant muscle fibrosis and complications associated with soft tissue injury.

Muscle injury could be dose limiting for IORT in some cases. For most retroperitoneal structures evaluated experimentally in the dog, 20 Gy IORT combined with 50 Gy EBRT appeared to be near the maximum tolerated dose.

Acknowledgments. This investigation was supported by PHS grant number CA29117 awarded by the National Cancer Institute, DHHS.

References

Calvo FA, Algarra SM, Azinovic I, Santos M, Escude L, Hernadez JL, Zornoza G, Voltas J (1989a) Intraoperative radiotherapy for recurrent and/or residual colorectal cancer. Radiother Oncol 15:133–140

Calvo FA, Sierrasesumaga L, Martin I, Santos M, Voltas J, Barian JM, Canadell J (1989b) Intraoperative radiotherapy in the multidisciplinary treatment of pediatric tumors. Acta Oncol 28:257–260

Chalkley HW (1943) Methods for quantitative morphologic analysis of tissue. J Natl Cancer Inst 4:47–53

Cotran RS, Kumar V, Robbins SL (1989) Disease of muscle. In: Cotran RS, Kumar V, Robbins SL (eds) Robbins pathologic basis of disease, 4th edn. Saunders, Philadelphia, pp 1363–1371

Gillette EL, Powers BE, McChesney SL, Withrow SJ (1988) Aortic wall injury following intraoperative irradiation. Int J Radiat Oncol Biol Phys 15:1401–1406

Gillette EL, Powers BE, McChesney SL, Park RD, Withrow SJ (1989) Response of aorta and branch arteries to experimental intraoperative irradiation. Int J Radiat Oncol Biol Phys 17:1247–1255

Hoekstra HJ, Sindelar WF, Kinsella TJ (1988) Surgery with intraoperative radiotherapy for sarcomas of the pelvic girdle: a pilot experience. Int J Radiat Oncol Biol Phys 15:1013–1016

Khan MY (1974) Radiation-induced changes in skeletal muscle: an electron microscopic study. J Neuropathol Exp Neurol 33:42–57

Kinsella TJ, Sindelar WF, DeLuca AM, Pezeshkpour G, Smith R, Maher M, Terrel R, Miller R, Mixon A, Harwell JF, Rosenberg SA, Glatstein E (1985) Tolerance of peripheral nerve to intraoperative radiotherapy (IORT): clinical and experimental studies. Int J Radiat Oncol Biol Phys 11:1579–1585

LeCouteur RA, Gillette EL, Powers BE, Child G, McChesney SL, Ingram JT (1989) Peripheral neuropathies following experimental intraoperative radiation therapy (IORT). Int J Radiat Oncol Biol Phys 17:583–590

McChesney Gillette SL, Gillette EL, Powers BE, Park RD, Withrow SJ (1989) Ureteral injury following experimental intraoperative radiation. Int J Radiat Oncol Biol Phys 17:791–798

Powers BE, Gillette EL, McChesney SL, LeCouteur RA, Withrow SJ (1989) Bone necrosis and tumor induction following experimental intraoperative irradiation. Int J Radiat Oncol Biol Phys 17:559–567

Powers BE, Gillette EL, McChesney Gillette SL, LeCouteur RA, Withrow SJ (1991) Muscle injury following experimental intraoperative irradiation. Int J Radiat Oncol Biol Phys 20:463–471

Remy J, Martin M, Lefaix JL, Daburon F (1986) Radiation induced fibrosis in pig muscle: pathological and cellular observations. Br J Cancer 53 [Suppl VII]:232–233

Schwenen MK, Altman KI, Schroder W (1989) Radiation-induced increase in the release of amino acids by isolated, perfused skeletal muscle. Int J Radiat Biol 55:257–269

Sindelar WF, Tepper J, Travis EL, Terrill R (1982) Tolerance of retroperitoneal structures to intraoperative radiation. Ann Surg 196:601–608

Sindelar WF, Hoekstra H, Restrepo C, Kinsella TJ (1986) Pathological tissue changes following intraoperative radiotherapy. Am J Clin Oncol 9:504–509

Tepper JE, Gunderson LL, Orlow E, Cohen AM, Hedberg SE, Shipley WU, Blitzer PH, Rich T (1984) Complications of intraoperative radiation therapy. Int J Radiat Oncol Biol Phys 10:1831–1839

Wegrowski J, Lafuma C, Lefaix JL, Daburon F, Robert L (1988) Modification of collagen and noncollagenous proteins in radiation-induced muscular fibrosis. Exp Mol Pathol 48:273–285
Zeman W, Solomon M (1971) Effects of radiation on striated muscle. In: Berdjis CC (ed) Pathology of irradiation. Williams and Wilkins, Baltimore, pp 171–185

An Experimental In Vivo Model in Mice to Evaluate the Change in Reservoir Function of the Urinary Bladder due to Irradiation Alone or Combined with Chemotherapy

F. Lundbeck

Danish Cancer Society, Department of Experimental Clinical Oncology, 8000 Aarhus C, and Institute of Experimental Clinical Research, and Department of Urology, University of Aarhus, Skejby Hospital, 8200 Aarhus N, Denmark

Introduction

Radiation damage to the urinary bladder is a serious matter in that any change in its reservoir function may have a major effect on the everyday life of the patient. Long-term bladder symptomatology following radiation therapy may be more frequent than generally realized – and seems always to give rise to fierce debates between radiotherapists and surgeons. The recorded evidence of serious radiation injury depends, of course, on whether the denominator is the *initial* number of patients or the *surviving* patients. For groups of fairly early cancers, where the survival is 60% or 70%, there will be only a low incidence, but if the survival is 25%–30% as in advanced bladder cancer, then the incidence will appear much higher. In a recent survey Kagan (1989) has found the serious complications of pelvic irradiation to total approximately 10%, and approximately 30% of these patients will have to undergo some form of surgery. The organs injured depend on the dose of external irradiation and whether brachytherapy has been performed as well. Ureteral and urethral injuries do occur, but mostly in concert with bladder injury sharing morbidity with rectum, sigmoid, and small intestine.

The exact mechanism and the sequence of events that lead to the sometimes deleterious effects to normal bladder tissue are still somewhat uncertain. Furthermore, data from clinical studies concerning late sequelae after radiotherapy are mostly qualitative rather than quantitative, and thus are seldom suited for thorough radiobiological analysis.

Experimental animal models are therefore needed in order to explore these matters. Hitherto only one experimental model has been described in which it was possible to monitor over a prolonged period of time changes in the reservoir function of the urinary bladder after irradiation alone or combined with cyclophosphamide (Edrees et al. 1988; Stewart et al. 1978). This mouse assay is based on the physiological voidings of the animals, the endpoint being the number of micturitions per milliliter per 24 h. The

Recent Results in Cancer Research, Vol. 130

assay is very reliable but rather time-consuming as the animals have to be observed during a 24-h period. Furthermore, for practical reasons it is only possible to investigate relatively few animals at a time.

In 1989 another mouse assay was published based on a direct assessment of the change in the passive biomechanical properties of the bladder over time (Lundbeck et al. 1989a), made possible by a simultaneous monitoring of the intravesical pressure–volume relationship.

Animal Model

Bladder Filling

All experiments were carried out on female $C_3D_2F_1$/Bom mice (C_3H/Tif♀ × DBA/2♂) obtained from Bomholtgaard Breeding and Research Center Ltd., Denmark. The mice were 12–14 weeks old at the start of the experiments, weighing 20–25 g. They were housed six per cage and given standard laboratory diet and tap water ad libitum.

At the beginning of each bladder-filling experiment the mice were anaesthetized (pentobarbital 60 mg/kg intraperitoneally). Shortly afterward an intravenous cannula (Viggo Venflon, 22G/0.8 mm outer diameter × 25 mm) was inserted through the urethra to ensure an empty bladder. The cannula was replaced by another fluid-filled cannula mounted on a fluid-filled catheter. This catheter was connected via a three-way stopcock to an infusion pump and a pressure transducer which in turn was connected to an ink jet recorder. The bladder filling was thereafter performed at an infusion rate of 0.1 ml/min using isotonic saline at room temperature. The infusion was stopped when leakage round the cannula occurred.

The described procedures do of course involve several possible sources of error. These include the effect of sedatives on the bladder and the urethral sphincter, the influence of a drop in body temperature due to the anaesthetics on the elastic properties of the bladder wall, the possible damage from repeated catheterizations on the urethra, the size of catheter, and the choice of infusion rate. These considerations have been dealt with in detail previously (Lundbeck et al. 1989a) and will not be discussed here.

Irradiation

Prior to each irradiation experiment the mice were anaesthetized and the bladder emptied transurethrally to ensure the position and size of the bladder. Thereafter, each mouse was restrained in a plastic cylinder snugly fitted into a lead box that allowed irradiation of the bladder only, shielding rectum and femurs. The irradiation was generated with a 250 kV constant potential. A detailed description of the irradiation set-up and the possible sources of error have been given elsewhere (Lundbeck et al. 1989b).

Endpoint

The endpoint selected for data evaluation was a 50% decrease in the estimated bladder volume at an intravesical pressure of 20 mmHg in relation to the control value of the same mouse (i.e. before treatment).

The Impact of Single-Dose Radiation on Bladder Reservoir Function

Applying a radiation dose of 20 Gy to the mouse bladder seemed to create significant variation in bladder capacity over time. Figure 1 thus shows the findings at three different times after treatment compared with control. The top curve represents the findings in the untreated, anaesthetized mouse. The

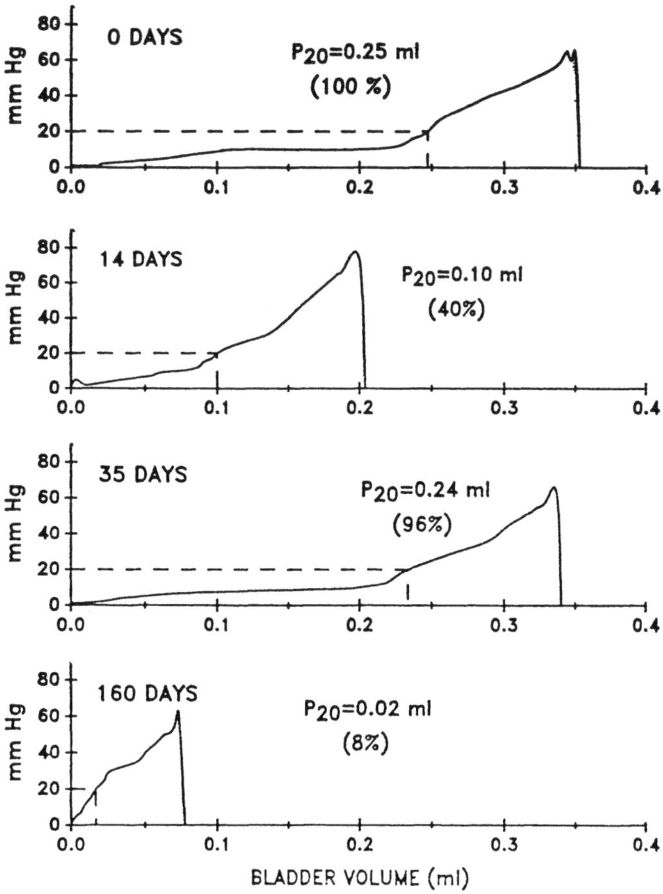

Fig. 1. The impact of a single-fraction radiation dose of 20 Gy on the reservoir function of the same mouse urinary bladder as a function of time after treatment. (From Lundbeck et al. 1989b, by permission of the publisher)

curve has a certain resemblance to the human counterpart in that it consists of three separate phases: an initial small rise (segment I), a long flat phase representing the compliance of the bladder wall (segment II), and a rising part (segment III) ending in leakage around the catheter. In a normal micturition encountered in the awake animal this third phase would be represented by a sudden spike (Yaksh et al. 1986), but because of the anaesthesia the increment in pressure reveals the distension of the connective tissue until the passive leakage point is reached.

The curve below represents the functional capacity of the same bladder 14 days after irradiation. It can be seen that the compliance of the bladder wall has vanished, leaving the animal with a low-volume irritated bladder. The same change in functional capacity is well known from the clinic when the small pelvis has been included in the irradiation field. This early damage results in pollakisuria and various levels of dysuria, sometimes necessitating a break in treatment. The early damage is, however, reversible and this finding is also demonstrated in the model (Fig. 1), where the bladder function is seen to have been restored to normal 35 days after treatment. The bottom curve in Fig. 1 illustrates the final and irreversible damage, demonstrated by the contracted bladder. Segment I and segment II are completely lost, and the animal is left with a severely diminished bladder capacity.

Early Bladder Damage

Calculating the percentage of mice responding from the number of mice available at each dose level within the first 30 days after irradiation (5–30 Gy) and performing a logit analysis (Suit and Wette 1967) revealed a dose–response curve as illustrated in Fig. 2. As seen from the curve, no animal responded at 5 Gy, but thereafter an increasing number did respond, culminating at 30 Gy, where a reduced bladder volume was encountered in all the mice in the group. The RD_{50} value (the radiation dose inducing a response in 50% of the animals) was estimated as 17.2 Gy (14.4–20.5 Gy; 95% confidence interval, CI). This is a much lower value than was found in a recent comparative study between the cystometry assay and the urination frequency assay (Stewart et al. 1991). In that study the RD_{50} value was calculated as 31.7 Gy (25.7–37.8 Gy; 95% CI) using the cystometry assay. The reason for this discrepancy is ascribed to the difference in mouse strain, the strain used in our laboratory being much more radiosensitive than the C_3H strain employed by Stewart. The uneven distribution of responding C_3H mice between the irradiation dose levels is reflected in the wide confidence interval. In the same study the RD_{50} value of the early damage was estimated as 25.2 Gy (22.4–28.1 Gy; 95% CI) using the frequency assay. This study was the first in which the early damage was detected using the urination frequency assay. This can be ascribed to several factors.

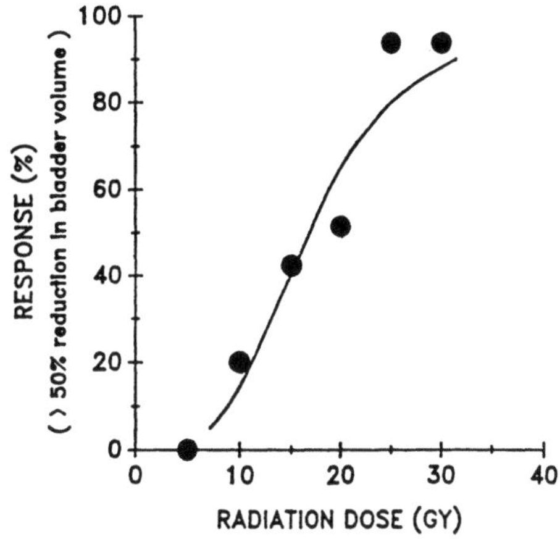

Fig. 2. Response in relation to radiation dose within the first 30 days after single-fraction radiation

First, the early damage is only of a few days' duration and thus the time between the bladder investigations should be fairly short and not at an interval of several weeks. Secondly, if the mouse strain for some reason is not particularly sensitive to bladder irradiation – as for example C_3H or the previously used CBA strains (Stewart et al. 1978) – then the early damage will be somewhat difficult to detect. Thirdly, in the previously chosen end-point the numbers of micturitions per milliliter per 24 h were presented as group mean values, and this probably underestimated the actual number of animals exhibiting early damage. In the last study (Stewart et al. 1991) this was changed to ≥6 spots per milliliter per 24 h (i.e. approximately 2× control, equivalant to a 50% decrease in bladder volume used in the cystometry value).

The exact mechanism for the early transient damage in the bladder after irradiation is not fully understood. Cell kinetic investigations (Stewart et al. 1980) after radiotherapy alone have shown an exceptionally slow turnover in the normal urothelium, and no change was noticed in proliferation until the late damage was about to be manifest. So the early damage leading to a hyperactive and irritated bladder is not due to cell death and sloughing of the urothelium such as is experienced after administering cyclophosphamide (Stewart 1985; Lundbeck and Stewart 1989). One might then assume there were some changes in the contractile mechanisms in the bladder, reflected in a decreased compliance. However, in a recent pharmacological in vitro study (Lundbeck and Sjögren 1992b) of the nerve and muscle functions in the mouse bladder wall, it was not possible to find any difference between bladder strips from irradiated (25 Gy) or from non-treated mouse bladders concerning the release mechanism of acetylcholine, cholinergic or non-cholinergic nerve activation, prostaglandin function or potassium channel activation.

Late Bladder Damage

The development of late damage as illustrated in the cystometry assay is demonstrated in Figs. 3 and 4 in two different ways.

In Fig. 3 the top curve illustrates the RD_{50} as a function of time. Thus logit analyses were performed at each bladder-filling experiment over time. It can be seen that not only do the mice treated with high-dose irradiation

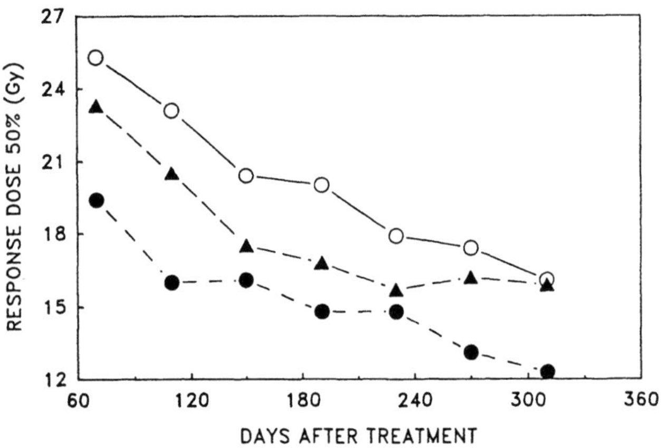

Fig. 3. RD_{50} for three selected groups at various time intervals after treatment. *Open circles*, radiation only (5–30 Gy); *triangles*, *cis*-DDP (6 mg/kg) administered 4 h before radiation (5–20 Gy); *filled circles*, *cis*-DDP (6 mg/kg) administered 15 min before radiation (5–20 Gy)

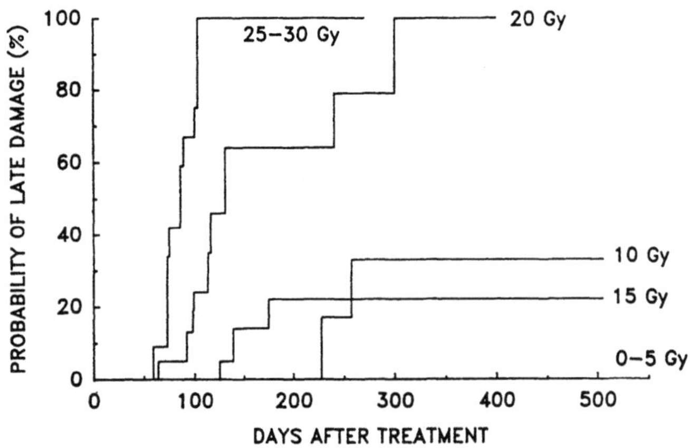

Fig. 4. Probability of developing late damage as a function of time at various dose points. Only mice surviving more than 30 days after radiation have been included

respond, but as time passes more and more mice respond also at lower dose levels. Time is thus the all-important factor in the development of late radiation damage.

Compared with the acute damage, the degree and time of appearance of the late event are dose dependent as shown in Fig. 4. This figure illustrates the probability of developing late damage estimated by the Kaplan–Meier method (Kaplan and Meier 1958) and compared by log rank test (Peto et al. 1977). It seems that the probability of developing late damage is dose dependent. A significant difference was found between the curves except for radiation doses of 10 Gy and 15 Gy. None of the animals in the control group responded ($n = 52$). This important characteristic feature of incidence and latency has been demonstrated by others (Stewart et al. 1978; Knowles and Trott 1987), although the theoretical conclusions from these studies have been questioned recently (Bentzen and Thames 1989).

The Combined Effect of *cis*-DDP and Radiation and the Impact of Varying the Time Interval Between the Two Treatment Modalities on Bladder Reservoir Function over Time

Experimental studies, both in vivo and in vitro, have suggested that *cis*-diamminedichloroplatinum II (*cis*-DDP) exerts a greater than additive effect on tumors when combined with radiation (Overgaard and Kahn 1981; Lelieveld et al. 1985). Recently it has been confirmed in the clinic that *cis*-DDP exerts a considerable effect on urogenital malignancies such as carcinoma of the testes, ovary, and bladder. Thus, for example, *cis*-DDP when combined with methotrexate, vinblastine, and doxorobicin, has yielded an approximately 30% complete response in patients with advanced carcinoma of the bladder (Sternberg et al. 1988). However, from a therapeutic point of view, a major aspect in treating malignant tumors is not supra-additivity of tumor cell kill but the achievement of enhanced tumor response without increased normal tissue morbidity. Established normal tissue assays have thus been used to investigate the effect of *cis*-DDP and radiation on early-reacting tissues such as skin (Overgaard and Kahn 1981) and intestinal crypt cells (Von der Maase 1986), or late-reacting tissues such as kidney (Stewart et al. 1986; Robbins et al. 1988; van Rongen et al. 1989), lungs (Von der Maase 1986), and the mouse rectum (Dewit et al. 1987). However, the results have been somewhat conflicting and will be discussed in relation to our recent investigation on normal mouse bladder reservoir function (Lundbeck and Overgaard 1992a).

In order to evaluate the impact on early and late damage of the interval between administration of *cis*-DDP and radiation, *cis*-DDP (6 mg/kg intraperitoneally) was administered from 336 h before to 336 h after irradiation as illustrated in Fig. 5.

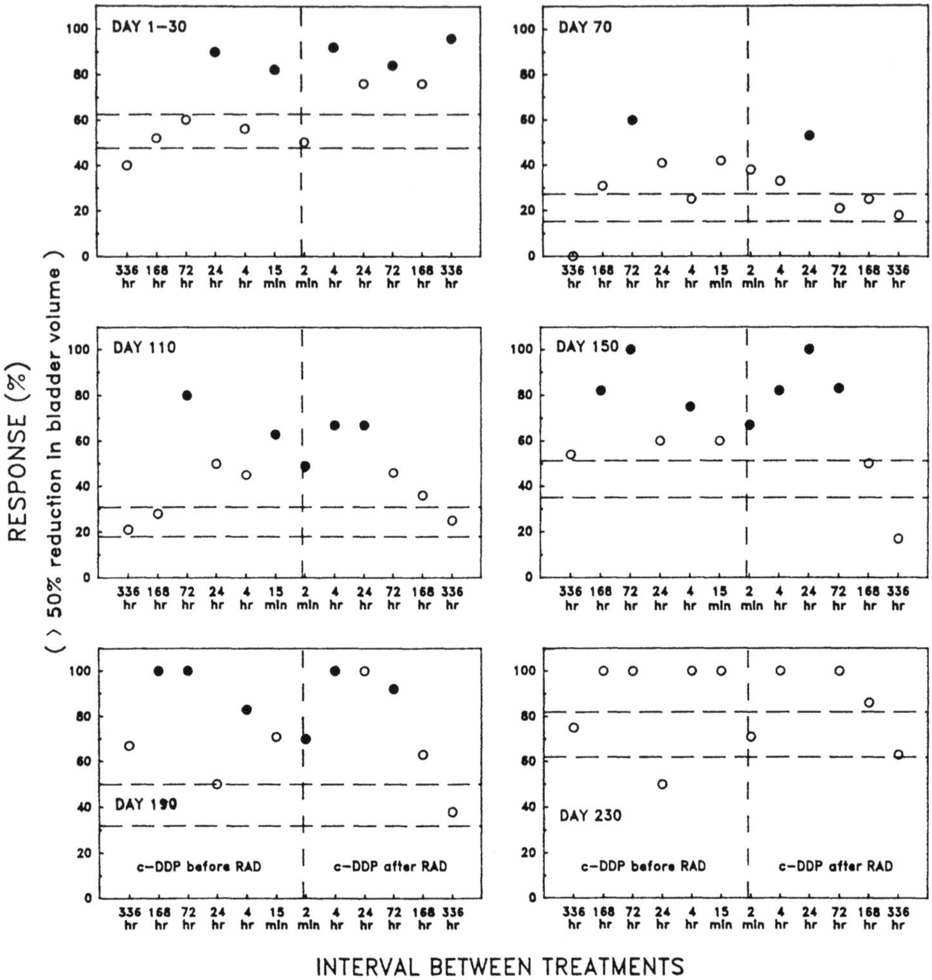

Fig. 5. Percentage of mice responding at selected time intervals after treatment. Points represent 20 Gy + *cis*-DDP 6 mg/kg at various time intervals in relation to radiation. The area between the *dashed lines* gives the percentage response after 20 Gy alone (±SD). *Filled circles*, significant difference from 20 Gy only ($p < 0.05$); *open circles*, no significant difference from 20 Gy only

Early Damage

The transient and reversible nature of the early damage is again demonstrated in Fig. 5, where 56% (49%–63%, 95% CI) of the animals treated with 20 Gy alone respond *within* 30 days after treatment. An increased response is seen in the groups treated with *cis*-DDP in the interval from 24 h before the 336 h after 20 Gy compared with the group treated with radiation alone. There were, however, two exceptions: groups treated 4 h before and 2 min after irradiation. None of the mice treated with *cis*-DDP alone (n = 11) or untreated control animals responded (n = 52). No animals either in the combined treatment groups or in the group given radiation alone responded *30 days after* treatment (data not shown), but thereafter an increase in response is seen.

The early damage indicated in this figure in the combined treatment groups occurs after a longer interval than was found by others in assays investigating early tissue damage after irradiation and *cis*-DDP. Thus the studies performed by von der Maase (1986) suggested an increased response after a much shorter interval, namely from 24 h before until simultaneous application of the two treatments. Luk et al. (1979), also investigating intestinal crypt cells, reported an increased response at an even shorter interval than von der Maase (1986), i.e. a few hours before until simultaneous treatment.

Contrary to these studies other investigations on similar relatively rapidly proliferating tissues have not revealed any effect due to *cis*-DDP when administered with radiation (Landuyt et al. 1986; Fu and Lam 1991) compared with radiation alone. Some of these discrepancies may be due to differences in animal strain, radiation doses, or skin scoring methods. But it is also important to consider the differences in selected endpoints. Thus as pointed out by Michalowski et al. (1984) and Overgaard and Matsui (1990), comparing results originating from a functional nonclonogenic assay with results from a clonal assay does entail some difficulties.

Late Damage

The development of late damage (as illustrated in Fig. 5) from 70 days until 230 days after treatment demonstrates an increased response in the combined treatment groups compared with the group receiving radiation alone. The effect was especially pronounced from 110 days after treatment onwards. This increase in number of responders suggests either a shorter time until response or genuine and more pronounced damage to the compliance capacity of the bladder wall in the combined treatment groups compared with the group receiving radiation alone. However, since the endpoint is qualitative rather than quantitative it is not possible at present to resolve this important issue.

In selected groups radiation was administered at different dose levels (Fig. 3). Thus the animals in the two combined treatment groups were irradiated in the range from 5 to 20 Gy. The reduction in the maximal doses from 30 Gy to 20 Gy was due to the toxicity previously seen (Lundbeck et al. 1989b) when there was significantly decreased survival in the 25 Gy and 30 Gy dose groups, it being assumed that adding *cis*-DDP to these doses would decrease survival even further.

Figure 3 illustrates two important differences in the effect of *cis*-DDP combined with radiation compared with the effect of radiation alone. First, there is an increased effect in the combined treatment groups reflected by a decreased RD_{50} compared with radiation alone. This is most pronounced in the group with a 15-min interval between the administration of *cis*-DDP and irradiation. The increased effect in the combined treatment groups compared with radiation alone can be expressed as the dose effect factor (DEF), defined as the ratio between the radiation dose producing a given effect when given alone and the isoeffect dose obtained when radiation is combined with *cis*-DDP. The DEF value was estimated at each time interval in both combined treatment groups and was found to range from 1.08 to 1.45. Secondly, from the parallel course of the combined treatment curves compared with the curve representing radiation alone, it can be assumed that in spite of the significant effect of *cis*-DDP on the response, radiation is the most important factor in the development of late damage.

Comparing Figs. 3 and 5 it may seem somewhat contradictory that administering *cis*-DDP 15 min before irradiation results in a significant decrease in RD_{50} during the whole observation period (Fig. 3) when this time interval only presents itself as significantly different from the group receiving radiation alone 110 days after treatment (Fig. 5). However, this apparent inconsistency can be ascribed to the difference in data analysis. There was only a fairly small number of animals available at 20 Gy in the combined treatment group compared with the group receiving radiation only. Estimation of a dose–response curve comprising several dose points, on the other hand, decreases the risk of a type 2 error considerably, provided that the confidence interval is reasonably tight.

The increased response seen after *cis*-DDP combined with radiation compared with radiation alone is consistent with studies performed on the mouse kidney (Stewart et al. 1986) that found DEF values from 1.1 to 1.3 when *cis*-DDP was administered either before or 2 weeks after irradiation. These findings and the present results are, however, in contrast to those of Dewit et al. (1987), who on examining stricture formation in the mouse rectum was unable to find any effect of *cis*-DDP. Those studies even showed an increased RD_{50} in the group irradiated only compared with the group treated with *cis*-DDP plus irradiation.

The exact mechanism by which *cis*-DDP seems to increase the radiation response of at least certain tissues is unclear. Since an increased response has been noticed whether the drug was administered before or after irradiation the term sensitization seems inappropriate. It has been suggested that the effect seen in kidney assays (Stewart et al. 1986; Robbins et al. 1988) was additive, since a dose-dependent effect by the drug could be clearly demonstrated. The toxic effect of *cis*-DDP in kidney is due to the damage inflicted on the tubular cells, and thus the toxicity seen in relation to bladder damage is distinctly different from this. Although both increased early and late damage could be demonstrated when the drug was combined with irradiation, no effect was seen when the drug was given alone. This may of course be due to a lack of sensitivity in the assay, but until further evidence concerning the effect of *cis*-DDP has been demonstrated it may be reasonable to describe the combined effect in the bladder only as "interaction" or perhaps "enhancement" (Steel 1979).

Fractionation Sensitivity of Late Radiation Damage Quantified by the α/β Ratio

It has been appreciated for a long time that cells and tissues are spared some damage when a radiation dose is fractionated, and thus this is the basis of all clinically applied external radiation therapy. However, it was only about 30 years ago that the importance of fraction size and number was made clear (Elkind and Sutton 1960; Fowler et al. 1963). A quantitative estimation of this pertinent concept of fractionation sensitivity was made possible by the introduction of the linear-quadratic (LQ) model (Douglas and Fowler 1976; Thames et al. 1982). This model can be used to describe an underlying dose–response curve if a plot of reciprocal dose for a given level of damage versus dose per fraction produces a straight line. The slope of this line is proportional to β and the intercept at the ordinate is proportional to α (Douglas and Fowler 1976). The α/β ratio has now been established for several normal tissues (for review see Thames and Hendry 1987).

Our fractionation studies suggested an α/β ratio at 5.8 Gy (3.6–8.8 Gy; 95% CI), which is at the upper end of the values for other late-responding tissues (Bentzen et al. 1992). The ratio is, on the other hand, in good agreement with that of Stewart et al. (1984), although it will be seen that the 95% confidence interval is much wider than those in our study. Thus using post-mortem bladder volumes as the endpoint the α/β ratio was estimated at 6.6 Gy (2.2–14.5 Gy; 95% CI), or 6.1 Gy (1.1–15.4 Gy; 95% CI) with urination frequency as the endpoint (after correction by an assumed relative biological effectiveness of 0.85 for 250 kVp X-rays relative to 1.8 MeV electrons). There may be at least three reasons for the considerably tighter confidence intervals seen in our study. First, the α/β ratio was estimated using direct methods (Thames et al. 1986). This provides a more reliable error estimate than does the reciprocal-dose technique used by Stewart et al. (1984) because it avoids the intermediate step of estimating the isoeffect doses. Secondly, Stewart's CBA mice seem less radiosensitive than the $C_3D_2F_1$ mice used in our laboratory (Stewart et al. 1991). Thirdly, of course, one should not neglect the difference in definition of endpoint as discussed in recent papers (Stewart et al. 1991; Edress et al. 1988).

Conclusion

The investigations described demonstrate that (1) repeated transurethral bladder filling in mice is a simple, minimally invasive method of investigating changes in the reservoir function of the mouse urinary bladder due to external irradiation alone or combined with *cis*-DDP, (2) the radiation dose determines the degree of acute response and the time of onset of the late response, (3) *cis*-DDP increases the acute and late damage to the urinary bladder when combined with irradiation, and (4) the mouse urinary bladder is one of the least sensitive late endpoints, with an α/β ratio of 5.8 Gy.

References

Bentzen SM, Thames HD (1989) Incidence and latency of radiation reactions. Radiother Oncol 14:261–262

Bentzen SM, Lundbeck F, Loft Christensen L (1992) Fractionation sensitivity and latency of late radiation injury to the mouse urinary bladder. Radiother Oncol (in press)

Dewit L, Oussoren Y, Bartelink H (1987) Early and late damage in the mouse rectum after irradiation and *cis*-diamminedichloroplatinum (II). Radiother Oncol 8:57–69

Douglas BG, Fowler JF (1976) The effect of multiple small doses of X-rays on skin reactions in the mouse and a basic interpretation. Radiat Res 66:401–426

Edrees G, Luts A, Stewart F (1988) Bladder damage in mice after combined treatment with cyclophosphamide and X-rays: the influence of timing and sequence. Radiother Oncol 11:349–360

Elkind MM, Sutton H (1960) Radiation response of mammalian cells grown in culture. I. Repair of X-ray damage in surviving Chinese hamster ovary cells. Radiat Res 13:556–593

Fowler JF, Morgan MA, Silvester JA, Bewley DK, Turner BA (1963) Experiments with fractionated X-ray treatment of the skin of pigs. I. Fractionation up to 28 days. Br J Radiol 36:188–196

Fu K, Lam KN (1991) Early and late effects of cisplatin and radiation at acute and low dose rates on mouse skin and soft tissues of the leg. Int J Radiat Oncol Biol Phys 20:327–332

Kagan AR (1989) Bladder, testicle, and prostatic irradiation injury. In: Vaeth JM, Meyer JL (eds) Radiation tolerance of normal tissues. Karger, Basel, pp 323–337

Kaplan EL, Meier P (1958) Nonparametric estimation from incomplete observations. J Am Stat Assoc 53:457–481

Knowles JF, Trott KR (1987) Experimental irradiation of the rat ureter: the effects of field size and the presence of contrast medium on incidence and latency of hydronephrosis. Radiother Oncol 10:59–66

Landuyt W, Ang KK, van der Schueren E (1986) Combinations of single doses and fractionated treatments of *cis*-dichlorodiammineplatinum (II) and irradiation: effects on mouse lip mucosa. Br J Cancer 54:579–586

Lelieveld P, Scoles MA, Brown JM, Kalman RF (1985) The effect of treatment in fractionated schedules with combination of X-irradiation and six cytostatic drugs on RIF-1 tumors and normal mouse skin. Int J Radiat Biol Phys 11:111–121

Luk KH, Ross GY, Phillips TL, Goldstein LS (1979) The interaction of radiation and *cis*-diamminedichloroplatinum (II) in intestinal crypt cells. Int J Radiat Oncol Biol Phys 5:1417–1420

Lundbeck F, Stewart FA (1989) Acute changes in the bladder reservoir function after irradiation or in combination with chemotherapy: a matter of mouse strain. Scand J Urol Nephrol 125[Suppl]:141–148

Lundbeck F, Djurhuus JC, Vaeth M (1989a) Bladder filling in mice: an experimental in vivo model to evaluate the reservoir function of the urinary bladder in a long term study. J Urol 141:1245–1249
Lundbeck F, Ulsoe N, Overgaard J (1989b) Cystometric evaluation of early and late irradiation damage to the mouse urinary bladder. Radiother Oncol 15:383–392
Lundbeck F, Overgaard J (1992a) Early and late changes in the normal mouse bladder reservoir function due to irradiation and *cis*-DDP. Br J Cancer 66:99–105
Lundbeck F, Sjögren C (1992b) A pharmacological in vitro study of the mouse urinary bladder at the time of acute change in bladder reservoir function after irradiation. J Urol 148:179–182
Michalowski A, Wheldon TE, Krik J (1984) Can cell survival parameters be deduced from non-clonogenic assays of radiation damage to normal tissues? Br J Cancer 49[Suppl VI]:257–261
Overgaard J, Kahn AR (1981) Selective enhancement of radiation response in C_3H mammary carcinoma by cis-platin. Cancer Treat Rep 65:501–503
Overgaard J, Matsui M (1990) Effect of radiation on glucose absorption in the mouse jejunum in vivo. Radiother Oncol 18:71–77
Peto R, Armitage P, Breslow NE et al. (1977) Design and analysis of randomized clinical trials requiring prolonged observation of each patient. II. Analysis and examples. Br J Cancer 35:1–39
Robbins MEC, Robinson M, Rezvani M, Golding SJ, Hopewell JW (1988) The response of the pig kidney to the combined effects of cisplatin and unilateral renal irradiation. Radiother Oncol 11:271–278
Steel GG (1979) Terminology in the description of drug–radiation interactions. Int J Radiat Oncol Biol Phys 5:1145–1150
Sternberg CN, Yagoda A, Scher HI, Watson RC, Herr HW et al. (1988) M-VAC (methotrexate, vinblastine, doxorubicin and cis-platin) for advanced transitional cell carcinoma of the urothelium. J Urol 139:461–469
Stewart F, Bohlken S, Begg A, Bartelink H (1986) Renal damage in mice after treatment with cisplatinum alone or in combination with X-irradiation. Int J Radiat Oncol Biol Phys 12:927–933
Stewart FA (1985) The proliferative and functional response of mouse bladder to treatment with irradiation and cyclophosphamide. Radiother Oncol 4:353–362
Stewart FA, Michael BD, Denekamp J (1978) Late radiation damage in the mouse bladder as measured by increased urination frequency. Radiat Res 75:649–659
Stewart FA, Denekamp J, Hirst DG (1980) Proliferation kinetics of the mouse bladder after irradiation. Cell Tissue Kinet 13:75–89
Stewart FA, Randhawa VS, Michael BD (1984) Multifraction irradiation of mouse bladders. Radiother Oncol 2:131–140
Stewart FA, Lundbeck F, Oussoren Y, Luts A (1991) Acute and late radiation damage in mouse bladder: a comparison of urination frequency and cystometry. Int J Radiat Oncol Biol Phys 21:1211–1219
Suit HD, Wette R (1967) Theoretical considerations on the influence of dose fractionation on effectiveness of radiation therapy. In: Conference on radiology and radiotherapy, monograph 24. National Cancer Institute, pp 225–242
Thames HD, Hendry JH (1987) Fractionation in radiotherapy. Taylor and Francis, London
Thames HD, Peters LJ, Withers HR, Fletcher GH (1982) Changes in early and late radiation responses with altered dose fractionation: implications for dose–survival relationships. Int J Radiat Oncol Biol Phys 8:219–226
Thames HD, Rozell ME, Tucker SL, Ang KK, Fisher DR, Travis EL (1986) Direct analysis of quantal radiation response data. Int J Radiat Biol 49:999–1009
Van Rongen E, van der Kogel AJ, Durham SK (1989) The influence of cisplatin and unilateral nephrectomy on the response of the rat kidney to irradiation. Int J Radiat Biol 55(4):661–677

Von der Maase H (1986) Experimental studies on interaction of radiation and cancer chemotherapeutic drugs in normal tissues and solid tumors. Radiother Oncol 7:47–68

Yaksh TL, Durant PAC, Brent CR (1986) Micturition in rats: a chronic model for study of bladder function and effect of anesthetics. Am J Physiol 251:R1177–R1185

Combined Chemo-Radiotherapy with Carboplatin, 5-Fluorouracil and Folinic Acid for Cancer of the Urinary Bladder: Acute and Late Side Effects

T. Wiegel[1], J. Lorenzen[1], W.-P. Brockmann[1], B. Lopez[2], R. Schwarz[1], and K.-H. Hübener[1]

[1] Department of Radiotherapy, University Hospital Hamburg-Eppendorf, W-2000 Hamburg, Fed. Rep. of Germany
[2] Department of Urology, General Hospital Hamburg-Eilbek, Fed. Rep. of Germany

Introduction

Conventional treatment of advanced bladder carcinoma included surgery, or preoperative irradiation combined with surgery. Results of cystectomy alone and irradiation/surgery for T3 tumors achieved 5-year survival rates up to 40% (Jacobi et al. 1983) and 40%–50% (van der Werf-Messing 1983). 5-Fluorouracil (5-FU), mitomycin C and cisplatin were shown to be useful as radiosensitizers in invasive bladder carcinoma. Rotman et al. (1987) and Russel et al. (1988) demonstrated an advantage for 5-year disease-free survival using irradiation and chemotherapy with 5-FU and mitomycin C. Sauer et al. (1988) and Shipley et al. (1984, 1985) reported similarly complete response rates with cisplatin and irradiation. However, cisplatin is a potentially more toxic drug, especially as regards its neurotoxicity and nephrotoxicity (Lelieveld et al. 1984).

In 1989 a clinical trial at the University Hospital of Hamburg-Eppendorf was started using carboplatin, 5-FU and folinic acid in combination with accelerated hyperfractionated irradiation up to 50.4 Gy to the pelvis and a boost up to 56.4 Gy to the bladder. The aim of this trial was to improve local control and survival rates using the proven advantage of 5-FU in combination with folinic acid and carboplatin, which has acceptable toxicity.

Material and Methods

Between October 1989 and November 1990 we treated 15 patients (9 women, 6 men, median age 66.4 years) with histologically confirmed invasive carcinoma of the urinary bladder with combined chemo-radiotherapy. Three patients were stage II (T2 NO MO), 4 patients stage III (T3 NO MO), and 8 patients stage IV (T4 NO MO, T1-3 N1-3 MO, any M1). Median follow-up was 13 months.

Recent Results in Cancer Research, Vol. 130

All patients were treated with 50.4 Gy in 4.5 weeks in 10 fractions per week (1.2 Gy per fraction) as a four-field box to the small pelvis and consecutively with a CT-planned tumor boost to the urinary bladder up to 56.4 Gy. Additionally, 5-FU was given in a dose of 350 mg/m^2 on days 1–10 as a continuous intravenous (i.v.) infusion, folinic acid in a dose of 200 mg/m^2 on days 1–10 as an i.v. infusion over 30 min, and carboplatin in a dose of 200 mg/m^2 on days 5 and 10 as an i.v. infusion over 30 min.

All side effects were classified according to the RTOG score (Radiation Therapy Oncology Group). The acute side effects for white blood cells (WBC), platelets, and hemoglobin (Hb) as defined by the RTOG are shown in Table 1. Demonstrated are the side effects for WBC, platelets and Hb, for the rectum, the bladder and the skin.

Results

Acute and late side effects were classified according to the RTOG score. Acute side effects are shown in Figs. 1 and 2. Two patients (13%) experienced acute grade III thrombopenia and anemia, 5 patients (33%) grade II leukopenia, and 7 patients (45%) grade I/II anemia. A total of 13 patients (93%) had acute side effects to the skin grade I and 1 patient grade II. For the rectum this rate was 20% (3) for grade I and 66% (10) for grade II. For the bladder 27% (4) had grade I and 13% (2) had grade II side effects. No grade III or IV effects for rectum, skin or bladder were observed.

Late side effects for platelets, WBC or Hb were not seen. For rectum (27%), bladder (20%) and skin (7%) only grade I side effects were seen. The late side effects are shown in Fig. 3.

Ten of 15 patients showed a complete response and 3/15 a partial response. Over a median follow-up of 13 months 5/15 developed a local progression and/or distant metastases. All 10 patients with complete response are living tumor-free.

Discussion

Results of conventional treatment for muscle-invading bladder carcinoma are unsatisfactory. Up to 50% of the patients can achieve 5-year survival

Table 1. RTOG score for acute side effects

	RTOG 1	RTOG 2	RTOG 3	RTOG 4
WBC	>4	3.0 to <4.0	2.0 to <3.0	1.0 to <2.0
Platelets	>100	75 to <100	50 to <75	25 to <50
Hb	>11	11 to 9.5	<9.5 to 7.5	<7.5 to 5.0

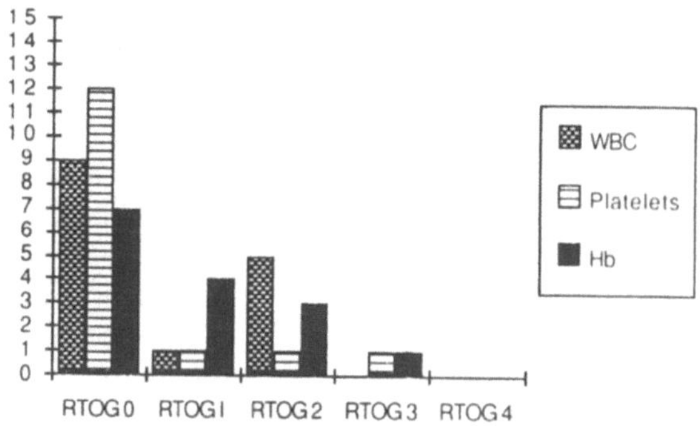

Fig. 1. Acute side effects for WBC, platelets and haemoglobin

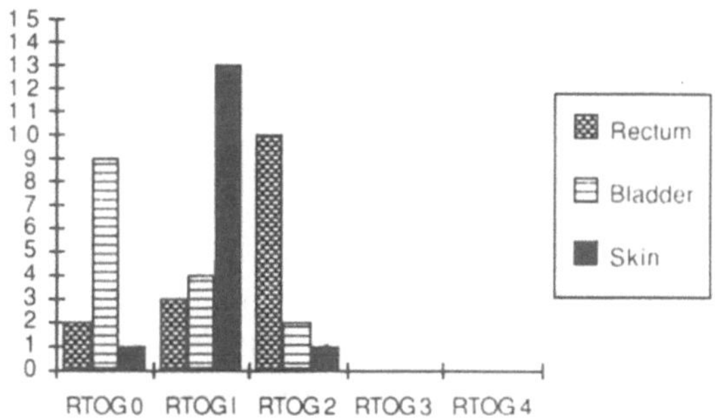

Fig. 2. Acute side effects for rectum, bladder and skin

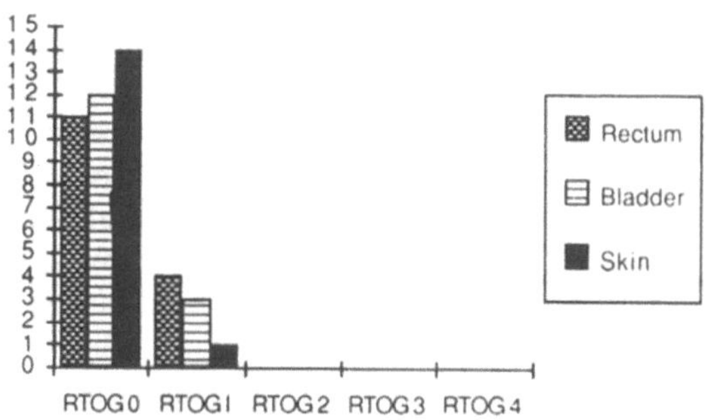

Fig. 3. Late side effects for rectum, bladder and skin

rates with cystectomy with or without irradiation (van der Werf-Messing 1983). Following cystectomy, sexual dysfunction and urinary diversion affect the quality of life. Therefore, improved survival and bladder preservation are important issues in new treatment programs.

Results of several studies for chemo-radiotherapy of bladder cancer using 5-FU with or without mitomycin C (Rotman et al. 1987; Russel et al. 1988), and cisplatin alone (Shipley et al. 1985; Sauer et al. 1988) or in combination with doxorubicin (Jakse et al. 1986) have been reported. Results or side effects of a combination of 5-FU, folinic acid and carboplatin with irradiation as described here have not been published.

Folinic acid modulates the effect of 5-FU, by prolonging the inhibitory effect of FdUMP, the active metabolite of 5-FU, to thymidilate synthetase. This effect is well documented in prospective randomized clinical trials in colorectal cancer, response rates being found that were up to 200% higher than using 5-FU alone (Arbuck 1989).

Carboplatin, a second-generation platinum complex, lacks neuro- and nephrotoxicity and is well tolerated by patients. However, using carboplatin as a single active agent, the effect in tumor cells is less than for cisplatin. When higher doses of carboplatin are given, similar effectiveness has been seen in vitro (Schwachöfer et al. 1991).

The aim of this trial was to use the well-documented effect of 5-FU, folinic acid and carboplatin with irradiation to improve survival time with acceptable toxicity.

Rotman et al. (1987) described the side effects of treatment with irradiation up to 65 Gy and concomitant 5-FU infusion in 19 patients. Acute complications were mild, but late side effects included 5 patients with hemorrhagic cystitis, 2 with contracted bladder, 3 with diarrhea, and 1 with rectal bleeding. This was similar to the side effects published by Russel et al. (1988). Marks et al. (1988) reported acute and late side effects using a combination of methotrexate, cisplatin and vinblastine (MCV) followed by cisplatin plus radiation therapy in 19 patients (irradiation up to 65 Gy). He noted dysuria in 68%, and in 36% there was mild bowel hyperactivity. Serious late side effects appeared in 2 patients. Sauer et al. (1988) reported on 41 patients treated with cisplatin and irradiation up to 50.4 Gy with encouraging results. There were mild to moderate acute side effects with good overall long-term treatment tolerance.

In our series acute side effects grade III with thrombopenia and anemia occurred in only 2 patients, but 66% of our patients had diarrhea requiring treatment (grade II). Six patients showed mild bladder side effects grade I/II. A total of 5 patients had mild late side effects (grade I) for rectum, bladder and skin. Over a median follow-up of 13 months no patient had serious complications. These results are similar to those when using 5-FU plus mitomycin C or cisplatin alone, but further evaluation and follow-up are necessary.

In conclusion, chemo-radiotherapy of invasive bladder carcinoma with 5-FU, folinic acid and carboplatin together with simultaneous accelerated hyperfractionated radiation therapy up to 56.4 Gy was tolerated well with acceptable toxicity.

References

Arbuck SG (1989) Overview of clinical trials using 5-fluorouracil and leucovorin for the treatment of colorectal cancer. Cancer [Suppl] 63:1036–1044

Jacobi GH, Klippel KH, Hohenfellner R (1983) Fifteen years' experience with radical cystectomy without preoperative radiotherapy or radiotherapy for bladder cancer. Aktuel Urol 14:63–70

Jakse G, Rauschmeier H, Fritsch E, Frommhold H, Marberger H (1986) Die integrierte Radiotherapie des lokal fortgeschrittenen Harnblasenkarzinoms. Actuel Urol 17:68–73

Lelieveld P, Vijgh WJF, Vildhuizen RW, van Velzen D, Putten LM, Atassi G, Danguy A (1984) Preclinical studies on toxicity, antitumor activity and pharmacokinetics of cis-platin and three recently developed derivates. Eur J Cancer Clin Oncol 20:1087–1104

Marks BL, Kaufman SD, Prout G, Heney NM, Griffin PP, Shipley WU (1988) Invasive bladder carcinoma: preliminary report of selective bladder conservation by transurethral surgery, upfront MCV chemotherapy and pelvic irradiation plus cisplatin. Int J Radiat Oncol Biol Phys 15:877–883

Rotman M, Macchia R, Silverstein M, Aziz H, Choi K, Rosenthal J, Braverman A, Laungani GB (1987) Treatment of advanced bladder carcinoma with irradiation and concomitant 5-fluorouracil infusion. Cancer 59:710–714

Russel KJ, Boileau MA, Ireton R (1988) Transitional cell carcinoma of the urinary bladder: histologic clearance with combined 5-FU chemotherapy and radiation therapy: preliminary results of a bladder-preservation study. Radiology 167:845–850

Sauer R, Schrott KM, Dunst J, Thiel HJ, Hermanek P, Bornhof C (1988) Preliminary results of treatment of invasive bladder carcinoma with radiotherapy and cisplatin. Int J Radiat Oncol Biol Phys 15:871–875

Schwachöfer JHM, Crooijmans RP, Hoogenhout J, Kal HB, Theeuwes AGM (1991) Effectiveness in inhibition of recovery of cell survival by cisplatin and carboplatin: influence of treatment sequence. Int J Radiat Oncol Biol Phys 20:1235–1241

Shipley W, Einstein AB, Soloway MS, Wajsman Z, Prout GR and the National Bladder Collaborative Group A (1984) Cisplatin and full dose irradiation for patients with invasive bladder carcinoma: a preliminary report of tolerance and local response. J Urol 132:899–903

Shipley W, Rose MA, Perrone TL, Mannix CM, Henry NM, Prout GR (1985) Full dose irradiation for patients with invasive bladder carcinoma: clinical and histological factors prognostic of improved survival. J Urol 134:679–683

Van der Werf-Messing B (1983) Carcinoma of the bladder treated by preoperative irradiation followed by cystectomy. Cancer 32:1084–1088

III. Radiation Effects on Lung and Heart

Radiopathology of the Lung: Experimental and Clinical Observations

M. Molls[1], Th. Herrmann[3], F. Steinberg[2], and H.J. Feldmann[2]

[1] Klinik für Strahlentherapie, Technische Universität, W-8000 München, Fed. Rep. of Germany
[2] Radiologisches Zentrum, Universitätsklinikum, W-4300 Essen, Fed. Rep. of Germany
[3] Radiologisches Zentrum, Medizinische Akademie, O-8019 Dresden, Fed. Rep. of Germany

Introduction

More than 40 cell types are found in the lung, most of which are considered to be relatively radioresistant. However, the lung is unable to tolerate large radiation doses since the organ as a whole has little regenerative capacity. Ionizing radiation causes immediate alterations at the biochemical, subcellular, and cellular level. Gross tissue injury associated with organ dysfunction is delayed: symptomatic pneumonitis occurs at about 1 to several months after irradiation, fibrosis after 6 months to 1 year.

The probability of developing symptomatic radiation pneumonitis depends on the total radiation dose, the temporal dose distribution (fractionation schedule, dose rate), and the irradiated lung volume. Especially in total body irradiation (TBI) prior to bone marrow transplantation, but also in conventional radiotherapeutic regimens, cofactors such as chemotherapy and infections may increase the risk of lung injury (Rubin and Casarett 1968; Coggle et al. 1986; Molls and van Beuningen 1991).

If pneumonitis is mild it may subside spontaneously as observed in experimental investigations. However, pneumonitis can be a very serious event, especially after irradiation of a large volume of the lung. The more severe reactions of the lung may progress so that fibrosis develops (Casarett 1980). Striation, mottling, and cloudiness constitute the radiographic picture of pneumonitis. Clinical characteristics are acute violent cough and shortness of breath which is the consequence of a disturbed balance between ventilation and perfusion and an impaired gas exchange. The main sequelae of radiation-induced fibrosis arise from shrinkage of the lung volume. A shift of the mediastinum toward the irradiated side may occur as well as pulmonary hypertension. Fibrosed lung is prone to infections, which may exacerbate cardiac problems. In large areas of fibrosis cystic or bronchiectatic

Recent Results in Cancer Research, Vol. 130

alterations can be found (Coggle et al. 1986; Molls and van Beuningen 1991). Our following brief review concentrates on the mechanisms in the development of radiation pneumonitis, relevant clinical data, and the difficulties in treating radiation-induced pulmonary injury.

Cellular Mechanisms in the Development of Radiation Pneumonitis

Despite many experimental efforts the pathogenesis of radiation pneumonitis remains a puzzle of cause and effect (Coggle et al. 1986). Lesions of the alveolar epithelium as well as of alveolar capillaries play an important role (Molls and van Beuningen 1991). According to Rubin and Casarett (1968) swelling of endothelium, congestion, thrombosis, increased vascular permeability, edema, fibrin exudation, diapedesis, and activation of fibroblasts are characteristic effects.

Recently we have published our own findings concerning the development of lung fibrosis. Using quantitative morphometric methods 11 weeks after irradiation of mice with single doses of 10, 12, or 14 Gy we found edema and a dose-dependent thickening of alveolar septa as well as an increase in the total collagen content. Concomitantly the alveolar surface was decreased (Kraus et al. 1991).

Van den Brenk (1971) assumed that damage to the epithelial cells is the most important causative factor. The alveoli are lined by an epithelium which consists of type I and type II pneumocytes. The type II cells represent the stem cell population for the type I pneumocytes. They also synthesize, store, and secrete the phospholipid and protein components of surfactant (Adamson and Bowden 1977; Evans et al. 1973, 1976; Travis 1987). It is not only the death and dysfunction of type II pneumocytes with the concomitant major alterations in levels of surfactant that may be decisive in the development of pneumonitis (van den Brenk 1971; Rubin et al. 1980; Naimark et al. 1970; Gross 1978). Other investigations suggest that necrosis and sloughing of type I cells, leaving denuded basement membranes and alveolar debris, also have a fundamental effect (Maisin 1970; Gross 1981; Adamson et al. 1970). Additionally, there are studies pointing out the important role of lymphocytes (Bennet et al. 1969) and the immune system (Madrazo et al. 1973).

In our own investigations we have counted macrophages, granulocytes, and lymphocytes obtained by bronchoalveolar lavage prior to and after TBI in bone-marrow-transplanted patients. Macrophages especially showed a time-dependent response to TBI, a significant decrease being followed by a later increase. The phagocytic activity of macrophages was tested after bronchoalveolar lavage of irradiated mice and TBI of patients. The human macrophages showed no changes whereas in mice the activity was decreased even 3 weeks after irradiation. Furthermore, macrophages expressed radiation-induced cytogenetic damage as revealed by formation of micronuclei (Steinberg et al. 1992; Steinberg et al., this volume). Macrophages but also mast cells release mediators such as prostaglandins, leukotrienes, and histamine. It has been hypothesized that these substances could be involved in early postradiation lung injury (Graham et al. 1990). It would therefore seem important to investigate the reaction of these cell types to irradiation.

Total Dose, Fractionation, Dose Rate, Repair

A direct assay of target cell response has not been developed. It is therefore difficult to define a representative endpoint that allows a dose–effect relationship for radiation-induced lung damage to be established. Philips and Margolis (1972) observed that mice died from pulmonary injury at 80–180 days after irradiation of the thorax. In general, the $LD_{50/180}$ values (dose required to kill 50% of animals between 80 and 180 days after irradiation) range from 10 to 14 Gy after application of a single acute X-ray dose. Values vary with species and strain (Wara et al. 1973; Field et al. 1976; Coggle et al. 1986; Travis 1987).

Upper half-body irradiation of 150 patients (TBI was administered in a small number of patients) with large single doses at a dose rate of 0.5–4.0 Gy/min yielded a dose–effect curve which showed a threshold for radiation pneumonitis at about 7.5 Gy, with a 5% actuarial incidence at approximately 8.2 Gy. An incidence of 50% and 90% was observed at 9.3 and 10.6 Gy respectively. Radiation was given mainly to relieve pain of advanced cancer using the upper half-body irradiation technique (Fryer et al. 1978; van Dyk et al. 1981). Clinical practice regarding administration of TBI prior to bone marrow transplantation differs widely between institutions: total lung doses range between 5 and 13 Gy; the radiation is given as a single dose or fractionated; and the dose rate may be rather low (<0.06 Gy/min) or high (0.1–0.5 Gy/min). Details have been reviewed recently (Molls and van Beuningen 1991).

A recent study in adults has generated a dose–response relationship between radiation-induced pulmonary damage and the estimated single-dose equivalent of fractionated radiotherapy schedules. Mah et al. (1987) measured the increase in lung density within the irradiated volume by computed tomography. Fifty-four patients with various malignancies of the thorax completed the prospective study. A 50% incidence of pulmonary damage was found for 1000 ± 40 ED (estimated single dose) units, which corresponds to 33 Gy in 15 fractions over 19 days (2.2 Gy per fraction). A lung dose of 24.7 Gy in 15 daily fractions yielded a comparatively low incidence of damage of 5%. Newton and Spittle (1969) treated adults with pulmonary metastases by irradiation of the total thorax with doses of 20 or 25 Gy given in daily fractions of 1.5 Gy. Survival of patients ranged between 1 and 85 months (mean 15 months). No early or late pulmonary complications were observed, whereas in 7 patients who received 30 Gy in daily fractions of 3 Gy, radiotherapy resulted in an unacceptable incidence of radiation pneumonitis. After lung irradiation of patients with macroscopic or suspected subclinical metastases with a dose of 20 Gy given in 10 fractions, no radiation pneumonitis occurred (Breur et al. 1978; Cox 1972). According to Phillips and Margolis (1972), the dose that will cause clinical pneumonitis in 5% of patients is about 26 Gy in 20 fractions.

The lung shows greater sparing from dose fractionation than do more rapidly proliferating tissues (Dutreix et al. 1979; Vegesna et al. 1985). $LD_{50/180}$ values increased with increasing time intervals between fractions. In mice the most dramatic changes occurred over the first few hours after the first X-ray treatment, due to repair of sublethal damage. For time intervals greater than 6 h the increase in $LD_{50/180}$ was less. This latter type of repair was considered to be a process of slow repair (Field and Hornsey 1974; Field 1977). Parkins and Fowler (1985) studied the fractionation response with low doses per fraction down to 1.1 Gy. Changes were assessed by $LD_{50/180}$ and breathing rate. Their findings were similar to those of Vegesna et al. (1985), and indicated that further significant sparing of X-ray-induced lung damage (both pneumonitis and fibrosis) could be observed when the dose per fraction was reduced from 1.6 Gy to approximately 1.1 Gy per fraction, even for 2 fractions per day with a 6 h interval. No such repair could be seen with fractionated fast neutrons.

The results of fractionation studies can be described by the linear-quadratic formula, the fractionation sensitivity being given by the α/β dose. Recently we have tabulated the α/β ratios for lung tissue which have been reported in the literature (Molls and van Beuningen 1991). Interestingly the α/β values obtained by experimental investigations are comparable with those obtained for humans: Herrmann et al. (1986a,b, 1987) reported a ratio of 3.7 Gy for pigs, van Dyk et al. (1989) a ratio of 3.3 Gy for humans. The relatively low α/β values indicate that the lung is a late-responding tissue in which the cell-killing mechanism is dominated by accumulation of reparable or β-type (multihit) injury. This means that in clinical fractionated radiotherapy the lung benefits from relatively low single doses.

Regarding the very special situation of clinical TBI, the multicenter study of the International Bone Marrow Transplant Registry yielded no evidence that fractionated irradiation reduced the risk of interstitial pneumonitis within the range of applied doses and in the schedules tested (Weiner et al. 1986). On the other hand a number of nonrandomized studies with smaller numbers of patients concluded that fractionation is beneficial when compared with single-dose TBI (Rohloff et al. 1987, 1988; Hübener et al. 1987; Ehninger et al. 1987; Molls et al. 1987; Pino et al. 1982; Vitale et al. 1983; Blume et al. 1987; Shank et al. 1983; Cosset et al. 1989).

The sparing effect of low-dose-rate irradiation has been found in a number of experiments. For dose rates of 1.1 Gy/min (mice) and 0.8 Gy/min (rats) the $LD_{50/180}$ values were 11 and 13.3 Gy, whereas for 0.08 Gy/min they were 20 Gy and 22.7 Gy respectively (Hill 1983; Lopez Cardozo et al. 1985). An effect of dose rate was also found when lung function was tested by measuring carbon monoxide uptake (Depledge and Barret 1982). The impairment of lung function increased with increasing dose rate over the range 0.02–1 Gy/min (in mice). Down et al. (1986) provided evidence for less dose sparing with single protracted dose of radiation at a dose rate of 0.05 Gy/min compared with a conventional fractionated schedule of 2 Gy per fraction. Only irradiation with dose rates as low as 0.02 Gy/min was comparable to fractionation. With regard to clinical TBI prior to bone marrow transplantation it was postulated that lowering the dose rate to below 0.05 Gy/min will shift the threshold for significant interstitial pneumonitis to 11–12 Gy (single dose) (Barrett et al. 1983).

Lung Volume, Cofactors, and the Risk of Pneumonitis in Clinical Radiotherapy

At a dose of 40 Gy given with conventional fractionation, morphological alterations of the lung can be expected in about 50% of the treated volumes. In most cases serious clinical symptoms will not arise if the irradiated lung volume is relatively small, i.e., less than about 20% of the total lung volume (Molls and van Beuningen 1991). After regimes which involve one third to one half of one lung, pneumonitis with nonproductive cough, spiking, fever, shortness of breath, and even respiratory distress will occur in about 10% of patients (Coggle et al. 1986).

The likelihood of radiation pneumonitis and factors associated with its development in breast cancer patients has been retrospectively investigated in 1624 patients. Patients were irradiated after conservative surgery with either tangential field alone ($n = 508$) or tangents with a third field to the supraclavicular or supraclavicular–axillary region ($n = 1116$). Seventeen patients with radiation pneumonitis were identified (1.0%). Radiation pneumonitis was diagnosed when patients presented with cough (15/17, 88%), fever (9/17, 53%), and/or dyspnea (6/17, 35%) and radiographic changes (17/17, 100%) following completion of radiotherapy. Radiographic infiltrates corresponded to treatment portals in all patients, and in 12 of the 17 patients returned to baseline within 1–12 months. Five patients had permanent scarring visible on chest radiographs. No patient had late or persistent pulmonary symptoms.

Interestingly, the incidence of radiation pneumonitis was correlated with a third field (irradiated volume) and the combined use of chemotherapy (different regimens: cyclophosphamide (CMF) without doxorubicin in 72%, doxorubicin without CMF in 4%, CMF plus doxorubicin in 14%, other drugs in 10%). Three percent (11/328) of patients treated with a three-field technique who received chemotherapy developed radiation pneumonitis compared with 0.5% (6/1296) of all other patients ($p = 0.0001$). When patients treated with a three-field technique received chemotherapy concurrently with radiation therapy the incidence of radiation pneumonitis was

8.8% (8/92), compared with 1.3% (3/236) for those who received sequential chemotherapy and radiation therapy ($p = 0.002$). The authors concluded that radiation pneumonitis following conservative surgery and radiation therapy for breast cancer is a rare complication, and that it is more likely to occur in patients treated with both a three-field technique and chemotherapy (Lingos et al. 1991). In respect of the lung volume irradiated by the three-field technique the investigation of Kaufmann et al. (1986) is of interest. The authors calculated from computed tomographic reconstructions for one lung an alveolar volume of 1346 ml. The values for the tangents, internal mammary portion, and supraclavicular field were 48 ml, 200 ml, and 300 ml respectively.

In radiotherapy for lung cancer and thoracic lymphomas the pattern of factors which increase the risk of pneumonitis is comparable to that in radiotherapy of breast cancer. In addition to total dose and fractionation schedule the probability of developing clinically significant radiation pneumonitis is dependent on the irradiated lung volume and cofactors such as chemotherapy. Details have been reviewed recently (Molls and van Beuningen 1991).

The clinical experience in the treatment of Hodgkin's disease shows that after application of the mantle field technique (linear accelarator) radiation-induced lung morbidity is relatively low (Kaplan 1972). Regarding functional alterations, slight and moderate restrictive disturbances of ventilation were found in 68% of patients, impairment of oxygen diffusion in 18%, and obstructive disturbances of ventilation in 7%. Severe functional changes were not observed. Interestingly, oxygen diffusion was impaired to a significantly greater extent among smokers than among nonsmokers (Slanina et al. 1977, 1982; Slanina 1977).

The risk of pneumonitis is comparatively high when concurrent radiotherapy and chemotherapy are given. Treatment of small cell lung cancer is a paradigmatic situation. A reduction in pulmonary toxicity can be achieved when chemotherapy is applied sequentially with radiotherapy or concomitantly for only a short time period of a few days (Choi and Carey 1976; Moore et al. 1978; Molls and van Beuningen 1991).

Recently Koga et al. (1988) reported that severe radiation pneumonitis was more often observed in elderly patients (70 years or more) with lung cancer than in younger ones (<70 years). In both age groups pneumonitis occurred earlier when the field size was 90 cm^2 or more. About one third of the patients also received chemotherapy.

It is well known that some cytotoxic drugs alone may cause acute and late pulmonary toxicity. Summaries have been published by Rosenow (1972), Philips et al. (1975), Weiss and Muggia (1980), Rubin (1984), Scheulen (1987), and Molls and van Beuningen (1991). Table 1 lists some of the most important chemotherapeutic substances and shows to what extent they may increase radiation damage to the lung under experimental conditions.

Table 1. Summary of experimental studies which provide evidence for drug-induced enhancement of lung morbidity[a] (from Molls and van Beuningen 1991)

		Enhancement for drug given			
Drug	Endpoint	Before	With	After	Reference[b]
Cyclo-phosphamide	Lethality		+++		1
	Lethality		+++		2
	Function	++	+++	++	3
Cisplatin	Lethality		–		2
	Function	–	–	–	4
	Function		–		2
Methotrexate	Lethality	–			1
	Lethality		–		2
	Function	+	–	–	4
	Function		–		2
Hydroxyurea	Lethality		–		5
Vincristine	Lethality		+		5
	Function	+	+	+	4
Actinomycin	Lethality	+	+++	–	5
	Lethality	–			1
	Function	–	+		4
Adriamycin	Lethality		+++		6
	Lethality	++			1
	Lethality		++	+	7
	Lethality		+++		2
	Function	–	+++	++	4
	Function		+++		2
Bleomycin	Lethality		–		5
	Lethality	++			1
	Lethality		++		2
	Function	++	++	+–	4
	Function		+++		2
Mitomycin C	Lethality		+++		2
	Function		+++		2
BCNU	Lethality		–		5
5-Fluorouracil	Lethality		–		2
	Function		–		2

[a] The extent to which the drug increased the damage over that produced by irradiation alone is indicated by approximate dose enhancement factors (DEF): +++ DEF above 1.4; ++ DEF 1.2–1.4 + DEF up to about 1.2; – no effect. Before: 7–28 days before irradiation. After: 7–28 days after irradiation.

[b] References: 1, Steel et al. 1979; 2, van der Maase et al. 1986; 3, Collis and Steel 1983; 4, Collis 1981; 5, Phillips et al. 1975; 6, Redpath et al. 1978; 7, Redpath et al. 1981 (from Steel 1988, with modifications).

Interestingly, in the experimental investigations methotrexate enhanced radiation-induced lung morbidity only to a comparatively low degree. However, one has to be aware that in methotrexate prophylaxis of graft-versus-host disease after TBI and bone marrow transplantation the risk of interstitial pneumonitis may be high (Deeg et al. 1988; Beelen et al. 1988; Molls et al. 1990). Cisplatin has only a slight effect on the radiation response of the lung. The experimental results are in accordance with our clinical experience of treating lung metastases of sarcoma patients, in whom radiotherapy was combined with a cisplatin-containing regimen (Zamboglou et al. 1988).

Prediction of Pulmonary Injury

Rubin et al. (1983, 1986) reported on observations in mice which provided evidence that alveolar surfactant release detected several days after irradiation may be an early biochemical marker predicting subsequent pneumonitis. The increases in surfactant and lethality were of comparable steepness over the dose range of about 12–15 Gy. However, doubt has been cast on this hypothesis (Down et al. 1988). A recent publication reported on investigations in patients. Maasilta et al. (1991) studied procollagen type III peptide concentration in serum, as well as fibronectin and plasminogen activation in bronchoalveolar lavage fluid during and following irradiation of human lung. The patients received high-dose irradiation either of the hemithorax for pleural mesothelioma ($n = 11$) or of individually shaped lung volumes for non-small-cell lung cancer ($n = 12$). The levels of plasmin and plasminogen activator in bronchoalveolar lavage fluid showed a tendency to be elevated in patients who developed severe radiation-induced lung injury.

With regard to conventional radiation therapy of the thoracic region, especially in patients with bronchial carcinoma, quantitative perfusion lung scanning and forced expiratory volume have been used to predict pulmonary function following lung irradiation (Rubenstein et al. 1988). From the serial follow-up observations it was concluded that such determinations can be of value in formulating a treatment plan for patients with significantly impaired pulmonary function.

Treating Pulmonary Injury

There are experimental but also clinical investigations suggesting that corticosteroids may reduce the morbidity and mortality of radiation-induced pneumonitis (Molls and van Beuningen 1991). In irradiated mice corticosteroids stimulated surfactant production, which prevented abnormalities in pulmonary mechanics and alveolar fluid surface tension (Gross 1980). A corticosteroid-induced augmentation of the enhanced reproductive activity of irradiated type II cells has also been described (Gross and Narine 1988).

Investigations by Evans et al. (1987) led to the hypothesis that the ability of dexamethasone to suppress the increased vascular permeability following irradiation could result in a long-term reduction in the incidence of fibrosis. Vascular permeability was significantly elevated in irradiated rat lung, heart, skin, and muscle between 19 and 26 days following irradiation of the thorax with 18 or 25 Gy. Dexamethasone was administered from 2 days before irradiation through the day of measurement. Shorter periods of steroid application were less effective in suppressing the response to irradiation. The same group (Graham et al. 1990) obtained comparable results after application of indomethacin, cromolyn, cyproheptadine, vitamin D_3, theophylline, and diethylcarbamazine, whereas substances such as captopril, penicillamine, and others had no significant effect on vascular permeability in the lung.

Clinically, application of steroids in a relatively large number of patients with the symptoms of pneumonitis was found to have no protective effect (Deeg et al. 1988). However, their withdrawal precipitated the radiation pneumonitis syndrome in a small number of cases (Freyer et al. 1978). In patients in whom symptoms of pneumonitis are mild and infections have been ruled out, treatment is not required. If, however, symptoms worsen, a course of corticosteroids has been recommended.

To establish the role of other therapeutic procedures such as substitution of phospholipids (surfactant) more experimental and clinical studies are needed. This is also true for the application of inhibitors of angiotensin converting enzyme, which have the potential to decrease radiation-induced pulmonary endothelial dysfunction and pulmonary fibrosis (Ward et al. 1988, 1989).

References

Adamson IYR, Bowden DH (1977) Origin of ciliated alveolar epithelial cells in bleomycin-induced lung injury. Am J Pathol 87:569–575

Adamson IYR, Bowden DH, Wyatt JP (1970) A pathway to pulmonary fibrosis: an ultrastructural study of mouse and rat following radiation to the whole body and hemithorax. Am J Pathol 58:481–498

Barret A, Depledge MH, Powles RL (1983) Interstitial pneumonitis following bone marrow transplantation after low dose rate total body irradiation. Int J Radiat Oncol Biol Phys 9:1029–1033

Beelen DW, Quabeck K, Graeven U, Sayer HG, Schaefer UW, Schmidt CG (1988) Influence of treatment-related factors on the results of allogeneic marrow transplantation for leukemia. J Cancer Res Clin Oncol 114 [Suppl]:144

Bennet DE, Million RR, Acherman LV (1969) Bilateral radiation pneumonitis, a complication of the radio-therapy of bronchogenic carcinoma. Cancer 23:1001–1018

Blume KG, Forman SJ, Snyder DS et al. (1987) Allogeneic bone marrow transplantation for acute lymphoblastic leukemia during first complete remission. Transplantation 43:389–392

Breur K, Cohen P, Schweisguth O, Hart AMM (1978) Irradiation of the lung as an adjuvant therapy in the treatment of osteosarcomas of the limbs. Eur J Cancer 14:461–471
Casarett GW (1980) Radiation histopathology. CRC Press, Boca Raton
Choi CH, Carey RW (1976) Small cell anaplastic carcinoma of the lung. Reappraisal of current management. Cancer 37:2651–2657
Coggle JE, Lambert BE, Moore SR (1986) Radiation effects in the lung. Environ Health Perspect 70:261–291
Collis CH (1981) The response of the lung to ionizing radiation and cytotoxic drugs. MD Thesis, University of Cambridge
Collis CH, Steel GG (1983) Lung damage in mice from cyclophosphamide and thoracic irradiation: the effects of timing. Int J Radiat Oncol Biol Phys 9:685–689
Cosset IM, Baume D, Pico JL, Shank B, Girinski T, Benhamou E, Briot E, Malaise E, Hayat M, Dutreix J (1989) Single dose versus hyperfractionated total body irradiation before allogeneic bone marrow transplantation: a non-randomized comparative study of 54 patients at the Institut Gustave-Roussy. Radiother Oncol 15:151–160
Cox JD (1972) Total pulmonary irradiation for metastases from testicular carcinoma. Radiology 105:163–167
Deeg HJ, Klingemann H-G, Phillips GL (1988) A guide to bone marrow transplantation. Springer, Berlin Heidelberg New York, p 120
Depledge MG, Barret A (1982) Dose rate dependence of lung damage after total body irradiation in mice. Int J Radiat Biol 41:325–334
Down JD, Easton DF, Steel GG (1986) Repair in the mouse lung during low dose rate irradiation. Radiother Oncol 6:29–42
Down JD, Coultas PG, Field SB (1988) Is surfactant release a reliable predictor of radiation pneumonitis? Int J Radiat Oncol Biol Phys 19:211–212
Dutreix J, Wambersie A, Coiretta M, Biosserie G (1979) Time factors in total body irradiation. Pathol Biol (Paris) 27:365–369
Ehninger G, Einsele H, Dopfer R, Waller HD (1987) The role of total body irradiation in conditioning adults for bone marrow transplantation. Strahlenther Onkol 163:210–211
Evans MJ, Cabral CJ, Stephens RJ, Freeman G (1973) Renewal of alveolar epithelium in the rat following exposure to NO_2. Am J Pathol 70:175–198
Evans MJ, Johnson CV, Stephens RJ, Freeman G (1976) Cell renewal in the lungs of rats exposed to low levels of ozone. Exp Morph Pathol 24:70–83
Evans ML, Graham MM, Mahler PA, Rasey JS (1987) Use of steroid to suppress vascular response to radiation. Int J Radiat Oncol Biol Phys 13:563–567
Field SB (1977) Early and late normal tissue damage after fast neutrons. Int J Radiat Biol Phys 3:203–210
Field SB, Hornsey S (1974) Damage to mouse lung with neutrons and X-rays. Eur J Cancer 10:621–627
Field SB, Hornsey S, Kutsutani Y (1976) Effects of fractionated radiation on mouse lung and a phenomenon of slow repair. Br J Radiol 49:700–707
Fryer CJH, Fitzpatrick PJ, Ridge WD, Doon P (1978) Radiation pneumonitis: experience following a large single dose of radiation. Int J Radiol Oncol Biol Phys 4:931–936
Graham MM, Evans ML, Dahlen DD, Mahler PA, Rasey JS (1990) Pharmacological alteration of the lung vascular response to radiation. Int J Radiat Oncol Biol Phys 19:329–339
Gross NJ (1978) Early physiologic and biochemical effects of thoracic x-irradiation on the pulmonary surfactant system. J Lab Clin Med 537–544
Gross NJ (1980) Radiation pneumonitis in mice: some effects of corticosteroids on mortality and pulmonary physiology. J Clin Invest 66:504–510

Gross NJ (1981) The pathogenesis-induced lung damage. Lung 159:115–125

Gross NJ, Narine KR (1988) Experimental radiation pneumonitis: corticosteroids increase the replicative activity of alveolar type 2 cells. Radiat Res 115:543–549

Herrmann T, Voigtmann L, Knorr A, Lorenz J, Johannsen U (1986a) The time-dose relationship for radiation-induced lung damage in pigs. Radiother Oncol 5:127–135

Herrmann T, Voigtmann L, Knorr A, Lorenz J, Johannsen U, Welker K (1986b) Fractionated lung irradiation in young pigs with 6.2 MeV neutrons and cobalt-60. Radiother Oncol 7:69–75

Herrmann T, Voigtmann L, Knorr A, Lorenz J (1987) Zum Reparaturverhalten der Lunge: experimentelle und klinische Ergebnisse. Strahlenther Onkol 163:370–377

Hill RP (1983) Response of mouse lung to irradiation at different dose rates. Int J Radiat Oncol Biol Phys 9:1043–1047

Hübener K-H, Schmidt B, Steidle B (1987) Clinical results of bone marrow transplantation in Tübingen after total body irradiation from the radiotherapeutical view. Strahlenther Oncol 163:214–216

Kaplan HS (1972) Hodgkin's disease. Harvard University Press, Cambridge, MA

Kaufman J, Gunn W, Hartz AJ, Fischer M, Hoffman R, Schlueter DP, Komanduri A (1986) The pathophysiologic and roentgenologic effects of chest irradiation in breast carcinoma. Int J Radiat Oncol Biol Phys 12:179–188

Koga K, Kusumoto S, Watanabe K, Nishikawa K, Harada K, Ebihara H (1988) Age factor relevant to the development of radiation induced pneumonitis in radiotherapy of lung cancer. Int J Radiat Oncol Biol Phys 14:367–371

Kraus R, Steinberg F, Rehn B, Bruch J, Streffer C (1991) Radiation-induced changes in lung tissue and development of fibrosis determined by quantitative morphometric methods. J Cancer Res Clin Oncol 117:27–32

Lingos TI, Recht A, Vicini F, Abner A, Silver B, Harris JR (1991) Radiation pneumonitis in breast cancer patients treated with conservative surgery and radiation therapy. Int J Radiat Oncol Biol Phys 21:355–360

Lopez Cardozo B, Zoetelief D, van Bekkum DW, Zurcher C, Hagenbeek A (1985) Lung damage following bone marrow transplantation: I. The contribution of irradiation. Int J Radiat Oncol Biol Phys 11:907–914

Maasilta P, Salonen EM, Vaheri A, Kivisaari L, Holsti LR, Mattson K (1991) Procollagen-III in serum, plasminogen activation and fibronectin in bronchoalveolar lavage fluid during and following irradiation of human lung. Int J Radiat Oncol Biol Phys 20:973–980

Madrazo A, Suzuki Y, Churg J (1973) Radiation pneumonitis. Arch Pathol 96:262–268

Mah K, van Dyk J, Keane T, Poon PY (1987) Acute induced pulmonary damage: a clinical study on the response to fractionated radiation therapy. Int J Radiat Oncol Biol Phys 13:179–188

Maisin JR (1970) The ultrastructure of the lung of mice exposed to a supra-lethal dose of ionizing radiation on the thorax. Radiat Res 44:545–564

Molls M, Bamberg M, Beelen DW, Mahmoud HK, Quast U, Schaefer UW (1987) Different TBI procedures in Essen: results and clinical considerations on the risk of leukemic relapse and interstitial pneumonitis. Strahlenther Onkol 163:237–240

Molls M, Quast U, Schaefer UW et al. (1990) Clinical results and the Essen concept of TBI. Radiother Oncol 18 [Suppl 1]:121–124

Molls M, van Beuningen D (1991) Radiation injury of the lung: experimental studies, observations after radiotherapy and total body irradiation prior to bone marrow transplantation. In: Scherer E, Streffer Ch, Trott K-R (eds) Medical radiology. Radiopathology of organs and tissues. Springer, Berlin Heidelberg New York, pp 369–404

Moore TN, Livingston R, Heilbrun L et al. (1978) An acceptable rate of complications in combined doxorubicin-irradiation for small cell carcinoma of the lung: a Southwest Oncology Group study. Int J Radiat Oncol Biol Phys 4:675–680
Naimark A, Newman D, Bowden DH (1970) Effect of radiation on lecithin metabolism, surface activity, and compliance of rat lung. Can J Physiol Pharmacol 48:685–694
Newton KA, Spittle MF (1969) An analysis of 40 cases treated by total body irradiation. Clin Radiol 20:19–22
Parkins CS, Fowler JF (1985) Repair in mouse lung of multifraction x-rays and neutrons: extension to 40 fractions. Br J Radiol 58:1097–1103
Phillips TL, Margolis L (1972) Radiation pathology and the clinical response of lung and oesophagus. Front Radiat Ther Oncol 6:254
Phillips TL, Wharam MD, Margolis L (1975) Modification of radiation injury to normal tissues by chemotherapeutic agents. Cancer 35:1678–1684
Pino Y, Torres JL, Bross DS, Lam WC, Wharam MD, Santos GW, Order SE (1982) Risk factors in interstitial pneumonitis following allogeneic bone marrow transplantation. Int J Radiat Oncol Biol Phys 8:1301–1307
Redpath JL, David RM, Colman M (1978) The effect of Adriamycin on radiation damage to mouse lung and skin. Int J Radiat Oncol Biol Phys 4:229–232
Redpath JL, Zabilansky E, Colman M (1981) The effect of Adriamycin on repair of sublethal damage and slow repair in irradiated mouse lung. Int J Radiat Biol 39:157–161
Rohloff R, Naujokat B, Bender C, Haas R, Kolb K-J (1987) Results and side effects after total body irradiation for bone marrow transplantation in the Munich group. Strahlenther Oncol 163:222–223
Rohloff R, Kolb K-J, Bender C, Haas R, Kantlehner R, Balk OA (1988) Methodik und Ergebnisse der Ganzkörperbestrahlung im Rahmen der Knochenmarkstransplantation. Radiobiol Radiother 29:289–290
Rosenow EC (1972) The spectrum of drug-induced pulmonary disease. Ann Intern Med 77:977–991
Rubenstein JH, Richter MP, Moldofsky PJ, Solin LJ (1988) Prospective prediction of post-radiation therapy lung function using quantitative lung scans and pulmonary function testing. Int J Radiat Oncol Biol Phys 15:83–87
Rubin P (1984) The Franz Buschke lecture. Late effects of chemotherapy and radiation therapy: a new hypothesis. Int J Radiat Oncol Biol Phys 10:5–34
Rubin P, Casarett GW (1968) Clinical radiation pathology. Saunders, Philadelphia
Rubin P, Shapiro DL, Finkelstein JN, Penney DP (1980) The early release of surfactant following lung irradiation of alveolar type II cells. Int J Radiat Oncol Biol Phys 6:75–77
Rubin P, Siemann DW, Shapiro D, Finkelstein J, VanHoutte P, Penney D (1983) Surfactant release as an early measure of radiation pneumonitis. Int J Radiat Oncol Biol Phys 9:1669–1673
Rubin P, Finkelstein JN, Siemann DW, Shapiro DL, VanHoutte P, Penney DP (1986) Predictive biochemical assays for late radiation effects. Int Radiat Oncol Biol Phys 12:469–476
Scheulen ME (1987) Reduction of pulmonary toxicity. Cancer Treat Rev 14:231–243
Shank B, Chu FCH, Dinsmore R et al. (1983) Hyperfractionated total body irradiation for bone marrow transplantation: results in seventy leukemia patients with allogeneic transplants. Int J Radiat Oncol Biol Phys 9:1607–1611
Slanina J (1977) Untersuchungen über somatische Spätschäden nach ausgedehnter Strahlentherapie. Ergebnisse von 135 Patienten mit Hodgkin'scher Erkrankung in Langzeitremission (Freiburger Kollektiv, Behandlungsjahre 1948–1974). Habilitationsschrift

Slanina J, Musshoff K, Rahner T, Stiasny R (1977) Long-term side effects in irradiated patients with Hodgkin's disease. Int J Radiat Oncol Biol Phys 2:1–19
Slanina J, Wannenmacher M, Bruggmoser G, Krüger H-U (1982) Die pulmonale Strahlenreaktion im Röntgenbild: Intensität und Häufigkeit röntgenmorphologischer Veränderungen der Lunge und des Mediastinums nach Mantelfeldbestrahlung mit 4-MeV Photonen und Satelitentechnik. Radiologe 22:74–82
Steel GG (1988) The search for therapeutic gain in the combination of radiotherapy and chemotherapy. Radiother Oncol 11:31–53
Steel GG, Adams K, Peckham MJ (1979) Lunge damage in C57B1 mice following thoracic irradiation: enhancement by chemotherapy. Br J Radiol 52:741–747
Steinberg F, Rehn B, Kraus R, Quabeck K, Bruch J, Beelen DW, Schaefer UW, Streffer C (1992) Activity testing of alveolar macrophages and changes in surfactant phospholipids after irradiation in bronchoalveolar lavage: experimental and clinical data. Environ Health Perspect (in press)
Travis L (1987) Relative radiosensitivity of the human lung. Adv Radiat Biol 12:205–238
van den Brenk HAS (1971) Radiation effects on the pulmonary system. In: Berdjis CC (ed) Pathology of irradiation. Williams and Wilkins, Baltimore, pp 569–591
van der Maase H, Overgaard J, Valth M (1986) Effect of cancer chemotherapeutic drugs on radiation-induced lung damage in mice. Radiother Oncol 5:245–259
van Dyk J, Keane TJ, Kan S, Rider WD, Fryer CJ (1981) Radiation pneumonitis following large single dose irradiation: a reevaluation based on absolute dose to the lung. Int J Radiat Oncol Biol Phys 7:461–467
van Dyk J, Mah K, Keane TJ (1989) Radiation-induced lung damage: dose–time–fractionation considerations. Radiother Oncol 14:55–69
Vegesna SL, Withers HR, Thames HD, Mason KA (1985) Multifraction radiation response of mouse lung. Int J Radiat Biol 47:413–422
Vitale V, Bacigalupo A, van Lint MT et al. (1983) Fractionated total body irradiation in marrow transplantation for leukemia. Br J Haematol 55:547–554
Wara WM, Phillips TL, Margolis LW, Smith V (1973) Radiation pneumonitis: a new approach to the deviation of time dose factors. Cancer 32:547–552
Ward WF, Kim YT, Molteni A, Solliday NH (1988) Radiation-induced pulmonary endothelial dysfunction in rats: modification by an inhibitor of angiotensin converting enzyme. Int J Radiat Oncol Biol Phys 15:135–140
Ward WF, Molteni A, Ts'ao C-H (1989) Radiation-induced endothelial dysfunction and fibrosis in rat lung: modification by the angiotensin converting enzyme inhibitor CL242817. Radiat Res 117:342–350
Weiner RS, Bortin MM, Gale RP et al. (1986) Interstitial pneumonitis after bone marrow transplantation. Ann Intern Med 104:168–175
Weiss RB, Muggia FM (1980) Cytotoxic drug-induced pulmonary disease. Am J Med 68:259–266
Zamboglou N, Fürst G, Pape H, Bannach B, Molls M, Schmitt G (1988) Ergebnisse der Ganzlungenbestrahlung und Chemotherapie im Vergleich zur Teillungenbestrahlung bei metastasierenden, undifferenzierten Weichteilsarkomen. Strahlenther Onkol 164:386–392

Diagnosis of Radiation-Pneumonitis

G. Sigmund[1], J. Slanina[2], and W. Hinkelbein[2]

[1] Department of Diagnostic Radiology, University of Freiburg, W-7800 Freiburg i. Br., Fed. Rep. of Germany
[2] Department of Radiotherapy, Radiologic Clinic, University of Freiburg, W-7800 Freiburg i. Br., Fed. Rep. of Germany

Introduction

The pulmonary radioreaction is an interstitial pulmonary inflammation, so-called pneumonitis, which to a certain degree has an intraalveolar exudative component. If the threshold of potential complete restitution is crossed, the pneumonitis will develop into pulmonary fibrosis (a scar) as a permanent residual (Gross 1977; Slanina et al. 1977; Westcott and Cole 1986; White 1975).

After radiotherapy has been completed patients are usually not sent to the X-ray department for diagnosis of pneumonitis but for follow-up of the underlying disease, i.e. lymphoma or other malignancy, or for other reasons such as unexplained symptoms. The task of the diagnostic radiologist is to identify the signs of a pulmonary radioreaction and to differentiate them from recurrent or intercurrent disease (Glazer et al. 1986; Heron et al. 1988; Lever et al. 1984). If the correct diagnosis of radiation pneumonitis or fibrosis is made, and other disease is ruled out, the patient will gain the important benefit of not having to undergo unnecessary diagnostic or therapeutic measures. In the case of a severe radioreaction the radiotherapist can immediately start treatment with corticosteroids.

The pulmonary radioreaction develops only in the irradiated volume. The distribution of the pneumonitic lesions therefore depends on the size, form, and arrangement of the radiation portals. Because of the highly standardized treatment of Hodgkin's lymphoma by the so-called mantle field, this situation is well suited to a study of the morphology and time course of the pulmonary radioreaction. Thus, the following results are mainly based on two studies of unselected patients followed up after mantle-field irradiation for Hodgkin's lymphoma. In one series only plain chest radiographs were taken; in the other both chest radiographs and computed tomography were performed. Details of the study protocols are given elsewhere (Slanina et al. 1982, 1988).

Recent Results in Cancer Research, Vol. 130

In mantle-field irradiation the paramediastinal and perihilar regions of the lung are fully involved, part of the lung apex, and only a little parenchyma near the axilla. Accordingly, in the frontal plane the pneumonitis will be visualized best in conventional plain radiography by a posterior–anterior view (Fig. 1a–d). On the other hand, the distribution of pulmonary changes in the transverse plane is best demonstrated by axial computed tomography, without any superposition (Fig. 2a,b).

Plain Radiographic Findings

Stage 0: Latency

During radiotherapy and even at the end of the treatment there is no visible change on plain chest radiography, though cellular damage can be assumed to have occurred at a submacroscopic level.

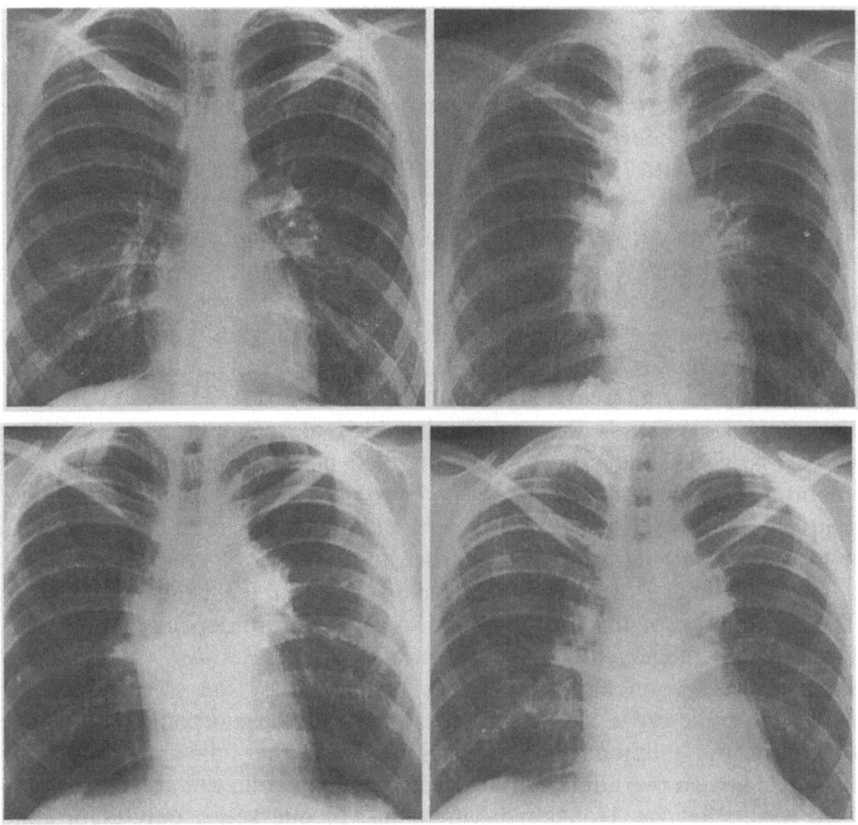

a b c d

Fig. 1.a–d Severe pulmonary radioreaction after mantle-field irradiation: **a** at the end of radiotherapy (RT): latency, **b** 15 weeks after beginning of RT: florid pneumonitis, **c** 22 weeks after beginning of RT: developing fibrosis, **d** 10 months after beginning of RT: stationary fibrosis.

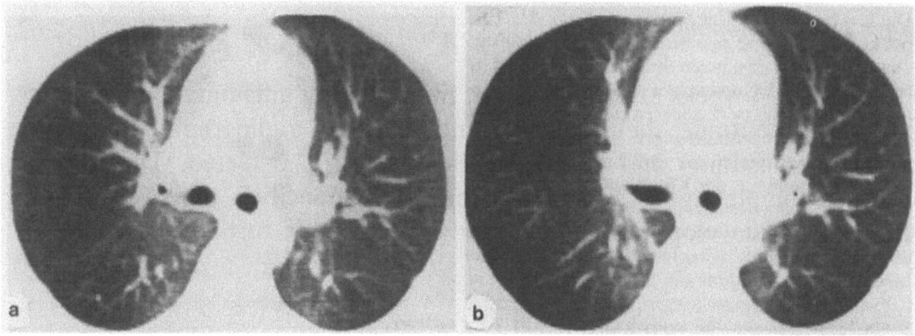

Fig. 2.a, b CT findings **a** 12 weeks after beginning of RT, Stage I: paramediastinal haziness, **b** 17 weeks after beginning of RT, Stage II: patchy consolidations predominate over the slowly vanishing haziness.

Stage I: Early Pneumonitis

After at least 6 weeks, and on average 12 weeks, after the start of radiotherapy the first signs of pneumonitis can be detected: a homogeneous slight opacity, best described by the term "haziness", in the paramediastinal and perihilar regions. This haziness causes the mediastinal contours to become blurred or unsharp. The histopathological substrate is considered to be interstitial edema (Gross 1977; White 1975). (It should be noted that the time schedule given here and in the following stages is subject to considerable individual variation, the standard deviation for any given value being about ±1 month (Slanina et al. 1982).)

Stage II: Florid (Acute) Pneumonitis

A highly active, flourishing radioreaction is seen between 15 and 20 weeks after the start of radiotherapy. It is characterized by partly patchy-confluent, partly streaky paramediastinal opacities which decrease to the periphery thus appearing as a corona radiata. The florid pneumonitis can be subdivided into two stages. Stage IIa, around 15 weeks after the start of radiotherapy, is when the visible changes reach their maximum intensity and volume. Stage IIb, around 20 weeks after the start of radiotherapy, marks the beginning of a retraction of the pneumonitis: the opacities get denser and better defined and start shrinking, and the pulmonary hili become distorted. Histopathological examinations at this stage have revealed exudation into the extravasal and interstitial spaces, partly in the alveoli, with desquamation of alveolar and epithelial cells. Hyaline membranes, lympho- and plasmacellular infiltration, and capillary thrombosis are also found. Later in stage IIb organization starts with increasing activity of fibroblasts (Gross 1977; White 1975).

Stage III: Developing Fibrosis

From 20 to 34 weeks after the start of radiotherapy inflammation decreases, fibroblasts continue their activity, and on plain radiographs contraction of the mediastinum and perimediastinal region is detected. The haziness vanishes completely, as do some of the patchy opacities; others shrink, get sharper, and develop into dense strands. The hili are further distorted.

Stage IV: Stationary Fibrosis

After 34 weeks (but in some individuals up to 1 year) after radiotherapy the fibrosis is fully developed: retraction has come to a standstill, the mediastinum reaching its final configuration. An increased translucency of the lung periphery and decreased pulmonary vascular markings may occur as sign of a compensatory emphysema. The hili are dense, sharply defined, retracted, and sometimes shifted cranially. Histopathologically, radiation fibrosis of the lung may be indistinguishable from fibrosis from other causes (Gross 1977; Lever et al. 1984; Nabawi et al. 1981; Westcott and Cole 1986; White 1975).

CT Findings

As in conventional plain radiography the pulmonary radioreaction also shows a typical morphology and time course on computed tomography (CT) (Frija et al. 1988; Glazer et al. 1986; Heron et al. 1988; Ikezoe et al. 1988; Libshitz and Shuman 1984; Mah et al. 1986; Nabawi et al. 1981; Pagani and Libshitz 1982; Slanina et al. 1988; Westcott and Cole 1986).

Stage 0: Latency

As on plain radiography there is also a latent period on CT when no changes are detectable, even with image postprocessing (windowing).

Stage I: Early Pneumonitis

About the same time as on plain radiography, possibly 1 week earlier, CT shows the first signs of early pneumonitis: a characteristic paramediastinal haziness, i.e. a homogeneous slight increase in lung density within the irradiated volume. The margins of the normal lung parenchyma are therefore straight and parallel.

Stage II: Florid (Acute) Pneumonitis

In florid pneumonitis a typical combination of this haziness with patchy infiltrations and partly confluent opacities is found on CT, again within the irradiated volume. The margins of the pulmonary changes are mostly straight and parallel, and conform with the radiation portals. However, the patchy infiltrations are not homogeneously distributed within the target volume, but tend to be localized to the paravertebral and perihilar regions, some being retrosternal. The reason for this remains unclear.

In stage IIb, florid pneumonitis with early retraction, the patchy consolidations predominate and the haziness slowly vanishes. Sometimes an air bronchogram may also be found, the radiation pneumonitis being considered the prototype of adhesive atelectasis: there is no obstruction of the bronchi but an adhesion and obliteration of the alveoli themselves (Naidich et al. 1984a).

Stage III: Developing Fibrosis

In developing fibrosis the haziness vanishes completely, and the patchy consolidations shrink and become better defined. The characteristic finding is the marked retraction of the affected area: the initially straight margins become convex or concave depending on the contour of the adjacent mediastinum or thoracic wall.

Stage IV: Stationary Fibrosis

Around 34 weeks after the start of radiotherapy the reaction ceases to be dynamic and stationary radiation-induced pulmonary fibrosis is established. The patchy consolidations have now developed into streaky ones, with connections to pleura and hili. The initially straight and parallel margins of the pulmonary radioreaction now show marked convex or concave distortion. This appearance remains very stable (as a scar), and only very rarely does further shrinkage occur. In individual cases calcifications may develop in the fibrosis.

Grading of the Pulmonary Radioreaction

CT gives the opportunity of applying a semiquantitative grading to the severity of the pulmonary radioreaction – florid pneumonitis as well as fibrosis. If pulmonary changes are found in up to 25% of continuous CT scans then this is judged a mild reaction. If changes are detected on more than 25% of CT scans this is defined as a moderate reaction. If the changes are not only seen in a lung window setting but are also readily detectable in a standard soft tissue window this indicates a severe reaction. For example, Fig. 3 shows the distribution of the severity of the pulmonary radioreaction in 36 patients after mantle-field irradiation. Here the plain radiographs were subjectively classified by comparison with reference radiographs. Since the grading of pneumonitis matched the grading of the fibrotic stages (for example, severe pneumonitis always resulted in severe fibrosis), the gradings at the different times were taken together.

A good agreement between the subjective classification by plain radiography and semiquantitative grading by CT is evident. Furthermore, the finding that about half the patients have only mild pulmonary radioreaction and about a third a moderate reaction is in good agreement with other data on mantle-field irradiation and with only mild to moderate clinical symptoms and pulmonary function tests (Slanina et al. 1977). Of course with higher doses, for example in the treatment of lung cancer, more severe reactions have to be expected (Ikezoe et al. 1988; Lever et al. 1984; Mah et al. 1986; Nabawi et al. 1981; Pagani and Libshitz 1982).

Mah and van Dyk have quantified the pulmonary radioreaction by measuring the density in Hounsfield units in regions of interest (Mah and van Dyk 1988). However, this is very time-consuming and not suitable for routine evaluation. In addition, in our experience and that of others (Naidich et al. 1984b) quantitative analysis of lung CT is no more sensitive than simple visual inspection, the human eye being a very accurate and fast "densitometer".

An advantage of CT over plain radiography is the good delineation of the pulmonary radioreaction after tangential field irradiation of the chest wall

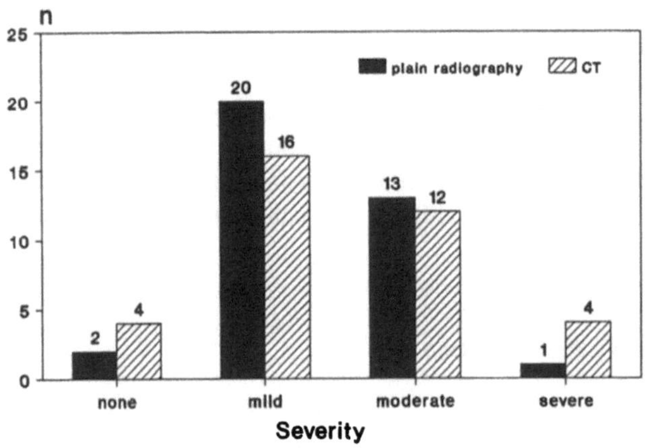

Fig. 3. Frequency of severity of pulmonary radioreaction after mantle-field irradiation for Hodgkin's disease (40–46 Gy; average of findings at 12, 17, and 37 weeks after radiotherapy; $n = 36$)

for mammary carcinoma (Coscina et al. 1986; Ikezoe et al. 1988; Mah et al. 1986; Shea et al. 1987). In plain radiography the oblique margin of the radioreaction leads to superposition in both the posterior-anterior and lateral views (Slanina et al. 1987).

MRI Findings

Preliminary experience with magnetic resonance imaging (MRI) of the pulmonary radioreaction indicates that the haziness seen on CT and plain radiography cannot be detected by standard MR spin-echo sequences due to the considerable motion of the lungs during scanning. However, a very high signal intensity on T2-weighted images is found in the patchy consolidations. With developing fibrosis signal intensity slowly decreases, but the fading of the signal seems to occur much slower than the shrinkage seen by morphology alone. Possibly this signal intensity pattern conveys extra information compared with morphology alone.

Two advantages of MRI are the visualization of great vessels without a contrast agent and the possibility of direct coronary or sagittal scans which may help in differentiating radioreaction from, for example, tumors of the chest wall or mediastinum. On the other hand, MRI is more inconvenient for the patient, and is even more expensive than CT. Therefore, more experience has to be gathered to define its role in the diagnostic work-up after irradiation.

Conclusions

For all techniques the important question to be answered is whether what is seen is simply a radioreaction or whether there is also a recurrence or nonrelated disease. The latter is, of course, the diagnosis if any mass or infiltration occurs outside the irradiated volume. It is also the diagnosis if an expansile lesion occurs at any time later than 20 weeks after the start of radiotherapy. By then the florid pneumonitis has reached its maximum, and the volume of the pulmonary radioreaction is decreasing by retraction of the fibrotic activity. After that time an expansile process cannot be attributed to the pulmonary radioreaction and is always suspect of recurrent or intercurrent disease. Possibly an increasing signal intensity on T2-weighted MR images or increasing gadolinium DTPA uptake may be another sign of recurrent disease. But we do not yet know whether this is already true after 20 weeks; rather it seems to take longer for this "signal conversion" than for the morphological retraction.

Plain radiography of the pulmonary radioreaction reveals a characteristic morphological appearance in the target volume, and a typical time course. The same is true for CT. Plain radiography has the advantage of an overview over the entire thorax in one single image: the caudocranial distortion of the hili and the configuration of the entire mediastinum are well depicted. Plain radiography is also easy to perform and easy to repeat; the technique is everywhere readily available and very cheap. It thus remains the radiological method of choice for the diagnosis of radiation pneumonitis and fibrosis in the follow-up of patients after irradiation involving the lung.

In CT the pulmonary radioreaction takes a similarly characteristic time course as in chest radiography, with corresponding distinguishable stages. On CT the typical radiation-induced changes are reducible to three basic patterns of opacification, that partly appear in combination and also show a characteristic spatial distribution. However, because of its cost and limited availability CT should only be used as an optional method in special situations such as when recurrent disease is suspected.

MRI using T2-weighted imaging demonstrates regions of high signal intensity in the lung parenchyma attributable to radiation pneumonitis. The role of MRI in the diagnosis of radiation pneumonitis has yet to be defined.

In the clinical setting it is important to know that after shrinkage has begun no new expansile mass or infiltration can be attributed to the pulmonary radioreaction. Instead, it must arouse the suspicion of another disease process, especially a recurrence.

References

Coscina WF, Arger PH, Mintz MC, Coleman BG (1986) CT demonstration of pulmonary effects of tangential beam irradiation. J Comput Assist Tomogr 10:600–602

Frija J, Fermé C, Baud L, Gisselbrecht C, Miot C, Fermand JP, Laval-Jeantet M (1988) Radiation-induced lung injuries: a survey by computed tomography and pulmonary function tests in 18 cases of Hodgkin's disease. Eur J Radiol 8:18–23

Glazer HS, Lee JKT, Levitt RG, Heiken JP, Ling D, Totty WG, Balfe DM, Emani B, Wasserman TH, Murphy WA (1986) Radiation fibrosis: differentiation from recurrent tumor by MR imaging. Work in progress. Radiology 156:721–726

Gross NJ (1977) Pulmonary effects of radiation therapy. Ann Intern Med 86:81–92

Heron CW, Husband JE, Williams MP, Cherryman GR (1988) The value of thoracic computed tomography in the detection of recurrent Hodgkin's disease. Br J Radiol 61:567–572

Ikezoe J, Takashima S, Morimoto S, Kadowaki K, Takeuchi N, Yamamoto T, Nakanishi K, Isaza M, Arisawa J, Ikeda H, Masaki N, Kozuka T (1988) CT appearance of acute radiation-induced injury in the lung. AJR 150:765–770

Lever AML, Henderson D, Ellis DA, Corris PA, Gilmartin JJ (1984) Radiation fibrosis mimicking local recurrence in small cell carcinoma of the bronchus. Br J Radiol 57:178–180

Libshitz HI, Shuman LS (1984) Radiation-induced pulmonary changes: CT findings. J Comput Assist Tomogr 1984;8:15–19

Mah K, van Dyk J (1988) Quantitative measurement of changes in human lung density following irradiation. Radiother Oncol 11:169–179

Mah K, Poon PY, van Dyk J, Keane T, Majesky IF, Rideout DF (1986) Assessment of acute radiation-induced pulmonary changes using computed tomography. J Comput Assist Tomogr 10:736–743
Nabawi P, Mantravadi R, Breyer D, Capek V (1981) Computed tomography of radiation-induced lung injuries. J Comput Assist Tomogr 5:568–570
Naidich DP, Zerhouni EA, Siegelman SS (1984a) Computed tomography of the thorax. Raven, New York, p 134
Naidich DP, Zerhouni EA, Siegelman SS (1984b) Computed tomography of the thorax. Raven, New York, p 205
Pagani JJ, Libshitz HI (1982) CT manifestations of radiation-induced change in chest tissue. J Comput Assist Tomogr 6:243–248
Shea WJ, deGeer G, Webb WR (1987) Chest wall after mastectomy. I. CT appearance of normal postoperative anatomy, post-irradiation changes, and optimal scanning techniques. Radiology 162:157–161
Slanina J, Musshoff K, Rahner T, Stiasny R (1977) Long-term side effects in irradiated patients with Hodgkin's disease. Int J Radiat Oncol Biol Phys 2:1–19
Slanina J, Wannenmacher M, Bruggmoser G, Krüger HU (1982) Die pulmonale Strahlenreaktion im Röntgenbild. (Pulmonary radioreaction demonstrated by X-ray pictures.) Radiologe 22:74–82 (In German, with English summary)
Slanina J, Maschitzki R, Wannenmacher M (1987) Die pulmonale Strahlenreaktion im Röntgenbild des Thorax nach Megavolttherapie bei Mammakarzinom. (Pulmonary reaction to radiation as seen on chest X-ray following megavolt therapy for carcinoma of the breast). Radiologe 27:181–191 (In German, with English summary)
Slanina J, Sigmund G, Hinkelbein W, Wenz W, Wannenmacher M (1988) Die pulmonale Strahlenreaktion nach Mantelfeldbestrahlung: Vergleich der Verlaufsstadien im konventionellen Röntgenbild und im Computertomogramm. (Radiation-induced pulmonary changes after mantle-field irradiation: comparison of consecutive stages in chest radiography and computed tomography.) Radiologe 28:20–28 (In German, with English summary)
Westcott JL, Cole SR (1986) Traction bronchiectasis in end-stage pulmonary fibrosis. Radiology 161:665–669
White DC (1975) An atlas of radiation histopathology. US Energy Research Development Administration, Government Printing Office, Washington, DC

Lung Effects after Total Body Irradiation of Mice and Bone Marrow Transplant Patients: Comparison of Experimental and Preliminary Clinical Data

F. Steinberg[1], K. Quabeck[2], B. Rehn[3], R. Kraus[3], M. Mohnke[2], U. Costabel[4], E. Kreuzfelder[5], M. Molls[6], J. Bruch[3], U.W. Schaefer[2], and C. Streffer[1]

[1] Institute of Medical Radiation Biology, University Clinic, Hufelandstr. 55, W-4300 Essen, Federal Republic of Germany
[2] Department of Bone Marrow Transplantation, University Clinic, Hufelandstr. 55, W-4300 Essen, Federal Republic of Germany
[3] Institute of Hygiene and Occupational Medicine, University Clinic, Hufelandstr. 55, W-4300 Essen, Federal Republic of Germany
[4] Department of Pneumology, University Clinic, Hufelandstr. 55, W-4300 Essen, Federal Republic of Germany
[5] Institute of Immunology, University Clinic, Hufelandstr. 55, W-4300 Essen, Federal Republic of Germany
[6] Department of Radiotherapy, University Clinic, Hufelandstr. 55, W-4300 Essen, Federal Republic of Germany

Introduction

In thoracic and total body irradiation (TBI) the lung represents a dose-limiting organ. In the setting of allogeneic bone marrow transplantation (BMT) TBI provides a high immunosuppressive and anti-tumor effect. However, up to 30% of patients develop interstitial pneumonitis which may partially be induced by radiation injury (Weiner et al. 1986; Beelen et al. 1987; Ettinger and Trulock 1991). In 95% of these patients interstitial pneumonitis is lethal. Its clinical course is comparable with the adult respiratory distress syndrome (ARDS) in polytrauma patients, which can develop dramatically and attain a stage which can no longer be controlled by therapy. The underlying pathomechanisms are still unknown. Bronchoalveolar lavage (BAL), especially measurements of surfactant and alveolar cells, may serve as an indicator of pulmonary injury or disease. BAL is a widely used method for investigating septic or polytraumatic shock induced ARDS (Henderson 1988; Kreuzfelder et al. 1988), severe infant respiratory distress syndrome (Collaborative Study 1988), effects of toxic drugs and dust on the lung (Bigby et al. 1985; Lemaire 1985), and radiation-induced changes in lung (Massilta et al. 1991; Molls et al. 1990; Rubin et al. 1983). It allows responses in the microenvironment of the alveolar system to be measured directly, which precede changes in the morphological structure (Kraus et al. 1990). However, this technique has not been generally used in association with TBI. Up to now, only a few, largely experimental animal

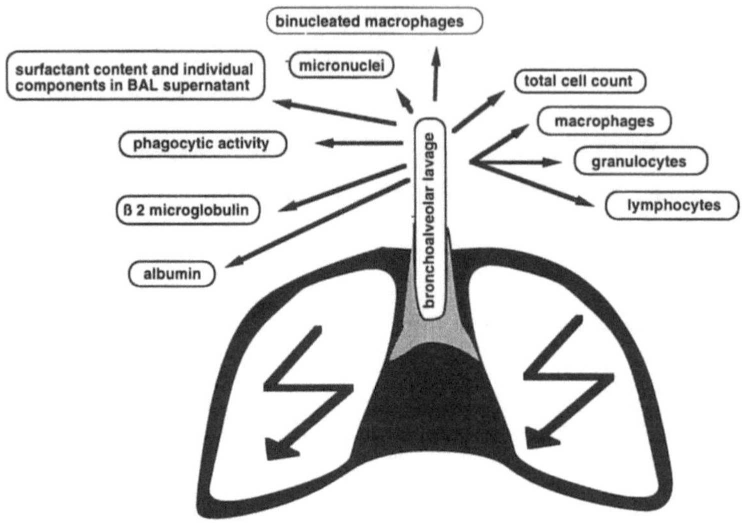

Fig. 1. Schematic drawing of all the parameters measured in the bronchoalveolar lavage of mice and patients

data are available on the interaction between surfactant, alveolar macrophage and pneumocyte type II cells.

This study presents the results of BAL after a single dose (10 Gy) of radiation to the lungs in mice, measurements being made of the total cell count (granulocytes, macrophages, and lymphocytes), the activity of macrophages after application of microbeads, and the sphingomyelin content as an important surfactant phospholipid fraction in the BAL indicative of cell death. Two proteins with different molecular weights (albumin and β2-microglobulin) were assayed as indicators of radiation-induced increased permeability of the endothelial and alveolar epithelium barrier (capillary leakage syndrome). The experimental data (Fig. 1) were compared with preliminary data from 12 BMT patients who received TBI and high doses of cyclophosphamide for conditioning.

Material and Methods

Radiation

A single dose of 10 Gy (1 Gy/min) was applied to the thorax of Heiligenberger mice (male, weight 28–35 g, $n = 40$) using an X-ray machine (Stabilipan,

Siemens, Erlangen, FRG) operating at 240 kV and 15 mA with a copper filter of 0.5 mm thickness. The focus skin distance was 47 cm. The animals were given 5 μg/g body weight pentobarbital intraperitoneally for anesthesia.

Patients received fractionated TBI of 4 × 2.5 Gy with lung shielding (lung dose 4 × 2.0 Gy) delivered by a ^{60}Co source. Cyclophosphamide 120 mg/kg body weight was given as conditioning therapy prior to BMT (Molls et al. 1990).

BAL and Cell Differentiation

Before irradiation and 7, 14, and 21 days after irradiation the mice were killed by intraperitoneal injection of barbiturate. The lung was washed with sterile ice-cold physiological saline (10 times with aliquots of 0.8 ml). Macrophages, lymphocytes, and granulocytes were counted. Cell viability after washing was greater than 95% as determined by Trypan blue dye exclusion (Steinberg et al. 1992).

BAL was performed on the patients under local anesthesia before and 1, 30, and 40 days after BMT using a flexible bronchoscope (Olympus, FRG) (0.9% saline solution with 10 fractions of 20 ml each) alternately in the lingula or the middle lobe. The cells were then examined as described above.

Macrophage Activity

For both mice and patients a total of 0.5×10^6 to 1×10^6 alveolar macrophages (2 ml cell suspension) were preincubated in plastic petri dishes. Fluorescent and carboxylated latex beads (2 μm in diameter) were added 1 h later. After a 2-h incubation the cells were fixed and examined microscopically. Phagocytic activity was defined as the percentage of cells showing phagocytosis. For details see Rehn et al. (1989).

BAL Protein

The concentrations of albumin (molecular weight 66 300 dalton) and β2-microglobulin (molecular weight 11 500 dalton) were estimated in the BAL fluid from the patients as parameters for capillary leakage and edema in lung by immunonephelometry and a radioimmunoassay, as recently described (Kreuzfelder et al. 1991).

Chromosomal Damage

To assess chromosomal damage BAL cell suspensions were mounted on glass slides by cytocentrifugation, air-dried and stained according to Pappenheim. In 2000 macrophages three parameters were estimated: macrophages with at least one micronucleus, binucleated marcophages without a micronucleus, and binucleated macrophages with at least one micronucleus.

Quantification of Surfactant Phospholipids

For both mice and patients phospholipids were measured after separation by high pressure liquid chromatography (HPLC) (Kontron, Munich, FRG). The total phospholipid content and sphingomyelin were extracted by the method of Folch et al. (1957) and pooled for each group of animals. For reference studies and calibration the phospholipids were purchased from Sigma (Munich, FRG).

Patients

Twelve patients (median age 38 years; range 19–51 years; 5 female, 7 male; 1 multiple myeloma, 6 chronic myelogenous leukemia, 2 acute lymphocytic leukemia, 3 acute myelogenous leukemia) received combined conditioning therapy with TBI and cyclophosphamide before BMT.

Statistical Evaluation

Calculations were carried out using the Statistical Analysis System (SAS, version 6; SAS Insitute, USA). Mean values ± SE are given. Unless otherwise stated results were statistically significant at $p < 0.05$.

Results

Differential Cell Count

Initial responses could be observed in the cellular microenvironment of the alveolar system 1 week after radiation. In the murine BAL fluid, the number of macrophages initially decreased up to 14 days after irradiation and then increased (Table 1a). Few granulocytes were found before irradiation in mice; after irradiation an increase was seen. The same tendency was observed in patients (Table 1b). An initial decrease in cells followed by an

Table 1. BAL total cell count, macrophages, granulocytes, and lymphocytes (cells/ml BAL) in (*a*) 10 Gy thorax-irradiated mice ($n = 10$) and (*b*) TBI (4×2.5 Gy) conditioned bone marrow transplant patients ($n = 12$)

(*a*) Differential cell count in mice

	Before irradiation	Time after irradiation		
		1 week	2 weeks	3 weeks
Total cell count ($\times 10^5$)	6.8 ± 0.7	3.8 ± 0.5*	4.5 ± 0.9*	6.7 ± 2.3
Macrophages ($\times 10^5$)	6.2 ± 0.7	3.4 ± 0.5*	3.1 ± 0.4*	4.8 ± 1.7
Granulocytes ($\times 10^4$)	0.1 ± 0.05	0.1 ± 0.05	0.8 ± 0.35*	1.1 ± 0.39*
Lymphocytes ($\times 10^4$)	0.4 ± 0.08	0.2 ± 0.05*	0.8 ± 0.17*	0.9 ± 0.24*

(*b*) Differential cell count in patients

	Before transplantation	Time after transplantation		
		1 day	30 days	40 days
Total cell count ($\times 10^5$)	1.3 ± 0.2	0.7 ± 0.1*	2.4 ± 1.3*	2.0 ± 0.7*
Macrophages ($\times 10^5$)	1.1 ± 0.0	0.7 ± 0.0*	2.0 ± 0.01*	1.6 ± 0.16*
Granulocytes ($\times 10^4$)	1.6 ± 0.5	0.2 ± 0.05*	3.6 ± 0.7*	3.5 ± 1.0*
Lymphocytes ($\times 10^4$)	0.03 ± 0.0	0.1 ± 0.0*	0.30 ± 0.0*	1.6 ± 0.5*

Values are mean ± SE

* Significantly different from control at $p \leqslant 0.05$

overshooting response with a tendency to normalize at 40 days after BMT was seen. The lymphocytes showed a slight but steady increase, whereas granulocytes were increased except 1 day after BMT.

Macrophage Activity

The phagocytic activity of the BAL macrophages in mice, measured as the number of cells with phagocytosed beads, showed a significant increase in the percentage of cells 2 weeks postradiation which normalized 3 weeks postradiation (Table 2a). The macrophage activity in patients was significantly higher before irradiation compared with mice (Table 2b). No significant changes were observed after BMT.

Chromosomal Damage

Chromosomal damage, measured as macrophages with micronuclei, binucleated macrophages, or binucleated macrophages with micronuclei (patients only) was at a very low level before irradiation in mice (Table 3a). Before

Table 2. Phagocytic activity in BAL macrophages (cells with phagocytosis in %) measured as percentage of cells showing phagocytosis after incubation of microbeads (2 μm in diameter) of (*a*) 10 Gy thorax-irradiated mice ($n = 10$) and (*b*) TBI (4 × 2.5 Gy) conditioned bone marrow transplanted patients ($n = 12$)

(*a*) Phagocytic activity of macrophages in mice

	Before irradiation	Time after irradiation		
		1 week	2 weeks	3 weeks
Macrophages (%)	37 ± 0.5	41 ± 12	48 ± 4*	36 ± 3

(*b*) Phagocytic activity of macrophages in patients

	Before transplantation	Time after transplantation		
		1 day	30 days	40 days
Macrophages (%)	89 ± 2	87 ± 2	87 ± 2	88 ± 1

Values are mean ± SE
* Significantly different from control at $p \leqslant 0.05$

Table 3. Cellular and chromosomal damage in BAL macrophages (cells in %) in (*a*) 10 Gy thorax-irradiated mice measured as binucleated cells and cells with micronuclei ($n = 10$) and (*b*) TBI (4 × 2.5 Gy) conditioned bone marrow transplant patients measured as cells with micronuclei, binucleated cells, and binucleated cells with micronuclei ($n = 12$)

(*a*) Chromosomal damage in macrophages of mice

	Before irradiation	Time after irradiation	
		2 weeks	3 weeks
Binucleated cells (%)	1.5 ± 0.5	9.8 ± 8	15 ± 7*
Cells with micronuclei (%)	0	9 ± 7*	12 ± 9*

(*b*) Chromosomal damage in macrophages of patients

	Before transplantation	Time after transplantation		
		1 day	30 days	40 days
Binucleated cells (%)	6.7 ± 0.6	7 ± 0.8	8.5 ± 0.9	8.2 ± 0.8
Cells with micronuclei (%)	0.7 ± 0.2	0.9 ± 0.3	1.7 ± 0.4*	1.3 ± 0.3
Binucleated cells with micronuclei (%)	0.4 ± 0.1	0.5 ± 0.1	1.2 ± 0.3*	1.4 ± 0.3*

Values are mean ± SE
* Significantly different from control at $p \leqslant 0.05$

irradiation no micronuclei were detectable. Two and 3 weeks after irradiation a significant increase was seen with a wide variance. When compared with a group of healthy volunteers (data not shown), a higher level of all three parameters was seen in patients before conditioning. After irradiation the values slightly increased in a time-dependent manner, but not significantly.

Surfactant Phospholipids

The changes induced by irradiation in the total added amount of surfactant expressed as the concentration of phospholipids are shown in Table 4. Sphingomyelin is used as a parameter for cell death. In mice, a decrease and then a slight increase in phospholipids was observed (Table 4a). Sphingomyelin was not detectable up to day 14. In contrast in patients even before conditioning sphingomyelin was measurable and showed a slight time-dependent increase.

Proteins

The high molecular weight protein albumin showed a slight, but not significant decrease 1 day after BMT and increased nearly threefold 40 days after

Table 4. Total surfactant phospholipids and surfactant sphingomyelin in BAL (μg/ml BAL) of (*a*) 10 Gy thorax-irradiated mice (n = 10) and (*b*) TBI (4 × 2.5 Gy) conditioned bone marrow transplant patients (n = 12)
(*a*) Surfactant phospholipids in mice

	Before irradiation	Time after irradiation		
		1 week	2 weeks	3 weeks
Phospholipids (μg/ml)	517 ± 79	290 ± 27	704 ± 24	767 ± 136
Sphingomyelin (μg/ml)	ND	0.01 ± 0*	0.9 ± 0.9*	2.2 ± 0.7*

(*b*) Surfactant phospholipids in patients

	Before transplantation	Time after transplantation		
		1 day	30 days	40 days
Phospholipids (μg/ml)	235 ± 29	260 ± 44	360 ± 73*	350 ± 44*
Sphingomyelin (μg/ml)	0.8 ± 0.4	1.0 ± 0.3	1.95 ± 1.2*	2.75 ± 1.3*

Values are mean ± SE. ND, not detectable
* Significantly different from control at $p \leqslant 0.05$

Table 5. Albumin and β2-microglobulin measured in BAL (mg/ml BAL) in TBI (4 × 2.5 Gy) conditioned bone marrow transplant patients (n = 12)

	Before transplantation	Time after transplantation		
		1 day	30 days	40 days
β2-microglobulin (mg/ml)	1.3 ± 0.1	1.15 ± 0.1	1.45 ± 0.1	1.55 ± 0.3*
albumin (mg/ml)	4.5 ± 0.7	3.8 ± 0.9	6.0 ± 1.4*	12 ± 7.2*

Values are mean ± SE
* Significantly different from control at $\leqslant p \leqslant 0.05$

BMT. This high value at 40 days was mainly due to 1 patient who died because of lung edema 51 days after BMT and had an albumin level of 83.6 mg/ml BAL. The changes in the low molecular weight protein β2-microglobulin showed the same but moderate tendency (Table 5). In serum, albumin decreased whereas β2-microglobulin showed a slight but not significant increase.

Discussion

This paper presents preliminary data from an elaborately planned study, the aim of which is to contribute to the understanding of the pathomechanism in interstitial pneumonitis after BMT. In order to find an answer to the question of whether irradiation is one of the main reasons for lung toxicity in BMT patients receiving TBI, this study compared BAL data obtained with idential methods in animals and patients (Molls et al., this volume). Important evidence that irradiation only partially contributes to lung toxicity emerges from the data of Wingard et al. (1988) and Beelen et al. (1987). They have seen a similarly high frequency of lung complications in BMT patients who were not irradiated but conditioned with busulfan and cyclophosphamide.

In the present study, significant differences between animals and patients *prior* to irradiation were seen with regard to the following parameters: chromosomal damage, macrophage activity and sphingomyelin concentration. An extensive pre-damage (previous therapies, effects of smoking, etc.) may already exist in patients. In general, the changes after irradiation are similar in animals and patients with one exception, namely macrophage activity. The number of BAL cells, mainly macrophages, lymphocytes, and granulocytes, changed in a time-dependent manner. The phagocytic activity of the macrophages showed a significant increase in mice after irradiation, but not in patients. The radiation-induced capillary leakage syndrome would tend to manifest itself in a higher permeability of the endothelial and alveolar epithelium barrier, which could be measured by an increase in both proteins in BAL. β2-microglobulin showed a slight increase compared with albumin, which increased nearly threefold. The comparative serum probes proved that the higher concentration in BAL is a lung-specific reaction (for interpretation see also Kreuzfelder et al. 1988). Perhaps the albumin permeability is disturbed selectively. Those effects have been extensively known in animals in terms of radiation effects (Graham et al. 1990). The contents of surfactant phospholipids and sphingomyelin (a parameter for cell death; Rehn 1991, unpublished data) were significantly increased. A very rapid response of the surfactant system has been described as early as 2h after irradiation with significant changes in fractions of individual phospholipids (Steinberg et al. 1992) showing extremely species-specific differences between mouse and rat (Hobusch et al. 1988). Similar findings could also be seen after total body irradiation of beagles (4.2 Gy ^{60}Co) (Quabeck and Rehn, personal communication, 1991). It must be pointed out here that the biological functions of individual surfactant components are poorly understood (Batenburg et al. 1984; Stratton 1984; Wright et al. 1987). There is an increased chromosomal damage in alveolar macrophages after irradiation which is known to be a well-defined biological parameter for radiation effects (Müller and Streffer 1988).

In conclusion, these comparative experimental and preliminary clinical data indicate (1) that BAL gives insights into the pathomechanism of radiation-induced lung damage, (2) that there are changes in alveolar surfactant, chromosomal damage, cell count, phagocytic activity of alveolar macrophages, and BAL proteins following TBI and allogeneic BMT, and (3) that an extensive pre-damage in patients may already exist at the time of BMT.

Acknowledgment. These studies were supported in part by the "Deutsche Krebshilfe", Bonn.

References

Batenburg JJ (1984) Biosynthesis and secretion of pulmonary surfactant. In: Robertson B, van Golde LMG, Batenburg JJ (eds) Pulmonary surfactant. Elsevier, Amsterdam, pp 237–270

Beelen DW, Quabeck K, Mahmoud HK, Schaefer UW, Becher R, Schmidt CG, Bamberg M, Quast U, Grosse-Wilde H, Haralambie E, Linzenmeier G, Stohmer B, Richter HJ, Hantschke D, Traenhard O, Henneberg-Quester K-B, Luboldt W (1987) Allogeneic bone marrow transplantation for acute leukaemia or chronic myeloid leukemia in the fifth decade of life. Eur J Cancer Clin Oncol 23:1665–1671

Bigby TD, Allen D, Leslie CD, Henson PM, Cherniack RM (1985) Bleomycin-induced lung injury in the rabbit. Am Rev Respir Dis 132:590–595

Collaborative European Multicenter Study Group (1988) An international randomized clinical trial of surfactant replacement therapy in severe neonatal respiratory distress syndrome. Pediatrics 82:683–691

Ettinger NA, Trulock EP (1991) Pulmonary considerations of organ transplantation. Am Rev Respir Dis 144:213–223
Folch J, Lees M, Stanley GHS (1957) A simple method for the isolation and purification of total lipids from animal tissue. J Biol Chem 226:497–509
Graham MM, Evans M, Dahlen D, Mahler P, Rasey J (1990) Pharmacological alterations of the lung vascular response to radiation. Int J Radiat Oncol Biol Phys 19:329–339
Henderson RF (1988) Use of bronchoalveolar lavage to detect lung damage. In: Gardner DE, Crapo JD, Massaro EJ (eds) Toxicology of the lung. Raven, New York, pp 239–267
Hobusch G, Steinberg F, Rehn B, Gono E, Bruch J, Streffer C (1988) Changes in bronchoalveolar lavage (BAL) after irradiation in Wistar rats. 7th annual meeting of the European Society for Therapeutic Radiology and Oncology, 7–9 Sept 1988, Den Haag, p 107
Kraus R, Steinberg F, Rehn B, Bruch J, Streffer C (1990) Radiation-induced changes in lung tissues and development of fibrosis revealed by quantitative morphometric methods. J Cancer Res Clin Oncol 117:27–32
Kreuzfelder E, Joka T, Keinecke HO, Obertacke U, Schmit-Neuerburg KP, Nakhosten JA, Paar D, Scheiermann N (1988) Adult respiratory distress syndrome as a specific manifestation of a general permeability defect in trauma patients. Am Rev Respir Dis 137:95–99
Kreuzfelder E, Obertache U, Newmann B, Thraenhart O (1991) Adult respiratory distress syndrome as a manifestation of a general permeability defect. In: Sturm JA (ed) Adult respiratory distress syndrome, Springer, Berlin Heidelberg New York, pp 257–264
Lemaire I (1985) Characterization of the bronchoalveolar cellular response in experimental Asbestosis. Am Rev Respir Dis 131:144–149
Maasilta P, Salonen E, Vaheri A, Kivisaari L, Holsti L, Mattson K (1991) Procollagen-III in serum, plasminogen activation and fibronectin in bronchoalveolar lavage fluid during and following irradiation of human lung. Int J Radiat Oncol Biol Phys 20:973–980
Molls M, Quast U, Schaefer UW, Szy D, Beelen DW, Quabeck K, Graeven U, Sayer HG, Bamberg M, Sack H (1990) Clinical results and the Essen concept of TBI. Radiother Oncol [Suppl]1:121–124
Molls M, van Beuningen D (1991) Radiation injury of the lung: experimental studies, observations after radiotherapy and total body irradiation prior to bone marrow transplantation. In: Scherer E, Streffer C, Trott K-R (eds) Radiopathology of organs and tissues. Springer, Berlin Heidelberg New York, pp 369–404
Müller WU, Streffer C (1988) Der Mikronukleustest. In: Dienstl F, Börner W, Messerschmidt O (eds) Strahlenschutz in Forschung und Praxis. Fischer, pp 259–275
Rehn B, Tong-Tong Z, Hobusch G, Bruch J (1989) The flushability of rat Alveolar Macrophages by bronchoalveolar lavage under normal and activated conditions. Sil Rep NRW 17:193–202
Rubin P, Siemann DW, Shapiro DL, Finkelstein JN, Penney DP (1983) Surfactant release as an early measure of radiation pneumonitis. Int J Radiat Oncol Biol Phys 9:1669–1673
Steinberg F, Rehn B, Kraus R, Hobusch G, Gono E, Bruch J, Streffer C, Schaefer UW (1992) Activity-test of alveolar macrophages, separation of 6 surfactant fractions after bronchoalveolar lavage and morphometrical determination of collagen content in X-irradiated mouse lung. Radiat Res (to be published)
Steinberg F, Rehn B, Kraus R, Quabeck K, Bruch J, Beelen DW, Schaefer UW, Streffer C (1992) Activity testing of alveolar macrophages and changes in sur-

factant phospholipids after irradiation in broncho-alveolar Lavage: experimental and clinical data. Environ Health Perspect 97:171–175
Stratton CJ (1984) Morphology of surfactant producing cells and of the alveolar lining layer. In: Robertson B, van Golde LMG, Batenburg JJ (eds) Pulmonary surfactant. Elsevier, Amsterdam, pp 68–118
Weiner RS, Bortin MM, Gale RP, Gluckmann E, Kay HEM, Kolb HJ, Hartz AJ, Rimm AA (1986) Interstitial pneumonitis after bone marrow transplantation: assessment of risk factors. Ann Intern Med 104:168–175
Wingard JR, Mellits ED, Sostrin MB, Yen-hung Chen D, Burn WH, Santos GW, Vriesendrop HM, Beschorner WE, Sara R (1988) Interstitial pneumonitis after allogeneic bone marrow transplantation: nine-year experience at a single institution. Medicine 67:175–186
Wright JR, Clements JR (1987) Metabolism and turnover of lung surfactant. Am Rev Respir Dis 136:426–444

Experimental Studies on the Pathogenesis of Damage in the Heart

S. Schultz-Hector

Institut für Strahlenbiologie, GSF, W-8042 Neuherberg, Fed. Rep. of Germany and Strahlenbiologisches Institut der LMU, W-8000 Munich, Fed. Rep. of Germany

Introduction

Radiation-induced heart disease has been observed in a significant number of patients following mediastinal radiotherapy of Hodgkin's disease or postoperative radiotherapy of breast cancer. Following higher radiation doses and especially following treatments delivering a particularly high dose to the anterior pericardium, a reversible exudative pericarditis can occur within the first 2–3 years (Pierce et al. 1969; Byhardt et al. 1975; Gottdiener et al. 1983; Greenwood et al. 1974; Applefeld and Wiernik 1983). A compilation of clinical data has shown that the incidence of pericarditis rises sharply with radiation dose to the anterior pericardium (Schultz-Hector 1991a). Since modern radiation techniques achieve a more homogeneous dose distribution, pericarditis has become a rare event and is no longer a major clinical concern (Carmel and Kaplan 1976; Watchie et al. 1987; Morgan et al. 1985). With increasing survival times, particularly in Hodgkin patients, late radiation effects on myocardial function have been observed. In a significant number of patients, left ventricular ejection fractions were reduced at 5–25 years postirradiation (Morgan et al. 1985; Burns et al. 1983; Savage et al. 1990; Gomez et al. 1983). Although these patients were asymptomatic, one has to assume that the cardiac reserve capacity, i.e., the ability to compensate for cardiac stress of other origin, is reduced in these patients. We therefore developed an animal model to study the pathogenesis of radiation-induced myocardial dysfunction.

Animals and Irradiation

All experiments reported in the following have been carried out in adult Wistar Neuherberg rats. Since the heart is surrounded by radiosensitive tissues, careful treatment planning is necessary for experimental heart

Recent Results in Cancer Research, Vol. 130

irradiation (Lauk et al. 1985). In the rat, esophagus and spinal cord can be completely avoided and the amount of lung tissue irradiated can be minimized by using a lateral beam. For localization of the heart, a thorax radiograph is taken on Polaroid film using the treatment machine at a reduced voltage, after the anesthetized rat has been fixed in the irradiation position. The irradiation field is then individually shaped by movable lead shields to encompass the entire heart. Irradiation of 300 kV X-rays was then delivered at a dose rate of 2 Gy/min.

Clinical Symptoms

Following single doses of 17.5 Gy or more, a very constant sequence of clinical symptoms is observed: After 100–120 days animals irradiated with ⩾20 Gy develop pleural or pericardial effusions. After very high doses of ⩾25 Gy these effusions increase rapidly in volume and animals have to be killed at this stage (Lauk et al. 1985). Following lower doses, the effusions are completely reversible, i.e., are resorbed within a few weeks. In these animals there follows a second clinically asymptomatic period of several weeks. Using radionuclide ventriculography, however, a reduction in cardiac output and left ventricular ejection fraction to about 65% of normal values can already be detected (Schultz-Hector et al. 1991a). Later, dyspnea on exertion, then dyspnea at rest as well as increasing apathy or subcutaneous edema gradually develop. Clinical symptoms of heart failure such as dyspnea at rest or subcutaneous edema are accompanied by a rapid deterioration in hemodynamic function, as well as in the general condition of the individual animal. This time course of experimental radiation-induced heart disease, characterized by an early phase of a reversible effusive pericarditis and a late phase of reduced left ventricular ejection fraction, is in good agreement will observations in dogs (Gavin and Gillette 1982; Gillette et al. 1985), but also in patients undergoing mediastinal radiotherapy (Pierce et al. 1969).

Survival and Dose Response

The latent time until manifestation of heart failure varies with radiation dose. Following a single dose of 25 Gy the average latency of heart failure is 220 days. With decreasing radiation dose this increases to 250 days after 20 Gy and 408 days after 17.5 Gy. In these dose groups, including 17.5 Gy, all treated animals do finally develop the described clinical symptoms of heart failure as well as very constant histopathological findings. After a lower dose of 15 Gy, however, only very minor clinical symptoms and histopathological changes are observed even after follow-up times approaching the animals' normal life span of 20 months. Therefore, the incidence of manifest radiation-induced heart disease shows a very steep dose response, while at doses higher than the ED_{100} the latent time of expression of heart failure is dose dependent.

Autopsy and Histopathology

The clinical diagnosis of congestive heart failure is confirmed at autopsy by observation of a pronounced liver congestion as well as serous pleural effusions. In animals killed with clinical symptoms of heart failure, histopathological changes in the heart are comparable for all dose groups.

The left ventricular wall thickness is reduced to about 85% of control values, and the left ventricular cavity is dilated. The most prominent finding at histological examination is a focal degeneration and necrosis of the myocardium. Foci are randomly distributed throughout the myocardium and cover about 23% of the entire left and right ventricular myocardium when heart failure is manifest. At the periphery of foci the typical cross striation of myocytes is lost. Toward the center of foci, the cytoplasm is gradually replaced by vacuoles, until only the empty sarcolemmal sheaths are left. Occasionally there are massive extravasations of erythrocytes, but an inflammatory infiltration or demarcation reaction does not occur. The absence of a significant phagocytic clearance reaction is further confirmed by the absence of any positive staining reaction for lysosomal enzymes such as acid phophatase or β-*n*-acetylglucosaminidase. Mitochondrial enzymes, such as cytochrome oxidase or succinate dehydrogenase, are completely lost from foci of degeneration (Fig. 1). However, this loss is clearly limited to severely degenerate myocytes. Even in the immediate vicinity of foci, enzyme activity is not visibly different from areas of unchanged myocardium or from control hearts. In contrast, endothelial marker enzymes, such as alkaline phosphatase or 5′-nucleotidase, are lost not only from areas of obvious tissue degeneration but also from the surrounding myocardium. At a light microscopic level, enzyme-negative capillaries appear morphologically intact (Fig. 2). In sequential serial tissue sections it is evident that the distribution of alkaline phosphatase and 5′-nucleotidase is identical even on a cell-to-cell basis. Thus three different zones can be morphologically distinguished in the irradiated heart:

1. There are always areas in which myocardial structure and endothelial enzyme activity are not distinguishable from untreated control hearts.
2. More than 50% of the myocardium is covered by enzyme-negative areas in which myocardial morphology is, however, unchanged.
3. Within these enzyme-negative areas there are foci of myocardial degeneration which cover about 23% of the entire myocardium.

First electron microscopic studies confirm the focality of these changes, showing areas of complete destruction as well as areas of fully intact ultrastructure in one and the same heart.

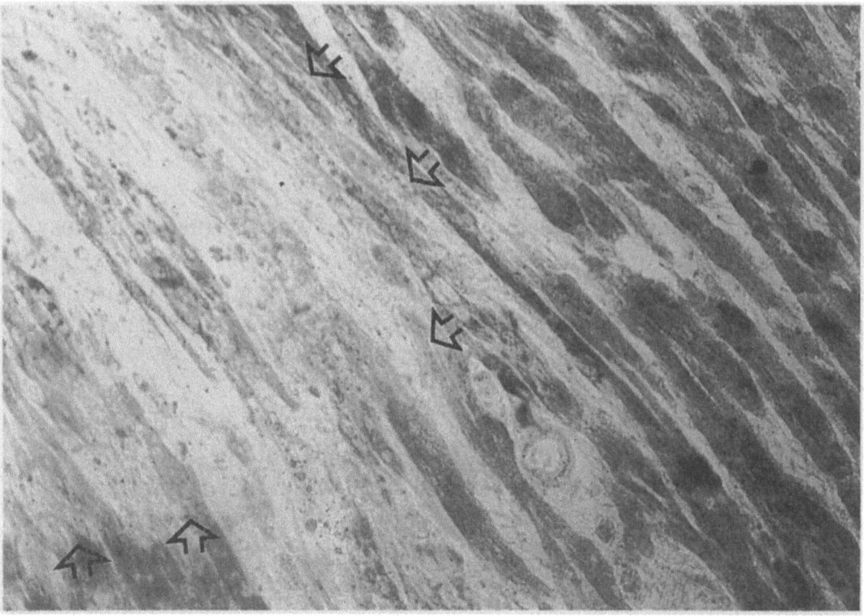

Fig. 1. Succinate dehydrogenase staining according to Lojda (1965) of the myocardium at 200 days after 20 Gy. Morphologically intact myocytes are intensively stained, while there is no enzyme reaction within the focus of degeneration (*arrows*)

Dose Fractionation

The described clinical symptoms and histopathological changes are not only observed after single doses but also after fractionated heart irradiation. However, the latent time to development of heart failure increases significantly with increasing number of dose fractions, indicating a very pronounced fractionation effect. Quantitative analysis of latent times of heart failure after irradiation in 1, 2, 4, or 10 fractions yields a low α/β ratio of 3.7 Gy (95% confidence interval 1.8–5.6). A quantitative comparison of typical changes in radiation-induced heart failure such as the decrease in ventricular wall thickness, the extent of myocardial degeneration, or the extent of alkaline phosphatase loss confirm that the cause of death is the same after single-dose or fractionated heart irradiation (Schultz-Hector et al. 1991b). Therefore, within the dose range studied, increasing total dose as well as increasing dose per fraction does accelerate the development of heart failure but does not appear to modify its pathogenesis. Once the disease is expressed and symptomatic, there is no difference between heart failure caused by a high or low dose of heart irradiation, i.e., by a single dose or a fractionated schedule. It therefore appeared appropriate to carry out pathogenetic studies after single doses of heart irradiation.

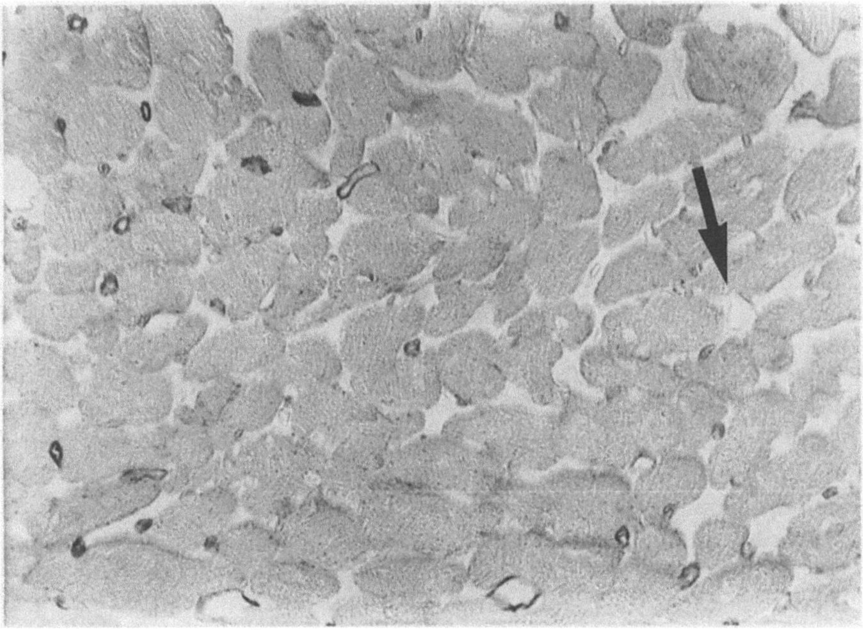

Fig. 2. Transition of an area of positive alkaline phosphatase staining of capillaries (*left*) to an enzyme-negative, but morphologically intact zone (*right*). In the enzyme-negative areas capillary structures are visible (*arrow*). The heart was perfusion fixed at 200 days after 20 Gy, embedded in glycol-methacrylate, and the alkaline phosphatase reaction carried out according to Burstone (1962)

Pathogenesis

The obvious cause of radiation-induced heart failure is the development of extensive myocardial degeneration. In proliferation kinetic studies in rats it was shown that proliferation of cardiomyocytes ceases by the age of 3 months (Engerman et al. 1967). Myocardial injury at a later age is compensated for by cellular hypertrophy but not by myocyte proliferation. Since it is generally assumed that cellular radiation injury is expressed at the time of mitosis, it is rather unlikely that myocardial degeneration should be a direct effect of irradiation on myocytes. The second most important cell population in the myocardium in terms of both tissue volume and function is the capillary endothelial cells. They are known to proliferate at a very low rate under resting conditions (Lauk and Trott 1990) and at a significantly increased rate when stimulated by injury (Haudenschild and Schwartz 1979) or ischemia (Pasyk et al. 1982). Therefore, capillary endothelial cells are the most likely target population of mitotically linked cell death in the heart. On the basis of sequential ultrastructural studies it has already been described that endothelial cell injury precedes radiation-induced myocardial changes (Morgenroth et al. 1967; Fajardo and Stewart 1971).

It has been demonstrated in several tissues, and has been accepted as a general principle, that irradiation leads to a quantitative cell loss from the actively proliferating target cell population in a tissue, which will cause clinically relevant tissue injury as soon as depletion exceeds a critical level. The latent time of these events should be correlated to the natural turnover time of the target cell population (Wheldon et al. 1982). If a similar sequence of events underlies radiation-induced myocardial degeneration, one would expect a radiation-induced loss of capillary endothelial cells followed by a compensatory wave of endothelial cell proliferation leading to further expression of radiation damage and finally to ischemic tissue breakdown. The latent time of these events should be correlated to resting endothelial cell turnover time. The spatial distribution of cell loss and of proliferative response should be homogeneous or random provided there is a homogeneous dose distribution in the tissue.

In order to test this hypothesis we carried out morphometric, enzyme histochemical, and proliferation kinetic studies. Most of the studies were carried out after 20 Gy, a relatively high dose causing heart failure in all treated animals, as well as after 15 Gy, which did cause morphological changes but no significant clinical symptoms of heart failure.

The development of myocardial degeneration with postirradiation time is represented in Fig. 3. At around 70 days after 20 Gy, first scattered foci of myocardial degeneration are detected, which then rapidly increase in size and number. Within 120 days they reach their maximum extent, covering around 23% of the entire myocardium. From this time onward the morphology changes very little, although heart failure occurs on average after only a further 130 days in this dose group. Following 15 Gy, a dose which

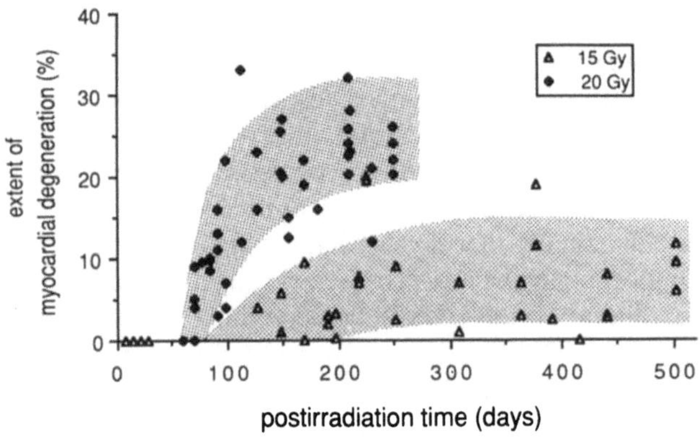

Fig. 3. Development of myocardial degeneration with postirradiation time after 15 or 20 Gy. Each symbol represents the extent of degeneration as a percentage of the entire section area analyzed from one heart

does not cause heart failure, myocardial degeneration affects significantly smaller proportions of the myocardium. However, it is noteworthy that once myocardial degeneration has occurred there is no recovery, even after an observation time of 500 days, which approaches the normal life span of the animal.

In perfusion-fixed hearts the volume density and length density of capillaries was determined in those areas where the myocardium was unchanged on light microscopy and where endothelial marker enzymes were positive. The volume density of capillaries is a measure of the maximal volume of blood that can be carried into the tissue. The length density is an estimate of the total length of capillaries per tissue volume and is thus related to the surface area of capillary walls available for the exchange of substrates. Following heart irradiation there is a diffuse reduction in the volume density as well as the length density of capillaries. After 20 Gy both parameters decrease rapidly to around 75% of control values within 35 days (Lauk 1987). At later time points the extent of alkaline phosphatase loss precludes a meaningful analysis in the remaining, grossly unchanged myocardium in this dose group. After 15 Gy a similarly steep loss of capillary volume density occurs in the first 50 days postirradiation that gradually leads to a minimum volume density of 50% of control levels at around 200 days (Fig. 4). Thereafter there appears to be some recovery; however, normal values are not attained. Length density of capillaries shows a similar time course of a steep drop within the first 50 days. After 15 Gy there appears to be some late but incomplete recovery (Fig. 5). It is remarkable that the latent time of capillary loss does not depend on radiation dose.

Apart from the structural loss of endothelial cells, there is a focal loss of the endothelial marker enzymes alkaline phosphatase and 5′-nucleotidase (Lauk 1987). Enzyme-negative areas in the myocardium are relatively well

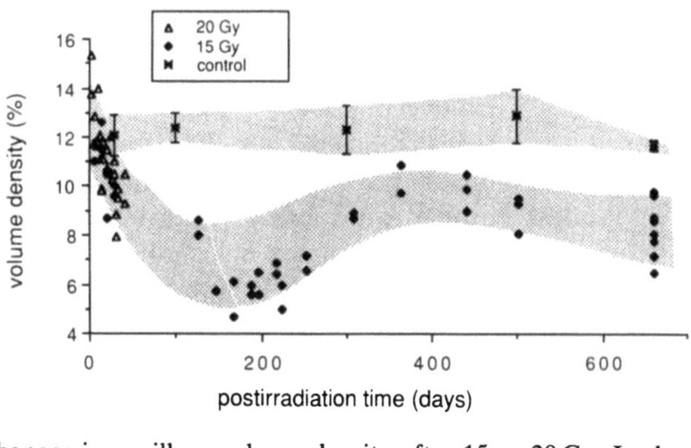

Fig. 4. Postirradiation changes in capillary volume density after 15 or 20 Gy. In the upper band means ± standard deviations of 4 or 5 age-matched control animals are shown, while irradiated animals are represented as single data points

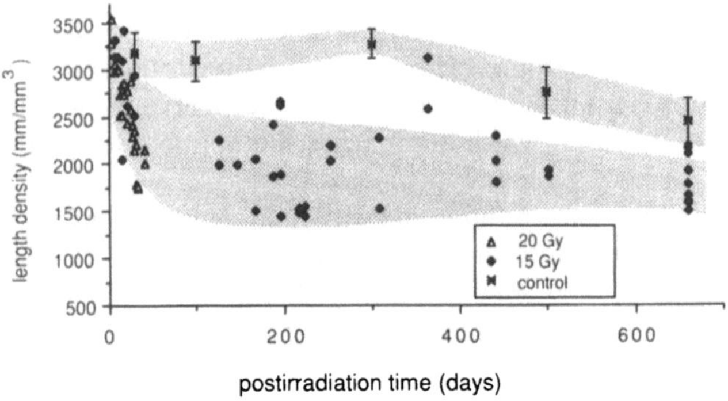

Fig. 5. Postirradiation changes in capillary length density after 15 or 20 Gy. In the upper band means ± standard deviations of 4 or 5 age-matched control animals are shown, while irradiated animals are plotted as single data points

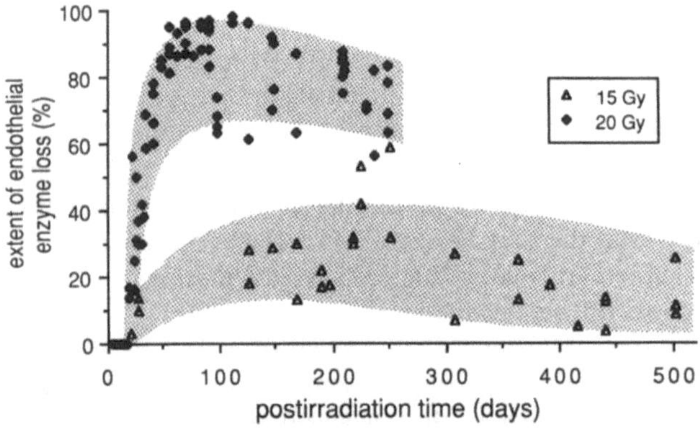

Fig. 6. Development of alkaline-phosphatase-negative areas with postirradiation time after 15 or 20 Gy. Each symbol represents the extent of enzyme loss as a percentage of the entire section area analyzed from one heart

defined and their extent can also be expressed as a percentage of the total myocardium. In sequential studies, represented in Fig. 6, first foci of enzyme loss become evident at 23 days postirradiation. After 20 Gy they already cover about 80% of the myocardium at 70 days, when myocardial degeneration starts to develop within these enzyme-negative areas. The time of onset of enzyme loss appears to be similar after 15 Gy, but the maximum extent is much lower. Again, there is no recovery of endothelial enzymes throughout the observation time of 500 days. These morphometric studies indicate that there is indeed a radiation-induced loss of myocardial capillaries, i.e., of endothelial cells, as would be expected in a proliferating cell population. Furthermore, there is a focal defect in endothelial cell function which precedes myocardial degeneration in these areas and increases in severity with dose.

The time course and spatial distribution of a radiation-induced proliferative response in a tissue show characteristic patterns which can help to identify possible target cell populations in that tissue. The proliferative activity can be studied by giving single or repeated injections of tritiated thymidine. Cells that have incorporated the label can then be identified in autoradiographs of tissue sections (Lauk and Trott 1990).

After a pulse label, only about 0.33% of capillary endothelial cells in the heart can be identified as being in S phase. Repeated labelling over various time periods yields increasing proportions of labelled endothelial cell nuclei. However, extrapolating these measured values to 100% labelled endothelial cells indicates a very long turnover time of around 420 days.

In 12 h labelling studies at various times after 20 Gy, a wave of increased endothelial cell proliferation is observed. The labelling index starts to rise above control levels at 49 days postirradiation. However, analyzing nuclei of alkaline-phophatase-positive and -negative endothelial cells separately reveals that this proliferative response is exclusively limited to enzyme-negative cells (Fig. 7). In areas of unchanged enzyme activity the normal endothelial cell proliferation is not disturbed by irradiation within the observation time of 150 days. These findings are in contrast to our hypothesis in two ways. First, the latent time of radiation-induced structural loss of capillaries as well as the wave of amplified endothelial cell proliferation is as much as an order of magnitude shorter than the natural turnover time of endothelial cells. It therefore appears unlikely that this proliferative

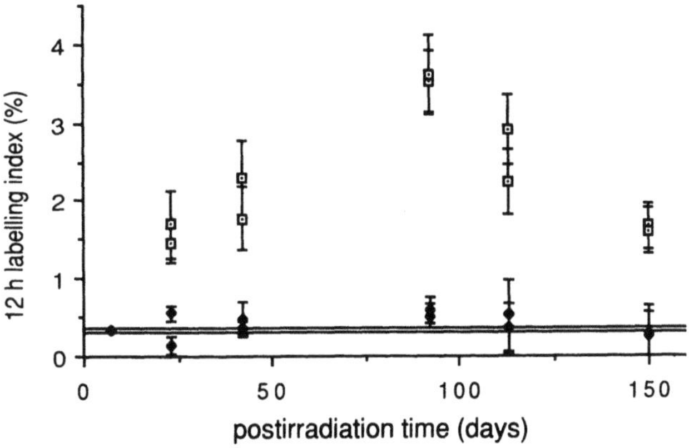

Fig. 7. Changes in 12h labelling index with postirradiation time in alkaline-phosphatase-positive (*filled symbols*) and -negative (*open symbols*) capillaries. Symbols represent single animals, error bars are 95% confidence intervals. The *horizontal band* represents the 95% confidence interval of the mean labelling index in age-matched control animals. (Data from Lauk and Trott 1990)

response would be triggered by radiation-induced endothelial cell death in mitosis. Furthermore, endothelial cell proliferation was not induced throughout the myocardium, but was linked to focal endothelial enzyme loss.

In agreement with findings in other late-reacting organs, radiation-induced cardiomyopathy is secondary to capillary damage. Although there is a quantitative loss of capillary endothelial cells, the generally assumed mechanism of mitotically linked depletion of target cells does not explain our findings. Obviously, specific cell functions are involved in the pathogenesis and have to be studied in detail in order to understand the mechanism of radiation damage.

Preliminary ultrastructural studies revealed a strongly positive alkaline phosphatase reaction in the abluminal cell membrane and in intracellular transport vesicles of endothelial cells, but also a positive reaction in pericytes, which are light microscopically indistinguishable from endothelial cells. The enzyme appears to play a key role in cardiac purine metabolism and control of regional blood flow (Dendorfer et al. 1987; Lauk et al. 1991). The ultrastructural correlate of radiation-induced alkaline phosphatase loss is currently being studied. Besides capillary marker enzymes, other regulatory mechanisms such as cardiac catecholamine metabolism and the myocardial adrenoceptor system have proved to be affected by heart irradiation (Lauk et al. 1989; Schultz-Hector 1991b; Schultz-Hector et al. 1991a). Thus a complex picture emerges of interactions between radiation-induced cell death and modulation of highly organ-specific regulatory cell functions. Further understanding of cardiac pathophysiology will be needed in order to integrate these observations into one coherent concept of pathogenesis of radiation-induced heart disease.

References

Applefeld MM, Wiernik PH (1983) Cardiac disease after radiation therapy for Hodgkin's disease: analysis of 48 patients. Am J Cardiol 51:1679–1681

Burns RJ, Bar-Shlomo B-Z, Druck MN, Herman JG, Gilbert BW, Perrault DJ, McLaughlin PR (1983) Detection of radiation cardiomyopathy by gated radionuclide angiography. Am J Med 74:297–302

Burstone MS (1962) Enzyme histochemistry and its application in the study of neoplasm. Academic, New York

Byhardt R, Brace K, Ruckdeschel J, Chang P, Martin R, Wiernik P (1975) Dose and treatment factors in radiation-related pericardial effusion associated with the mantle technique for Hodgkin's disease. Cancer 35:795–802

Carmel RJ, Kaplan HS (1976) Mantle irradiation in Hodgkin's disease: an analysis of technique, tumour eradication and complications. Cancer 37:2813–2825

Dendorfer A, Lauk S, Schaff A, Nees S (1987) New insights into the mechanism of myocardial adenosine formation. In: Gerlach E, Becker EF (eds) Topics and perspectives in adenosine research. Springer, Berlin Heidelberg New York, pp 171–187

Engerman RL, Pfaffenbach D, Davis MD (1967) Cell turnover in capillaries. Lab Invest 17:738–743
Fajardo LF, Stewart JR (1971) Capillary injury preceding radiation-induced myocardial fibrosis. Radiology 101:429–433
Gavin PR, Gillette EL (1982) Radiation response of the canine cardiovascular system. Radiat Res 90:489–500
Gillette EL, McChesney SL, Hoopes PJ (1985) Isoeffect curves for radiation-induced cardiomyopathy in the dog. Int J Radiat Oncol Biol Phys 11:2091–2097
Gomez GA, Park JJ, Panahon AM, Parthasarathy KL, Pearce J, Reese P, Bakshi S, Henderson ES (1983) Heart size and function after radiation therapy to the mediastinum in patients with Hodgkin's disease. Cancer Treat Rep 67:1099–1103
Gottdiener JS, Katin MJ, Borer JS, Bacharach SL, Green MV (1983) Late cardiac effects of therapeutic mediastinal irradiation. Assessment by echocardiography and radionuclide angiography. N Engl J Med 308:569–588
Greenwood RD, Rosenthal A, Cassady R, Jaffe N, Nadas AS (1974) Constrictive pericarditis in childhood due to mediastinal irradiation. Circulation 50:1033–1039
Haudenschild CC, Schwartz CU (1979) Endothelial regeneration. II. Restitution of endothelial continuity. Lab Invest 41:407–418
Lojda Z (1965) Remarks on histochemical detection of dehydrogenases. II. Intracellular localization. Folia Morphol 13:84–96
Lauk S (1987) Endothelial alkaline phosphatase activity loss as an early stage in the development of radiation-induced heart disease in rats. Radiat Res 110:118–128
Lauk S, Trott K-R (1990) Endothelial proliferation in the rat heart following local heart irradiation. Int J Radiat Biol 57:1017–1030
Lauk S, Kiszel Z, Buschmann J, Trott K-R (1985) Radiation induced heart disease in rats. Int J Radiat Oncol Biol Phys 11:801–808
Lauk S, Böhm M, Feiler G, Geist BJ, Erdmann E (1989) Increased number of cardiac adrenergic receptors following local heart irradiation. Radiat Res 119: 157–165
Lauk S, Dendorfer A, Nees S (1991) Isolierung reiner myokardialer Kapillaren (K) und Diskriminierung der enthaltenen Endothelzellen (EZ) und Perizyten (P) in der Gewebekultur. Z Kardiol 80 [Suppl 3]:117
Morgan GW, Freeman AP, McLean RG, Jarvie BH, Giles RW (1985) Late cardiac, thyroid and pulmonary sequelae of mantle radiotherapy for Hodgkin's disease. Int J Radiat Oncol Biol Phys 11:1925–1931
Morgenroth K, Junge-Hülsing G, Hauss WH (1967) Über Veränderungen am Rattenherzen nach gezielter Röntgenbestrahlung. Strahlentherapie 133:610–620
Pasyk S, Schaper W, Schaper J, Pasyk K, Miskiewicz G, Steinseifer B (1982) DNA synthesis in coronary collaterals after coronary artery occlusion in conscious dog. Am J Physiol 242:H1031–H1037
Pierce RH, Haferman MD, Kagan AR (1969) Changes in the transverse cardiac diameter following irradiation for Hodgkin's disease. Radiology 93:619–624
Savage DE, Constine LS, Schwartz RG, Rubin P (1990) Radiation effects on left-ventricular function and myocardial perfusion in long term survivors of Hodgkin's disease. Int J Radiat Oncol Biol Phys 19:721–727
Schultz-Hector S (1991a) Heart. In: Scherer E, Streffer C, Trott K-R (eds) Radiopathology of organs and tissues. Springer, Berlin Heidelberg New York, pp 347–368
Schultz-Hector S (1991b) Radiation-induced heart disease: review of experimental data on dose response and pathogenesis. Int J Radiat Biol (to be published)
Schultz-Hector S, Böhm M, Blöchel A, Dominiak P, Erdmann E, Müller-Schauenburg W, Weber A (1991a) Radiation-induced heart disease: morphology, changes in catecholamine synthesis and content, β-adrenoceptor density and hemodynamic function in an experimental model. Radiat Res (to be published)

Schultz-Hector S, Sund M, Thames HD (1991b) Fractionation response and repair kinetics of radiation-induced heart failure in the rat. Radiother Oncol (to be published)

Watchie J, Coleman N, Raffin T, Cox R, Rauibitschek A, Fahey T, Hoppe R, Venkessel A (1987) Minimal long-term cardiopulmonary dysfunction following treatment for Hodgkin's disease. Int J Radiat Oncol Biol Phys 13:517–524

Wheldon TE, Michalowski AS, Kirk J (1982) The effect of irradiation on function in self-renewing normal tissues with different proliferative organisation. Br J Radiol 55:759–766

Myocardial Infarction after Irradiation in Hodgkin's Disease: A Review

H. Joensuu

Department of Oncology and Radiotherapy, Turku University Central Hospital, 20520 Turku, Finland

Introduction

Hodgkin's disease can be effectively treated with irradiation, and the role of radiation therapy is well established in the management of early-stage Hodgkin's disease. About 80% of patients with stage I or II Hodgkin's disease who are free from constitutional symptoms will live free from relapse for 10 years from the diagnosis if treated with irradiation alone (Hoppe et al. 1982; Mauch et al. 1988). As the cure rate has increased, late complications of irradiation have become increasingly important.

Before the 1960s and even up to the 1970s, the heart was considered to be relatively resistant to doses of irradiation that were used in clinical radiotherapy. Now radiation-related acute and delayed pericarditis, pancarditis, cardiomyopathy, myocardial fibrosis, and functional valvular and conduction defects are established entities (Byhardt et al. 1975; Tötterman et al. 1983; Stewart and Fajardo 1984), but controversial views on the potential role of irradiation in the genesis of myocardial infarction continue to be expressed. The relationship of coronary artery disease (CAD) to irradiation has been considered to be rare (Kinsella et al. 1982) and questionable (Fajardo 1977; Stewart and Fajardo 1984), and it has been suggested that CAD in particular should not be an important consideration when planning a course of radiotherapy (Fajardo 1977).

An important hypothesis of the pathogenesis of atherosclerosis proposes that "injury" to the endothelium is the initiating event (Ross and Glomset 1976). All four principal cells involved in atherosclerosis – endothelium, smooth muscle, platelets, and monocyte/macrophages – either contain or can synthesize and release growth factors, and it is thus possible that "injury" or other stimuli can induce growth-factor release. A modified response-to-injury hypothesis of atherosclerosis suggests that at least two pathways may lead to formation of smooth-muscle proliferative lesions in the intima. The first pathway involves the monocyte and is demonstrated in

Recent Results in Cancer Research, Vol. 130

hypercholesterolemia. The second pathway involves direct stimulation of endothelium, and may be important in diabetes, hypertension, cigarette smoking, or other circumstances associated with increased incidence of atherosclerosis (Ross 1986). There is no definite evidence that cancer per se predisposes to CAD, but cardiac metastases can cause CAD via tumor emboli, extrinsic compression, or ostial obstruction (Kopelson and Herwig 1978).

Theoretically, all agents capable of producing an injury to the endothelial cells of the coronary arteries could be risk factors for CAD and myocardial infarction. In this article evidence for irradiation-related myocardial infarction is reviewed, and its relationship to the irradiation technique in Hodgkin's disease is discussed.

Evidence for Radiation-Related Myocardial Infarction

The evidence that therapeutic irradiation may cause CAD and myocardial infarction comes mainly from experimental studies, case reports, autopsy studies, studies of cohorts of patients who have undergone cardiac testing years after irradiation, and clinical series of patients who have received chest irradiation.

Experimental Studies

A considerable amount of work has been done to examine the effect of irradiation on the genesis of atherosclerosis in animal models. The results obtained in these studies may not, however, be directly applied to humans because of the many differences between the species, the diet, and other factors, such as smoking. Furthermore, large fractions, even one large single fraction, have often been used to irradiate animals, which is unlike the clinical situation. It is also not clear whether the age of the animals at the time of irradiation, and the follow-up times chosen, are really valid for clinical conclusions.

In experimental studies irradiation has caused both micro- and macrovasculopathy. In the New Zealand white rabbit maintained on a normal diet and irradiated with either a 18–83 Gy single dose or fractionated irradiation to the heart, three phases of irradiation-induced cardiac injury were observed (Stewart et al. 1968; Fajardo and Stewart 1970). A transient acute phase was seen within a few hours to days from irradiation, and was characterized by a neutrophilic infiltrate involving all layers of the heart. This was followed by a latent phase that lasted from 2 to 70 days, when no significant lesions could be seen in light microscopy. In the late stage, beyond 70 days, there was progressive pericardial and myocardial fibrosis and pericardial effusion. Although no changes were seen by light microscopy during the latent phase, electron microscopy revealed ultrastructural damage to the endothelial cells of blood capillaries, which varied from luminal projections of cytoplasm to cell necrosis and rupture of the capillary wall (Fajardo and Stewart 1973). These changes obstruct the capillary lumen and cause the formation of thrombi, leading to the reduction of the relative number of the capillaries compared with myocytes, and finally to ischemia and fibrosis.

Lindsay et al. (1962) irradiated localized segments of the abdominal aorta of 18 dogs, kept presumably on their normal diet, with X-rays in doses ranging from 15 to 55 Gy. Atherosclerosis developed at the irradiated sites, and was significantly more severe than that which occurred in nonirradiated control sites in the abdominal aorta; it resembled the arteriosclerotic lesions that occur naturally in old dogs. Gold (1961) reported marked atherosclerotic lesions in the coronary arteries in 27% of Wistar rats kept on a high-fat diet and irradiated at weekly intervals to a total dose of about 25 Gy to the thorax, whereas no such marked lesions were seen in the nonirradiated control group also fed a high-fat diet. Amromin et al. (1964) found that X-rays given in 5-Gy weekly fractions to a total dose of 25 Gy to the heart in the rabbit were responsible only for rare areas of medial degeneration and intimal proliferation of the major epicardial arteries, but if the rabbits were exposed to high-cholesterol diets in addition to irradiation, diffuse severe atherosclerotic lesions were produced. Similarly, Kirkpatrick (1967) could reproduce in the ears of rabbits foam cell lesions similar to those observed in the vessels of irradiated tissues in man by combining local X-ray irradiation and hyperlipidemia, but fibrous plaques were formed in irradiated vessels if the animals had normal serum lipid levels.

Typical coronary atherosclerosis of the type seen in man is not produced in some animal species such as the rabbit by irradiation alone when the animals are kept on their normal diet (Fajardo 1977), but the above studies and others (Artom et al. 1965; Bradley et al. 1981) suggest that irradiation coupled with a diet rich in cholesterol and lipids is capable of causing accelerated atherosclerosis. Such a diet may be consumed by patients receiving cardiac irradiation. Heart irradiation has been shown to induce endothelial cell proliferation and increased labelling of endothelial cells with tritiated thymidine (Lauk and Trott 1990), a finding which is compatible with the modified response-to-injury hypothesis of atherogenesis (Ross 1986).

Case Reports

Many case reports on myocardial infarction following radiotherapy have been published since 1957 (Pearson 1957). It has been pointed out that from the many thousands of patients surviving many years after irradiation of the heart, few cases of CAD have been reported (Steward and Fajardo 1978). On the other hand, it may be argued that because CAD may occur incidentally in irradiated patients older than 40, an attempt to publish such a case may result in a failure. Furthermore, the correct diagnosis may not always have been reached, especially if the patient is young, because myocardial infarction is not easily suspected in patients aged 30 or less (Ali et al. 1976; Leong et al. 1979; Applefeld and Wiernik 1983; Burns et al. 1983; Joensuu 1989).

There are at least 17 published cases where CAD has occurred in patients irradiated for Hodgkin's disease and who have been younger than 30 when the symptoms of CAD first appeared, and at least 22 other cases where it has been found in patients aged from 30 to 39 (Tables 1 and 2). Still more cases in young patients with no published details exist (Donaldson and Kaplan 1982; Burns et al. 1983; Hancock et al. 1988); patients older than 40 at diagnosis are not discussed here (Nakhjavan et al. 1984; McEniery et al. 1987). Probably the youngest reported case was of a boy who was irradiated for Hodgkin's disease at the age of 6, and died from myocardial infarction at the age of 12 (Tötterman et al. 1983).

Young patients with radiation-related CAD are often male (male to female ratio about 3:1, Tables 1 and 2), they usually lack a positive family

Table 1. Patients aged under 30 at the time of coronary artery disease manifestation treated with chest rediotherapy for Hodgkin's disease

Case	Source	Sex/Age[b]	Diagnosis[a]	Dose (Gy)	Interval from RT to CAD/MI (yr)
1	Tötterman et al. (1983)	M/12	MI, fatal	29	6
2	Cohn et al. (1967)	M/15	MI, fatal	40	1 (16 mo)
3	Angelini et al. (1985)	F/18	MI, fatal	40	9
4	Voelker et al. (1987)	M/18	MI	45	3
5	Prentice (1965)	M/19	MI, fatal	33	3
6	Yahalom et al. (1983)	F/19	MI	44	2
7	Huff and Sanders (1972)	M/21	MI, fatal	35	1 (9 mo)
8	Rasmussen et al. (1978)	M/21	MI, fatal	37	1 (16 mo)
9	Carlson et al. (1991)	M/22	MI	41	4
10	Ali et al. (1976)	M/24	CAD	35	5
11	Joensuu (1989)	M/25	MI	43	4
12	Schechter (1975)	F/27	MI	?	7
13	Gottdiener et al. (1983)	F/27	MI	≤40	5
14	Radwaner et al. (1987)	F/27	MI, fatal	46	8
15	Joensuu (1989)	M/28	MI, fatal	41	1 (9 mo)
16	Dunsmore et al. (1986)	F/28	MI	40	9
17	Murphy (1977)	M/29	Sudden coronary death	?	2

Male to female ratio = 11:6
Age range = 12–29 years (median 22 years)
Dose range = 29–46 Gy (median 40 Gy)
Interval from irradiation to first symptoms: range 9 months 9–years (median 4 years)

MI, myocardial infarction; CAD, coronary artery disease
[a] Age, age at first symptoms of CAD/MI

Table 2. Patients aged 30–39 years at the time of coronary artery disease manifestation treated with chest radiotherapy for Hodgkin's disease

Case	Source	Sex/Age[b]	Diagnosis[a]	Dose (Gy)	Interval from RT to CAD/MI (yr)
18	McEniery et al. (1987)	M/30	CAD	?	13
19	Tötterman et al. (1983)	M/31	CAD	42	10
20	Dollinger et al. (1966)	M/31	MI	14	0 (2 mo)
21	Dunsmore et al. (1986)	M/31	MI	44	12
22	McEniery et al. (1987)	M/31	MI	?	5
23	Pohjola-Sintonen et al. (1987)	M/31	MI	42	10
24	Rodgers (1976)	M/32	MI	43	6
25	Miller et al. (1983)	M/32	CAD	35	4
26	McEniery et al. (1987)	F/32	CAD	45	14
27	McReynolds et al. (1976)	M/33	Sudden coronary death	50	8
28	Leong et al. (1979)	M/34	MI, fatal	45	8
29	Tracy et al. (1974), Ringrose (1974)	F/35	CAD	51	2
30	Iqbal et al. (1977)	M/35	MI	38	1
31	Simon et al. (1984)	F/35	CAD	?	?
32	Mittal et al. (1986)	M/35	MI	40	6
33	Dunsmore et al. (1986)	M/36	MI	41	4
34	Tenet et al. (1986)	M/36	CAD	30	10
35	Gustavsson et al. (1990)	F/36	MI, fatal	40	4
36	Gustavsson et al. (1990)	M/36	CAD	42	?
37	Annest et al. (1983)	M/37	MI	28	13
38	Annest et al. (1983)	M/38	CAD	33	16
39	Gustavsson et al. (1990)	M/39	MI	38	14

Male to female ratio = 9:2
Age range = 30–39 years (median 34.5 years)
Dose range = 14–51 Gy (median 41 Gy)
Interval from irradiation to first symptoms: 2 months–16 years (median 8 years)

CAD, coronary artery disease; MI, myocardial infarction; RT, radiotherapy
[a] Age, age at first symptoms of CAD/MI

history of early CAD, blood cholesterol is usually within the normal limits and there is no hyperlipidemia, but they often are or have been smokers (Table 3). The interval between irradiation and the appearance of symptoms of CAD or myocardial infarction varied from a few months to 16 years. Radiation-associated CAD appears to be characterized by a high incidence of left main coronary artery and right ostial coronary disease (Tommaso et al. 1984; McEniery et al. 1987). Coronary artery bypass surgery has been shown to be a feasible method of treating radiation-related CAD (Iqbal et al. 1977; Ali et al. 1976; Applefeld and Wiernik 1983; Annest et al. 1983; Dunsmore et al. 1986; Tenet et al. 1986; Carlson et al. 1991).

Table 3. Family history, hyperlipidemia, and smoking in young patients with Hodgkin's disease and with radiation-related coronary artery disease

Risk factor	Cases number[a]	*n*
Family history of coronary artery disease		
Present	15, 18, 22, 29, 30, 36, 38	7
Absent	2, 3, 5, 6, 7, 8, 10, 12, 14, 20, 23, 25, 26, 27, 28, 32, 34, 37, 39	19
Not known	1, 4, 9, 11, 13, 16, 17, 19 21, 24, 31, 33, 35	13
Hyperlipidemia		
Present	4, 16, 24, 25, 27, 29, 36	7
Absent	1, 2, 3, 5, 6, 7, 9, 10, 11, 12, 14, 15, 19, 20, 22, 23, 26, 28, 30, 32, 34, 37, 38	23
Not known	8, 13, 17, 18, 21, 31, 33 35, 39	9
Smoking		
Smoker	4, 8, 9, 11, 15, 18, 21, 24, 25, 27, 29, 30, 32, 36, 37, 39	16
Nonsmoker	1, 6, 12, 14, 16, 22, 26, 28, 34, 38	10
Not known	2, 3, 5, 7, 10, 13, 17, 19, 20, 23, 31, 33, 35	13

[a] Case number refers to the sources shown Tables 1 and 2

Although in some cases (Mittal et al. 1986) the irradiation technique appears to have been in line with the modern recommendations for mantle irradiation, in the great majority of the above case reports it was not, or the details on the irradiation technique are lacking. Irradiation has been given from the anterior portal of the mantle field only (McReynolds et al. 1976; Annest et al. 1983; Gottdiener et al. 1983; Tötterman et al. 1983), which will result in a large cardiac dose, as does also anterior weighting of radiation (Ali et al. 1976; Iqbal et al. 1977; Annest et al. 1983). The use of large daily fractions (Iqbal et al. 1977; Yahalom et al. 1983) and the failure to treat both the anterior and posterior portals of the mantle field daily to reduce the so-called edge effect (Ali et al. 1976; Dunsmore et al. 1986; Joensuu 1989) are also likely to increase the rate of cardiac complications. Linear accelerators are now usually used to irradiate the mantle field. They have higher energy and less rapid dose fall-off in the tissue than does ^{60}Co, and they produce a lower epicardial dose for a given midline dose. ^{60}Co was used to treat many of the cases with precocious CAD (Tracy et al. 1974; Ali et al. 1976; Iqbal et al. 1977; Gottdiener et al. 1983; Dunsmore et al. 1986; Gustavsson et al. 1990).

There are also several reports where irradiation has been related to occlusion of large arteries, such as the subclavian (Loeffler 1975; Budin et al. 1976), carotid (Levinson et al. 1973; Silverberg et al. 1978), axillary and iliac arteries (Butler et al. 1980), and the aorta (Ormerod 1976).

Apart from smoking, the lack of risk factors for CAD in irradiated young patients with CAD gives strong support to the hypothesis that radiotherapy has been involved in the development of precocious CAD. Furthermore, in several case reports severe angiographic or histological changes have been seen in coronary arteries but not in arteries outside the radiation portal (Prentice 1965; Dollinger et al. 1966; Cohn et al. 1967; Leong et al. 1979). Although the published case reports strongly suggest that irradiation is a risk factor for myocardial infarction, there is currently little information available from case reports to suggest that radiotherapy given in line with the modern recommendations would cause significant CAD. Finally, a few of the patients with precocious CAD have been treated with cancer chemotherapy also, either with a regimen that contains doxorubicin (Schechter and Jones 1975; Mittal et al. 1986; Tenet et al. 1986; Voelker et al. 1987; Joensuu 1989) or does not (Prentice 1965; Leong et al. 1979; Radwaner et al. 1987), or contains unspecified agents (Angelini et al. 1985).

Autopsy Findings

Brosius et al. (1981) described in detail the autopsy findings of 16 patients aged 15 to 33 years at death who had received mediastinal irradiation 5–144 months before death, and 10 control subjects matched for age and sex. Only 6 of the 16 patients had clinical evidence of cardiac dysfunction, but at necropsy all had anatomical evidence of cardiac abnormality including fibrous thickening of pericardium, mural and valvular endocardium, and interstitial myocardial fibrosis. One patient had a healed myocardial infarction at necropsy; another patient who died suddenly was shown at necropsy to have died as the result of severe coronary artery narrowing. In the 16 patients 16 of the 64 major epicardial coronary arteries were narrowed >75% in cross sectional area, as compared with only 1 of the 40 major arteries among the 10 control subjects.

The intimal plaques in the patients were largely composed of fibrous tissue; little lipid was present. However, while there was no difference in the composition of the intimal lesions between the irradiated patients and the controls, in the irradiated hearts a striking loss of smooth muscle cells was seen from the media, and the adventitia were often densely thickened by fibrous tissue. Other authors have also found the coronary artery plaques associated with radiation to be fibrotic (Dollinger et al. 1966; McReynolds et al. 1976; Simon et al. 1984; Dunsmore et al. 1986), whereas still others have described them to be atherosclerotic or atheromatous (Prentice 1965; Cohn et al. 1967; Huff and Sanders 1972; Murphy 1977; Rasmussen et al. 1978; Leong et al. 1979; Angelini et al. 1985; Radwaner et al. 1987). In a few studies no severe occlusion has been found on coronary arteriography in a patient with radiation-related angina (Miller et al. 1983) or myocardial infarction (Yahalom et al. 1983), and the presence of coronary artery spasm has been suggested in these cases.

In the study by Brosius et al. (1981) the patients were treated with techniques now considered as unacceptable (anterior-only portals, anterior wall doses ranging from 40 to 89 Gy, multiple courses of radiotherapy), and 3 patients received doxorubicin. However, in 4 cases the anterior and posterior wall of the heart received <42 Gy. Anatomical changes were detected in these cases also, but no information on fractionation was provided.

Thus, autopsy findings of frequent fibrous changes in the coronary arteries of the irradiated patients, together with similar changes found elsewhere in the heart, provide evidence that irradiation may cause CAD and myocardial infarction, but more information is needed on the cardiac effects of radiotherapy when modern treatment techniques have been used.

Frequency of Myocardial Infarction in Clinical Series

More than one case of myocardial infarction has been encountered in relatively small series of young patients irradiated for Hodgkin's disease (Pohjola-Sintonen et al. 1987, Gustavsson et al. 1990). In our own series (Joensuu 1989), two young men aged 25 and 28 at the time of myocardial infarction were seen in a small series consisting only of 47 patients younger than 40 at the time of irradiation. This was clearly more than the expected number assessed from the available statistics on the incidence of myocardial infarction in Finland ($p = 0.003$ or smaller). Irradiation was given with a linear accelerator to about 40 Gy in daily fractions of less than 2 Gy and equally weighted fields, which were treated on alternate days. Annest et al. (1983) found five (18%) cases with severe CAD in a series of 29 irradiated patients with lymphoma or thymoma, who had survived 10 or more years after irradiation. Two of the five patients were younger than 40 at onset of ischemic symptoms. Mediastinal irradiation had been given with anterior or anterior weighted fields.

Boivin and Hutchison (1982) analyzed the reports of 957 patients diagnosed with Hodgkin's disease in the Harvard Joint Center for Radiation Therapy and the Massachusetts General Hospital in 1942–1975. Mortality from CAD in patients who had received irradiation for Hodgkin's disease to the lower mediastinum (dose not specified) was compared both with the rate in nonirradiated subjects seen in the center at the same time, and to the expected number of deaths from CAD in the general population. The cause of death was obtained from death certificates. After adjustment for interval of observation, age, stage, and B symptoms, they found the relative death rate in CAD to be 1.5 times greater in irradiated than in non-irradiated subjects, a figure that did not differ significantly from unity (95% confidence limits 0.59–3.7). The group of nonirradiated patients differed greatly from the irradiated patients especially as regards stage and age distribution, and only 63 (26%) patients in the nonirradiated group had been followed up for 5 years or longer. Of more interest is their finding of 2.1 times greater mortality in the irradiated group compared with the general population (95% confidence limits 1.0–3.9) – and death certificates may underestimate the frequency of coronary deaths, especially in young patients.

Although the above series provide evidence that mediastinal irradiation may increase the frequency of myocardial infarction, there are large series where modern techniques of irradiation have been used and no excess of death from myocardial infarction has been seen. In the Stanford series (Hancock et al. 1988) that included 326 patients with median follow-up exceeding 14 years, only 9 patients died from acute myocardial infarction 2–19 years after therapy, which did not exceed mortality due to acute myocardial infarction in the general population. However, 5 patients died from myocardial infarction between 33 and 43 years of age and had no known cardiac risk factors, and Donaldson and Kaplan (1982) from the same center found 2 cases with premature CAD among 120 pediatric patients who had received high-dose mantle-field irradiation. Investigators from the Joint Center for Radiation Therapy (Boston, MA) found only 3 cases of fatal myocardial infarctions among 315 patients who were treated with mantle irradiation given with modern techniques and with a median follow-up time of 9 years (Mauch et al. 1988). All the 3 cases were older than 40, and 2 of them had significant risk factors for arteriosclerotic heart disease.

For every patient who dies from radiation-related myocardial infarction there are probably cases of non-fatal CAD and of silent ischemia, and a long follow-up period may be needed for such cases to become manifest. Yet the data suggest that radiation-related myocardial infarction is rare if mediastinal irradiation is given with equally weighted, individually contoured fields treated daily with a linear accelerator, the daily midplane doses ranging from 150 to 200 cGy (Carmel and Kaplan 1976; Hoppe et al. 1982).

Myocardial Infarction in Clinical Series Studied for Cardiac Function

Cohorts of patients have been evaluated for cardiac function a few years following chest irradiation for Hodgkin's disease. Some of these studies are listed in Table 4, but studies with few details on the irradiation technique (Burns et al. 1983) or those that also include patients without lymphoma are not included (Perrault et al. 1985). At least one study has developed out of the case of a young patient who succumbed to myocardial infarction

Table 4. Cohorts investigated for cardiac function after chest irradiation for Hodgkin's disease

Source	*n*	Age range at study (yr)	Time interval from RT (yr)	Cardiac evaluation	Coronary artery disease
Single anterior mantle portal or anterior weighting					
Applefeld and Wiernik (1983)	48	18–68	3–14	Echocardiography, radionuclide ventriculography, cardiac catheterization	6 CAD (2 MI)
Gottdiener et al. (1983)	25	25–59	5–15	ECG, radionuclide cineangiography, echocardiography	1 MI, 1 CAD
Pohjola-Sintonen et al. (1987)	28	12–38	>5	ECG, chest radiograph, echocardiography, bicycle exercise test	2 MI
Equally weighted AP: PA portals in most patients					
Gomez et al. (1983)	55	21–60	3–10	Chest radiograph, ^{99m}Tc ventriculography	No CAD diagnosed
Morgan et al. (1985)	25	18–35	5–16	ECG, chest radiograph ^{201}Tl scintigraphy, ^{99m}Tc ventriculography, echocardiography	No CAD diagnosed, Tl scintigraphy normal in all
Green et al. (1987)	28	11–27	1–15	ECG, chest radiograph, echocardiography	No CAD diagnosed
Kadota et al. (1988)	12	13–27	7–12	ECG, chest radiograph, echocardiography, bicycle exercise test	No CAD diagnosed
Gustavsson et al. (1990)	26	21–45	10–20	exercise ECG, CT, ^{201} Tl scintigraphy, echocardiography, Doppler cardiography	2 MI, 1 CAD; Tl scintigraphy normal in 9/23
Savage et al. (1990)	16	mean, 34	3–22	exercise ECG, ^{201} Tl scintigraphy, ^{99m} Tc cardiography	No CAD detected, Tl scintigraphy normal in 12/12

AP: PA, anterior–posterior, posterior–anterior; CAD, coronary artery disease; MI, myocardial infarction; RT, radiotherapy

(Pohjola-Sintonen et al. 1987) and, therefore, the results of these studies may not be directly generalized to all patients irradiated for Hodgkin's disease.

Among the 263 patients investigated in the studies listed in Table 4, myocardial infarction or CAD was diagnosed in 13 (5%) cases. However, in studies where irradiation was carried out through an anterior portal only, or where an anteriorly weighted treatment plan was used, CAD was seen more commonly (10/101, 10%) than in studies where equally weighted anterior and posterior portals had been used (3/162, 2%, $p = 0.003$, chi-square test). This finding should be interpreted with caution, since the series of both Applefeld and Wiernik (1983) and Gottdiener et al. (1983) contain patients who were older than 50 at the time of cardiac evaluation, whereas all but 1 of the series where treatment consisted of equally weighted portals contain only patients younger than 50. Furthermore, some patients have been followed up only for a few years, and the methods of cardiac evaluation have been variable. With the exception of the series investigated by Pohjola-Sintonen et al. and Gustavsson et al., which both had a high frequency of cardiac abnormalities, the series contain patients also treated with chemotherapy. Thyroid function has rarely been evaluated, although patients with mantle radiotherapy seldom have completely normal thyroid function, which may contribute to CAD in these patients (Morgan et al. 1985; Gustavsson et al. 1990).

The series with anteriorly weighted therapy also report a high frequency of cardiac complications other than CAD. As many as 46 (96%) of the 48 patients investigated by Applefeld and Wiernik (1983) had cardiac disease discovered, which included cases of pericarditis (24 patients), abnormal hemodynamic response to fluid challenge (14 patients), CAD (6 patients), and ventricular dysfunction (2 patients). In the study by Morgan et al. (1985) a subcarinal shield was inserted after 30 Gy, and Green et al. (1987) used a low midplane mediastinal dose in their pediatric series (median 31 Gy). Both of these series report a low frequency of cardiac complications compared with studies where the median cardiac dose was 35 Gy or greater (Applefeld and Wiernik 1983; Gomez et al. 1983; Gottdiener et al. 1983; Pohjola-Sintonen et al. 1987; Kadota et al. 1988; Gustavsson et al. 1990). In addition to anterior weighting and a large total dose delivered, irradiation of a large volume of the heart has been found to be associated with decreased cardiac performance (Savage et al. 1990).

Other Evidence

Information on the effect of radiotherapy on cardiovascular mortality can be obtained from randomized trials in which one arm is treated with chest irradiation and the other is not. This kind of evidence is lacking in Hodgkin's disease, but there are such data available from adjuvant irradiation of breast cancer following mastectomy, and they are briefly discussed here.

Jones and Ribeiro (1989) recently reported the long-term results of the Manchester trial in England, where 1461 patients with operable breast cancer were randomized after radical mastectomy to receive either postoperative radiotherapy (709 patients) or a watching policy (752 patients) with radiotherapy reserved for local recurrence. The authors report a significant increase in cardiovascular mortality after 15 years of follow-up in patients treated with radiotherapy compared with those not treated. Mortality caused by myocardial infarction was not compared between the two arms, but acute myocardial infarction was a common cause of death in the series, second only to death from breast cancer.

Similarly, in the Oslo trial in Norway (Høst et al. 1986) an increase in the number of cardiac deaths was observed in patients who received postoperative radiotherapy after Halsted's radical mastectomy (and ovarian radiation). A significant increase in the number of deaths caused by myocardial infarction was observed in stage I patients treated with ^{60}Co irradiation; most of the infarctions were seen in patients treated for cancer of the left breast. The follow-up time ranged from 11 to 20 years, and the increased mortality from causes other than breast cancer became apparent only after the first 5 years of follow-up. Haybittle et al. (1989) found excess mortality from causes other than breast cancer among 1376 women treated with adjuvant postoperative radiotherapy following simple mastectomy as compared with 1424 women treated with simple mastectomy alone. The follow-up time ranged from 13 to 18 years. The excess mortality resulted from deaths from new malignancies and cardiac disease. It became evident during the second decade of follow-up, and was mainly seen in women who had tumors of the left breast and who had been treated with orthovoltage radiotherapy.

Orthovoltage or ^{60}Co radiotherapy and a large fraction size were used in these trials, and other criticisms can be made (Levitt and Fletcher 1991). Yet they provide evidence that mediastinal irradiation may cause excess mortality from cardiac disease and myocardial infarction. They, together with other studies (Applefeld et al. 1981; Annest et al. 1983), also suggest that a long follow-up period from 5 to 15 years may be needed for radiation-related heart disease to become manifest. Again, cardiac complications appear to be fewer and the treatment benefit greater if more modern irradiation techniques are used in adjuvant irradiation for breast cancer (Wallgren et al. 1986; Haybittle et al. 1989).

Conclusions

Experimental data, case reports on precocious myocardial infarction in young patients with no or a few risk factors for CAD, autopsy studies, cardiac evaluation of cohorts of patients irradiated for Hodgkin's disease, clinical series, and data from randomized trials on adjuvant treatment of breast cancer all provide evidence that cardiac irradiation is a risk factor for CAD and myocardial infarction. The exact mechanisms of radiation-related CAD are not established, and additional factors, such as a diet rich in lipids, smoking, and concomitant and earlier diseases may play a role. There is evidence that the frequency of radiation-related CAD is greatly dependent on the technique of irradiation used. At present, the major portion of the evidence on radiation-related CAD comes from patients irradiated with techniques not considered appropriate today (Corn et al. 1990).

Recommendations

The hazards of radiotherapy need to be weighted against the benefits. Recent results show that prolonged survival with apparently good quality of life can be achieved in the majority of patients with early stage Hodgkin's disease treated with radiotherapy alone. The heart and the coronary arteries must be recognized to be sensitive to irradiation. Irradiation should preferably be given with a linear accelerator and using a small daily fraction size (<2 Gy/fraction). Both the anterior and the posterior portals should be treated daily. Shielding of the heart with a subcarinal block inserted at about 30 Gy total dose should be considered whenever possible (Carmel and Kaplan 1976), as well as shielding of the cardiac apex. The shrinking field technique should be considered to minimize the volume of the heart irradiated to a high dose.

Although the role of other risk factors for arteriosclerosis in the genesis of radiation-related CAD remains obscure, discontinuing tobacco smoking, dietary counseling, and control of hypertension, thyroid dysfunction, and obesity may be of value in the prevention of radiation-related CAD. More data are required on the cardiac effects of modern irradiation methods, and autopsy studies, prospective cohort studies with careful assessment of the cardiac function, and results from clinical series with long follow-up are needed.

References

Ali MK, Khalil KG, Fuller LM, Leachman RD, Sullivan MP, Loh KK. Gamble JF, Shullenberger CC (1976) Radiation-related myocardial injury: management of two cases. Cancer 38:1941–1946

Amromin GD, Gildenhorn HL, Solomon RD, Nadkarni BB, Jacobs ML (1964) The synergism of x-irradiation and cholesterol-fat feeding on the development of coronary artery lesions. J Atheroscler Res 4:325–334

Angelini A, Benciolini P, Thiene G (1985) Radiation-induced coronary obstructive atherosclerosis and sudden death in a teenager. Int J Cardiol 9:371–373

Annest LS, Anderson RP, Li W, Hafermann MD (1983) Coronary artery disease following mediastinal radiation therapy. J Thorac Cardiovasc Surg 85:257–263

Applefeld MM, Wiernik PH (1983) Cardiac disease after radiation therapy for Hodgkin's disease: analysis of 48 patients. Am J Cardiol 51:1679–1681
Applefeld MM, Cole JF, Pollock SH, Sutton FJ, Slawson RG, Singleton RT, Wiernik PH (1981) The late appearance of chronic pericardial disease in patients treated by radiotherapy for Hodgkin's disease. Ann Intern Med 94:338–341
Artom C, Lofland HB, Clarkson TB (1965) Ionizing radiation, atherosclerosis, and lipid metabolism in pigeons. Radiat Res 26:165–177
Boivin J-F, Hutchison GB (1982) Coronary heart disease mortality after irradiation for Hodgkin's disease. Cancer 49:2470–2475
Bradley EW, Zook BC, Casarett GW, Rogers CC (1981) Coronary arteriosclerosis and atherosclerosis in fast neutron or photon irradiated dogs. Int J Radiat Oncol Biol Phys 7:1103–1108
Brosius FC, Waller BF, Roberts WC (1981) Radiation heart disease: analysis of 16 young (aged 15 to 33 years) necropsy patients who received over 3500 rads to the heart. Am J Med 70:519–530
Budin JA, Casarella WJ, Harisiadis L (1976) Subclavian artery occlusion following radiotherapy for carcinoma of the breast. Radiology 118:169–173
Burns RJ, Bar-Shlomo B-Z, Druck MN, Herman JG, Gilbert BW, Perrault DJ, McLaughlin PR (1983) Detection of radiation cardiomyopathy by gated radionuclide angiography. Am J Med 74:297–302
Butler MJ, Lane RHS, Webster JHH (1980) Irradiation injury to large arteries. Br J Surg 67:341–343
Byhardt R, Brace K, Ruckdeschel J, Chang P, Martin R, Wiernik P (1975) Dose and treatment factors in radiation-related pericardial effusion associated with the mantle technique for Hodgkin's disease. Cancer 35:795–802
Carlson RG, Mayfield WR, Normann S, Alexander JA (1991) Radiation-associated valvular disease. Chest 99:538–545
Carmel RJ, Kaplan HS (1976) Mantle irradiation in Hodgkin's disease: an analysis of technique, tumor eradication, and complications. Cancer 37:2813–2825
Cohn KE, Stewart JR, Fajardo LF, Hancock EW (1967) Heart disease following irradiation. Medicine 46:281–298
Corn BW, Trock BJ, Goodman RL (1990) Irradiation-related ischemic heart disease. J Clin Oncol 8:741–750
Dollinger MR, Lavine DM, Foye LV (1966) Myocardial infarction due to postirradiation fibrosis of the coronary arteries. JAMA 195:316–319
Donaldson SS, Kaplan HS (1982) Complications of treatment of Hodgkin's disease in children. Cancer Treat Rep 66:977–989
Dunsmore LD, Loponte MA, Dunsmore RA (1986) Radiation-induced coronary artery disease. J Am Coll Cardiol 8:239–244
Fajardo LF (1977) Radiation-induced coronary artery disease. Chest 71:563–564
Fajardo LF, Stewart JR (1970) Experimental radiation-induced heart disease. Am J Pathol 59:299–316
Fajardo LF, Stewart JR (1973) Pathogenesis of radiation-induced myocardial fibrosis. Lab Invest 29:244–257
Gold H (1961) Production of atherosclerosis in the rat: effect of X-ray and a high-fat diet. Arch Pathol 71:268–273
Gomez GA, Park JJ, Panahon AM, Parthasarathy KL, Pearce J, Reese P, Bakshi S, Henderson ES (1983) Heart size and function after radiation therapy to the mediastinum in patients with Hodgkin's disease. Cancer Treat Rep 67:1099–1103
Gottdiener JS, Katin MJ, Borer JS, Bacharach SL, Green MV (1983) Late cardiac effects of therapeutic mediastinal irradiation. N Engl J Med 308:569–572
Green DM, Gingell RL, Pearce J, Panahon AM, Ghoorah J (1987) The effect of mediastinal irradiation on cardiac function of patients treated during childhood and adolescence for Hodgkin's disease. J Clin Oncol 5:239–245

Gustavsson A, Eskilsson J, Landberg T, Svahn-Tapper G, White T, Wollmer P, Akerman M (1990) Late cardiac effects after mantle radiotherapy in patients with Hodgkin's disease. Ann Oncol 1:355–363
Hancock SL, Hoppe RT, Horning SJ, Rosenberg SA (1988) Intercurrent death after Hodgkin disease therapy in radiotherapy and adjuvant MOPP trials. Ann Intern Med 109:183–189
Haybittle LJ, Brinkley D, Houghton J, A'Hern RP, Baum M (1989) Postoperative radiotherapy and late mortality: evidence from the Cancer Research Campaign trial for early breast cancer. Br Med J 298:1611–1614
Hoppe RT, Coleman CN, Cox RS, Rosenberg SA, Kaplan HS (1982) The management of stage I–II Hodgkin's disease with irradiation alone or combined modality therapy: the Stanford experience. Blood 59:455–465
Høst H, Brennhovd IO, Loeb M (1986) Postoperative radiotherapy in breast cancer: long-term results from the Oslo study. Int J Radiat Oncol Biol Phys 12:727–732
Huff H, Sanders EM (1972) Coronary-artery occlusion after radiation. N Engl J Med 286:780
Iqbal SM, Hanson EL, Gensini GG (1977) Bypass graft for coronary arterial stenosis following radiation therapy. Chest 71:664–666
Joensuu H (1989) Acute myocardial infarction after heart irradiation in young patients with Hodgkin's disease. Chest 95:388–390
Jones JM, Ribeiro GG (1989) Mortality patterns over 34 years of breast cancer patients in a clinical trial of post-operative radiotherapy. Clin Radiol 40:204–208
Kadota RP, Burgert EO, Driscoll DJ, Evans RG, Gilchrist GS (1988) Cardiopulmonary function in long-term survivors of childhood Hodgkin's lymphoma: a pilot study. Mayo Clin Proc 63:362–367
Kinsella TJ, Fraass BA, Glatstein E (1982) Late effects of radiation therapy in the treatment of Hodgkin's disease. Cancer Treat Rep 66:991–1001
Kirkpatrick JB (1967) Pathogenesis of foam cell lesions in irradiated arteries. Am J Pathol 50:291–309
Kopelson G, Herwig KJ (1978) The etiologies of coronary artery disease in cancer patients. Int J Radiat Oncol Biol Phys 4:895–906
Lauk S, Trott K-R (1990) Endothelial cell proliferation in the rat heart following local heart irradiation. Int J Radiat Biol 57:1017–1030
Leong ASY, Forbes IJ, Ruzic T (1979) Radiation-related coronary artery disease in Hodgkin's disease. Aust NZ J Med 9:423–425
Levinson SA, Close MB, Ehrenfeld WK, Stoney RJ (1973) Carotid artery occlusive disease following external irradiation. Arch Surg 107:395–397
Levitt SH, Fletcher GH (1991) Trials and tribulations: do clinical trials prove that irradiation increases cardiac and secondary cancer mortality in breast cancer patients? Int J Radiat Oncol Biol Phys 20:523–527
Lindsay S, Kohn HI, Dakin RL, Jew J (1962) Aortic arteriosclerosis in the dog after localized aortic x-irradiation. Circ Res 10:51–60
Loeffler RK (1975) Subclavian artery occlusion following radiation therapy. Invest Radiol 10:391–393
Mauch P, Tarbell N, Weinstein H, Silver B, Goffman T, Osteen R, Zajac A, Coleman CN, Canellos G, Rosenthal D (1988) Stage IA and IIA supradiaphragmatic Hodgkin's disease: prognostic factors in surgically staged patients treated with mantle and paraaortic irradiation. J Clin Oncol 6:1576–1583
McEniery PT, Dorosti K, Schiavone WA, Pedrick TJ, Sheldon WC (1987) Clinical and angiographic features of coronary artery disease after chest irradiation. Am J Cardiol 60:1020–1024
McReynolds RA, Gold GL, Roberts WC (1976) Coronary heart disease after mediastinal irradiation for Hodgkin's disease. Am J Med 60:39–45

Miller DD, Waters DD, Dangoisse V, David P-R (1983) Symptomatic coronary artery spasm following radiotherapy for Hodgkin's disease. Chest 83:284–285
Mittal B, Deutsch M, Thompson M, Lee Dameshek H (1986) Radiation-induced accelerated coronary arteriosclerosis. Am J Med 81:183–184
Morgan GW, Freeman AP, McLean RG, Jarvie BH, Giles RW (1985) Late cardiac, thyroid, and pulmonary sequelae of mantle radiotherapy for Hodgkin's disease. Int J Radiat Oncol Biol Phys 11:1925–1931
Murphy GK (1977) Cancer and the coroner. JAMA 237:786–788
Nakhjavan FK, Yazdanfar S, Friedman S (1984) Percutaneous transluminal angioplasty for stenosis of the ostium of the right coronary artery after irradiation for Hodgkin's disease. Am J Cardiol 53:341–342
Ormerod LP (1976) Acquired coarctation of the aorta: a long term complication of irradiation. Br Med J 2:977
Pearson HES (1957) Coronary occlusion following thoracic radiotherapy: 2 cases. Proc R Soc Med 50:516
Perrault DJ, Levy M, Herman JD, Burns RJ, Bar Shlomo B-Z, Druck MN, Wu WQ, McLaughlin PR, Gilbert BW (1985) Echocardiographic abnormalities following cardiac radiation. J Clin Oncol 3:546–551
Pohjola-Sintonen S, Tötterman K-J, Salmo M, Siltanen P (1987) Late cardiac effects of mediastinal radiotherapy in patients with Hodgkin's disease. Cancer 60:31–37
Prentice RTW (1965) Myocardial infarction following radiation. Lancet 2:388
Radwaner BA, Geringer R, Goldmann AM, Schwartz MJ, Kemp HG (1987) Left main coronary artery stenosis following mediastinal irradiation. Am J Med 82:1017–1020
Rasmussen S, Dossing M, Walbom-Jorgensen S (1978) Coronary heart disease: a possible risk in megavoltage therapy? Acta Med Scand 203:237–239
Ringrose TL (1974) Radiation-"induced" coronary artery disease. JAMA 230:961–962
Rodgers DL (1976) Precocious myocardial infarction after radiation treatment for Hodgkin's disease. Chest 70:675–677
Ross R (1986) The pathogenesis of atherosclerosis: an update. N Engl J Med 314:488–500
Ross R, Glomset JA (1976) The pathogenesis of atherosclerosis. N Engl J Med 295:369–377
Savage DE, Constine LS, Schwartz RG, Rubin P (1990) Radiation effects on left ventricular function and myocardial perfusion in long term survivors of Hodgkin's disease. Int J Radiat Oncol Biol Phys 19:721–727
Schechter JP, Jones SE (1975) Myocardial infarction in a 27-year-old woman: possible complication of treatment with VP-16-213 (NSC-141540), mediastinal irradiation, or both. Cancer Chemother Rep 59:887–888
Silverberg GD, Britt RH, Goffinet DR (1978) Radiation-induced carotid artery disease. Cancer 41:130–137
Simon EB, Ling J, Mendizabal RC, Midwall J (1984) Radiation-induced coronary artery disease. Am Heart J 108:1032–1034
Stewart JR, Fajardo LF (1978) Cancer and coronary artery disease. Int J Radiat Oncol Biol Phys 4:915–916
Stewart JR, Fajardo LF (1984) Radiation-induced heart disease: an update. Prog Cardiovasc Dis 27:173–194
Stewart JR, Fajardo LF, Cohn KE, Page V (1968) Experimental radiation-induced heart disease in rabbits. Radiology 91:814–817
Tenet W, Missri J, Hager D (1986) Radiation-induced stenosis of the left main coronary artery. Cathet Cardiovasc Diagn 12:169–171
Tommaso CL, Applefeld MM, Scherlis L, singleton RT (1984) Incidence and etiology of isolated left main coronary artery stenosis. Chest 86:284 (abstract)

Tötterman KJ, Pesonen E, Siltanen P (1983) Radiation-related chronic heart disease. Chest 83:875–878

Tracy GP, Brown DE, Johnson LW, Gottlieb AJ (1974) Radiation-induced coronary artery disease. JAMA 228:1660–1662

Voelker W, Schuler U, Ehninger G, Jacksch R, Mauser M, Steidle B, Karsch KR (1987) Vorderwandinfarkt bei einem 18järigen patienten mit M. Hodgkin. Dtsch Med Wochenschr 112:1216–1219

Wallgren A, Arner O, Bergström J, Blomstedt B, Granberg P-O, Räf L, Silfverswärd C, Einhorn J (1986) Radiation therapy in operable breast cancer: results from the Stockholm trial on adjuvant radiotherapy. Int J Radiat Oncol Biol Phys 12:533–537

Yahalom J, Hasin Y, Fuks Z (1983) Acute myocardial infarction with normal coronary arteriogram after mantle field radiation therapy for Hodgkin's disease. Cancer 52:637–641

IV. Radiation Induced Sequelae of the Central Nervous System (CNS) and the Eye

Experimental Radiation Damage of the Central Nervous System

W. Calvo

Institut für Arbeits- und Sozialmedizin der Universität Ulm,
Albert-Einstein-Allee 11, W-7900 Ulm, Fed. Rep. of Germany

Introduction

Delayed radionecrosis, occurring in humans late after exposure of the brain to X-irradiation, has been reported since the very early use of X-rays for therapeutic purposes. The numerous experiments designed to elucidate the pathogenesis of radionecrosis pointed out changes occurring in either the stroma or the parenchyma of the tissues as the primary cause of late effects of ionizing radiation.

Recent studies by Calvo et al. (1987, 1988), by Hopewell et al. (1989), and by Reinhold et al. (1990) described a combined effect of the ionizing radiation on the vessels of the brain and their satellite astrocytes as the initial changes during the latent period preceding necrosis. The present article discusses and extends the information gained by the abovementioned authors, who form part of a group of scientists at European research centers who are jointly studying the late effects of ionizing radiation, under the name of the European Late Effects Project. Dr. Hopewell has described earlier in this volume (see Hopewell et al. "Microvasculature and Radiation Damage") the effects on the choroid plexus of rats; I shall describe here the changes to the white matter of the same animals.

Materials and Methods

Bilateral irradiation of the brain was carried out on anesthetized 3-month-old female Sprague–Dawley rats. Shielding ensured that the brain alone was irradiated. Radiation was from two parallel-opposed 250 kV X-ray units, operating at 15 mA, with 0.5 mm copper and 1.0 mm aluminum filters. The doses used were 17.5, 20, 22.5, or 25 Gy at a dose rate of 1.2 Gy/min. Observations were at 1, 12, 26, 39, and 52 weeks after irradiation on groups of 6–8 animals at each dose level, plus a comparable group of age-matched control rats.

Coronal sections of complete brain hemispheres at the level of the optic chiasma were stained by means of routine and special histological techniques. Selected brain areas were evaluated by electron microscopy. The main parameters measured were blood vessel changes, qualitative and quantitative glial changes, and the presence of necrosis. Endpoints such as paralysis or death of the animals are easy to observe but can only be ascertained after necrosis of the brain or the spinal cord has already destroyed its vital centers or the pathways responsible for the transmission of stimuli from these centers to the muscles. Therefore, such endpoints cannot be used to study the initial changes appearing in the central nervous system (CNS) before necrosis is established. For this reason we preferred to rely on the study of the initial morphological changes occurring in the brain during the latent period preceding necrosis. Such a study is time-consuming and requires a great effort on the part of the observer, but is clearly the best procedure for the interpretation of the pathogenesis of radionecrosis of the CNS.

Results

According to our observations on the time-related effects of X-irradiation in the brain of rats it is possible to categorie effects as early (before 6 months), intermediate (6–9 months), or late (beyond 9 months) after low single doses of 20, 22.5, or 25 Gy.

Early Effects

The first morphological changes observed in the irradiated brain consist of slight edema which appears to be limited to the perivascular space of dilated vessels of the fimbria, hippocampus, and corpus callosum (Fig. 1). Some lymphocytes and a few monocytes can occasionally be found in that space. Edema and vascular dilatation can be observed by 1 month after irradiation, but edema diminishes by the sixth month. A reduction in the number of endothelial cell nuclei also occurs before the sixth month.

Intermediate Effects

Intermediate effects occurring between the sixth and ninth months postirradiation consist in a number of spectacular changes abruptly appearing in the white matter before demyelination and necrosis take place (Figs. 2 and 3). We studied those changes in various areas of the brain, observing and

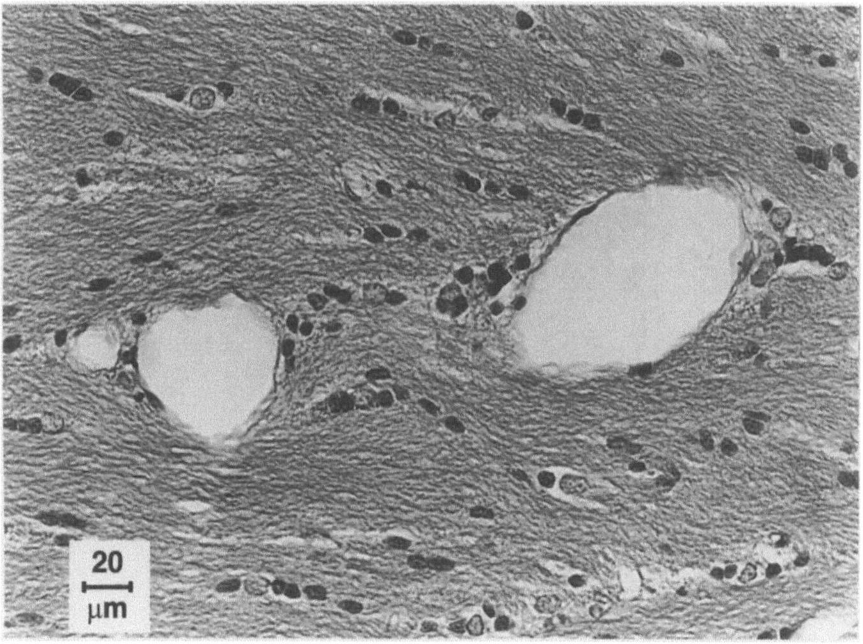

Fig. 1. Vasodilatation in well-myelinated fimbria of a rat 6 months after local X-irradiation with a dose of 25 Gy. Glial cells and nerve fibers still normal. Hematoxylin and eosin

quantitating the following parameters: (1) dilatation of blood vessels, (2) thickening of the blood vessel wall, (3) enlargement of endothelial cell nuclei, and (4) hypertrophy of perivascular astrocytes. The incidence of these four factors was highly correlated and, collectively, they were referred as a "tissue injury unit" (TIU). Such changes increased in incidence and severity until demyelination and necrosis ensued. Table 1 shows the difference in the time of appearance of the TIU and necrosis in the fimbria after irradiation of the rat brain with single X-ray doses of 20, 22.5, or 25 Gy. The TIU precedes necrosis by several weeks and is dose and time dependent. In the absence of any of the four changes which form the TIU, there was no necrosis within the whole period of observation (52 weeks) when the brain was irradiated with 22.5 or 25 Gy. Vessel changes such as telangiectasia were seen from 1 to 2 years after irradiation with 20 Gy, but some of the elements characteristic of the TIU were missing and necrosis was absent.

In addition to the abovementioned gliovascular changes, perivascular edema and proliferation of endothelial cell nuclei in some capillaries, with consequent reduction of the vessel lumen, may have contributed to cause ischemia and, therefore, anoxia, to which the neural parenchymal elements are known to be very sensitive.

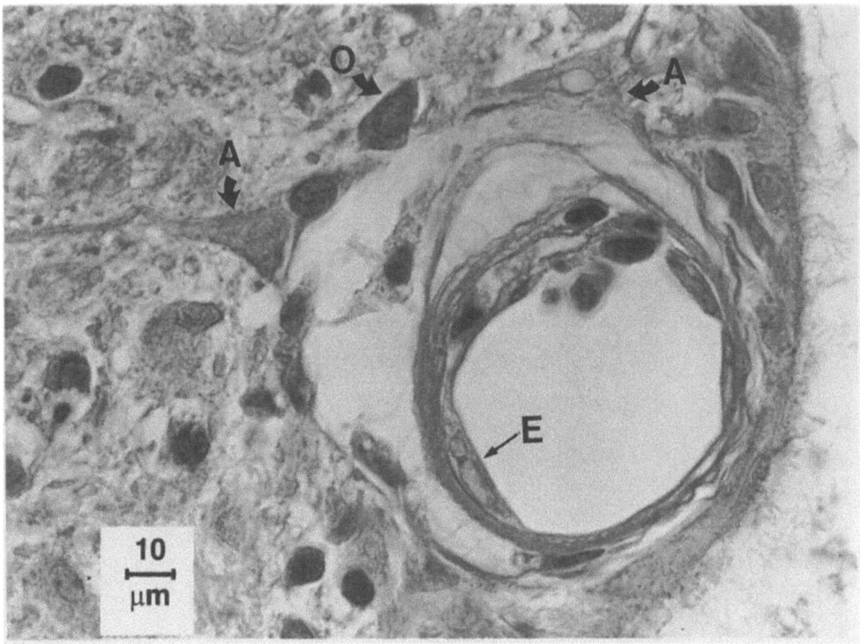

Fig. 2. Fimbria of a rat 9 months after 25 Gy. four changes characterizing the TIU are present: a dilated blood vessel with thickened wall, enlargement of endothelial cell nucleus (*E*), and hypertrophy of astrocytes (*A*). In addition, there is hypertrophy of oligodendrocytes (*O*) and perivascular edema. Luxol-PAS-hematoxylin

During the development of the intermediate changes there was no diminution in either the number of glial cells, the number of astrocytes, or the number of oligodendrocytes present in the fimbria or in the corpus callosum.

Late Effects

Late effects appear from the ninth to the twelfth month after doses of 22.5 or 25 Gy. Most of the late changes seem to be a consequence of the early and intermediate effects described above and, therefore, could be considered as a combination of degenerative and reactive phenomena.

The most evident late effects are the necrotic changes in the white matter. In the rat brain they appear first in the fimbria around the ninth month. About 3 months later, necrosis commences in the corpus callosum and in the capsula interna. Necrosis can be found in most of the white matter areas of the brain 12 months after 25 Gy. The superficial cortex and the meninges appeared to be much better preserved, even at the end of our observation

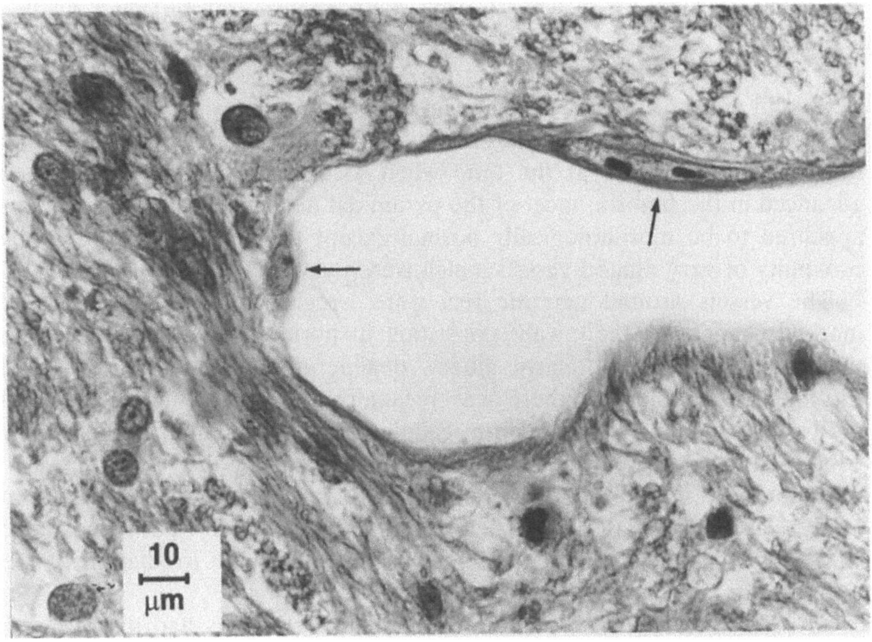

Fig. 3. Fimbria of a rat 9 months after 25 Gy. Giant endothelial cell nuclei (*arrows*) with enormous nucleoli are seen in the wall of extremely dilated blood vessel. Luxol-PAS-hematoxylin

Table 1. Latent period for the appearance of the combined changes defined as a tissue injury unit (TIU) and for necrosis in the fimbria of 50% of animals ($LP_{50} \pm SE$) after local irradiation of the rat brain with single doses of 20, 22.5, and 25 Gy of X-rays

Dose (Gy)	LP_{50} (weeks) after irradiation	
	TIU	Necrosis
20.0	Incomplete	Absent
22.5	33.1 ± 1.2	48.7 ± 2.9
25.0	24.8 ± 1.4	35.9 ± 2.6

period of 52 weeks. Only the deeper layers of the cortex appeared damaged, and then in areas intimately related to focal necrosis developed in the corpus callosum.

Necrosis appeared as well-circumscribed round or oval areas in the white matter in the vicinity of vessel changes, while most of the neurons originating the myelinated tracts were still morphologically normal.

Recent necrotic areas were traversed by numerous interlacing swollen axons ending in knobs as seen in regenerating nerves (Fig. 4). This finding was interpreted as a sign of abortive regeneration of neuronal processes located in areas of the irradiated brain away from necrosis. For the fimbria, the neurons originating the efferent (myelinated) nerve fibers are located in the hippocampus and, at the time when focal necrosis was already well advanced in the fimbria, most of the pyramidal neurons of the hippocampus appeared to be morphologically normal except for the few located in the proximity of very dilated vessels which were pyknotic or had disappeared.

The vessels around necrotic foci were irregulary dilated and showed marked changes in their walls consisting in fibrinoid necrois, collagenous thickening, splitting of elastic fibers, degeneration of muscle cells, and thrombosis; occasionally there was recanalization of the lumen. Marked perivascular edema with moderate cellular perivascular infiltration, mostly composed of lymphocytes and monocytes, was also present.

Granulocytes were found rarely. Small extravasations of blood were seen in areas around the lateral ventricle 12 months after 25 Gy, but hemorrhage was not a distinct component of the lesions caused by irradiation of the brain in rats.

In more advanced necrotic areas, all neural elements had disappeared. Myelin, axons, oligodendrocytes, and astrocytes were absent in the center of

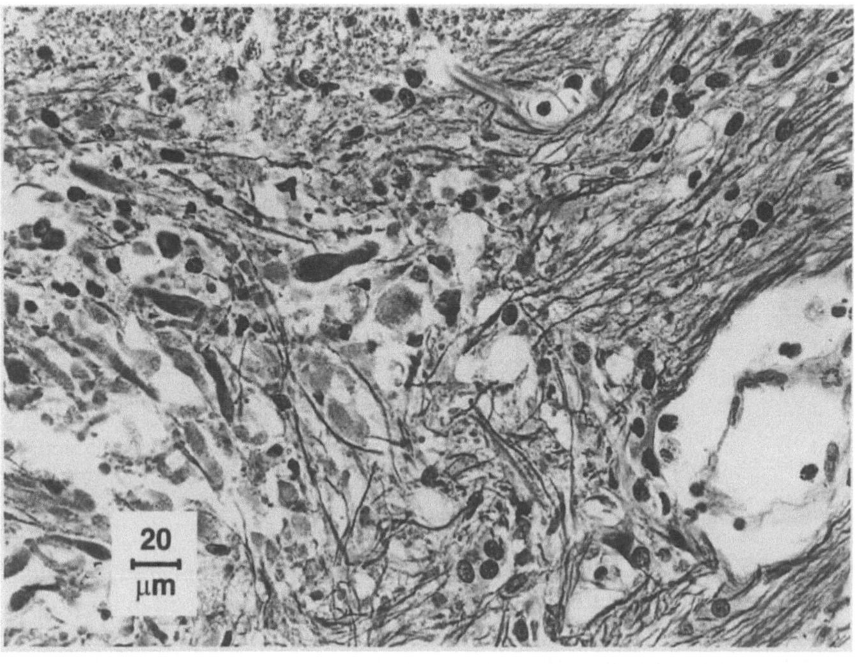

Fig. 4. Capsula interna of a rat 12 months after 25 Gy. There are swollen axons in an early necrotic area, edema, and perivascular infiltration. Holmes silver impregnation

necrotic areas. The blood vessels either disappeared or were present as walls lacking endothelial and muscle cells. The lumen was empty or thrombotic. The center of necrotic areas became invaded by phagocytes which dissolved the debris and produced liquefaction of the necrotic tissue, leaving pseudocysts.

Around the necrosis, in contrast, there was a mixed tissue composed of glial and vascular elements. The astrocytes and the oligodendrocytes were hypertrophic, with abnormal nuclei and cytoplasm. The presence of polynuclear and polynucleolar cells as well as the occasional mitosis found in both cell types was interpreted as an indication of reactive phenomena, probably induced by decaying products of the necrotic brain tissue.

An active microglial reaction can be seen also in areas adjacent to necrosis and even at a certain distance away, but was not a substantial component of the brain lesions.

An overview of the radio-induced morphological changes observed in the fimbria of rats irradiated with single X-ray dose of 22.5 Gy is given in Table 2.

Table 2. Radiation-induced morphological changes in the rat brain: observations in the fimbria after a single X-ray dose of 22.5 Gy

Time after irradiation	Vascular changes	Parenchymal changes
Early (within 6 months)	Minimal: Slight vesseel dilatation Occasional perivascular lymphocyte and monocyte infiltration Reduction of endothelial cell nuclei, slight edema	PAS-positive grains in astrocytes Lack of glial reaction
Intermediate (6–9 months)	Marked: Wide dilatation Thickening of walls Enlargement of endothelial nuclei Moderate edema	Reactive: Hypertrophy of astrocytes
Late (beyond 9 months)	Maximal: Muscle cell degeneration Marked fibrosis Fibrinoid degeneration Thrombosis Hemorrhage Marked edema Perivascular infiltration	Degenerative and reactive: Demyelination Focal necrosis Perifocal glial reaction Activation of microglia Loss of nerve fibers Abortive regeneration of axons Liquefaction of brain tissue Pseudocyst formation

Pathogenesis

The sequential study of the locally X-irradiated brain of rats with doses within the therapeutic range indicates that the CNS suffers morphological changes which manifest between the time of irradiation and the development of necrosis. Such changes begin as dilatation of vessels and perivascular edema in which fluid, some lymphocytes, and monocytes may be present. A few weeks later the vessel walls become thickened, their endothelial cells enlarge, and their satellite astrocytes suffer marked hypertrophy. As a consequence of such changes, the nutrition and the oxygen supply of the tissue are impaired and necrosis of the nerve cells is the likely consequence. A preponderance of white matter necrosis may be attributed to the marked differences in vascular density, which is much lower in the white than in the gray matter of the brain. Hyperplasia of astrocytes, present in the vicinity of necrosis may be a reactive phenomenon. Necrohormones and catabolites produced during degeneration of the nerve fibers stimulate proliferation of cells in the vicinity of necrotic areas. Necrosis appears always related to vessel changes and begins as small round or oval areas surrounded by morphologically normal tissue – a characteristic that points to vessel damage as the primary cause of necrosis of the CNS.

The swelling and the bulbous axon knobs which traverse the areas of necrosis in their initial stage, are changes similar to those produced by mechanical injury such as compression or sectioning of nerves, and were interpreted as the start of regenerative development of neuronal processes.

Hypertrophy and hyperplasia of oligodendrocytes at the edge of the initial necrotic areas seem to be the contribution of the myelin-forming cells to the regeneration of axons.

Complete regeneneration was not possible due to the increase in severity of the vessel changes, which became fibrotic and even thrombotic at later times after irradiation, causing total necrosis in their vicinity.

All nerve cell structures degenerated in old necrotic areas, and their debris was removed by phagocytes which later disappeared, leaving empty spaces.

The degenerative process is progressive and ends by destroying further areas until total brain necrosis ensues.

Discussion

Discrepancies in the reports describing the effects of irradiation on the CNS seem to be due to the use of different species, doses, dose rates, and field sizes, and to the types of parameters observed in each experiment. Therefore, our findings will be compared here with those reported by authors who used a similar methodology. In this way it will be possible to avoid analyzing the numerous papers with conflicting ideas already published in the literature that contain extensive analysis of the pathogenesis of delayed radiogenic injury in the nervous system. A comprehensive analysis of that type has been done by Zeman and Samorajski (1971) and by Haymaker et al. (1968), who reviewed 267 publications relating to the effects of irradiation on the nervous system.

Choice of Animals

Monkeys should have been used in studies comparing the effects of experimental procedures in animals with those produced by their use in human therapy, but the study of the possible changes occurring in the brain during the latent asymptomatic period preceding paralysis or death required the use of hundreds of animals. The cost of such experiments using monkeys was prohibitive. The fact that much cheaper animals such as rats could show morphological changes in the irradiated brain similar to those described in humans after the therapeutic use of irradiation was the reason for the decision to use rats in our experiments.

Females were chosen instead of animals of both sexes because the brain of female rats ceases to increase in size when they become adult (Hopewell 1971), while that of males continues to grow. Adult animals were used to avoid changes due to the destruction of the proliferative stem cells that exist in the paraventricular areas during the growing period of rats.

Doses

Single dose levels around 20 Gy were selected for our experiments on the basis that the induced effects in animals should be similar to those observed in the human brain after a full course of fractionated radiation therapy. The effect of the single X-ray doses at the level of 20–25 Gy was thought to be comparable to the effects of 60 Gy given as fractionated doses in 6 weeks (Reinhold 1974). Application of a higher dose will result in more extensive tissue damage, but it is questionable whether this is relevant to human therapy (Reinhold and Hopewell 1980). Hopewell and Wright (1970) observed that a dose of 20 Gy produced vascular lesions only, while doses of 30–40 Gy resulted in the death of the animals before vascular lesions could develop.

According to the abovementioned reasoning regarding the choice of animal species, sex, age, and irradiation conditions in our experiments, we believe we have matched the conditions existing in radiotherapy of adult humans; it could therefore be expected that the knowledge derived from our study could be used to elucidate the pathogenesis of the delayed injury suffered by the CNS in humans after ionizing irradiation.

Morphological Findings

Some of our findings confirm and extend those in the literature. Brain edema is a common reaction to toxic and physical insults. It appears to be associated with white matter necrosis and can be found early after ionizing irradiation. Its intensity varies in different species. In monkeys and dogs is marked and widespread, while in rodents it is less pronounced. Discrete edema was present in most of our rats within 3 months after irradiation and always around slightly dilated blood vessels. Edema diminished from the third to the sixth month and increased markedly shortly before the beginning of white matter demyelination, being maximal from the ninth to the twelfth month, in connection with necrotic areas.

Vasogenic edema is a consequence of the breakdown of the blood brain barrier (BBB; Klatzo 1967). We did not explore the changes in the BBB. Caveness et al. (1974) studied its damage in monkeys by measuring the cerebral spinal fluid pressure after X-irradiation with a dose of 3500 rads and found an abrupt brain swelling 18–36 weeks after irradiation caused by extravasation of fluid into the brain parenchyma. By means of the injection of Evans blue dye and electroencephalography, Remler et al. (1986) demonstrated the breakdown of the BBB as an effect of α-particle irradiation of the brain of rats. They concluded from their study that endothelial cell damage could be the main mechanism mediating the late radiation damage because the function of the BBB is a property of the vessel and not of the glia.

According to Rubinstein et al. (1962) extracellular edema leads to a secondary response by astrocytes. In our irradiated rats edema, vasodilatation, and loss of endothelial cells occurred early after irradiation, and the astrocyte reaction could be considered secondary to the early blood vessel changes.

Blood Vessel Changes

A decrease in the number of endothelial cells in the walls of capillaries and veins was one of the earliest morphological changes found after irradiation. It was observed in the vessels of the lung and mesentery and was quantified in the choroid plexus by Calvo et al. (1987) and in the pig skin by Archambeau et al. (1984). The reduction in the number of endothelial cells was associated with an abortive attempt at regeneration (Hopewell 1983), during which time groups of endothelial cells narrowed and even occluded the vessel lumen of many arterioles. The same process was observed in the capillaries of the choroid plexus by Calvo et al. (1987). The presence of mitotic figures demonstrated that the groups of endothelial cells resulted from active cell proliferation rather than from condensation by the shrinkage of tissue. Occlusion or narrowing of the vessel lumen is likely to produce a deficit in the oxygenation and nutrition of the nervous tissue and to be instrumental to the development of necrosis, since not only neurons but also axons are extremely sensitive to anoxia, as pointed out by Leone and Ochs (1978).

Vascular changes in the brain of rats after a moderate dose of X-rays (20 Gy) have been investigated by Reinhold and Hopewell (1980) using an angiographic method. The authors demonstrated a gradual development of focal telangiectasis which starts 12 months after irradiation in the vicinity of the lateral ventricles and continues over 2 years, during which time the animals behaved quite normally. An increase in the dose to 25 Gy produced a shortening of the time for the development of vascular abnormalities (Reinhold and Hopewell 1980). On the basis of a study of rats irradiated with X-ray doses in the same range as those used in our experiments (1300–2500 rads) Yoshii and Phillips (1982) found dose-dependent vessel damage between 41 and 87 weeks after irradiation. In their opinion, brain damage depends on the development of changes that originate in the blood vessels. Radiation myelopathy seems also to be preceded by vessel changes (Reinhold et al. 1984). Plotnikova et al. (1988) suggseted, therefore, using drugs to protect the microvasculature, hoping to increase the tolerance of the brain to local irradiation.

Electron microscopic studies of the vessels of irradiated brain tissue demonstrated a thickening of the basement membranes (Cervós-Navarro 1964; Blakemore and Palmer 1982). Such lesion was also observed by McDonald and Hayes (1967) in connection with perivascular edema. Endothelial cell damage seems to be effected primarily by the free radicals resulting from the ionizing irradiation. Cerebral vessels denuded by the loss of endothelial cells may induce platelet aggregation leading to thrombosis.

Glial Cells

A study of the glial population by Calvo et al. (1988) demonstrated a lack of reduction in the number of astroctyes prior to the development of necrosis. Instead of a reduction, hypertrophy of astrocytes, which appears during the changes preceding demyelination and necrosis, was associated with moderate hyperplasia. Hypertrophy and hyperplasia constitute the usual response of astrocytes to nervous tissue injury (Hortega and Penfield 1927; Rubinstein et al. 1962; Blakemore 1971). Zeman and Samorajski (1971) found that delayed degenerative changes in neuroglia cells are always present in the irradiated human brain. Furthermore, Arnold and Bailey (1954) described monstrous forms in the glial cells of the irradiated brain of primates. A number of astrocytes showing nuclear and cytoplasmic monstrosity were present near necrotic areas in our rats 12 months after a dose of 25 Gy (Calvo, Hopewell, Reinhold and Yeung, unpublished observations).

No significant changes were found in the relative number of oligodendrocytes near but not adjacent to necrotic areas. Within areas of necrosis all glial cells had disappeared, while in the adjacent areas the numbers of oligodendrocytes showed large variations. Groups of hypertrophic cells and even mitotic figures represented an active reaction to necrosis (Calvo et al. 1988). The very low correlation between the number of glial cells and the occurrence of demyelination in our experiments supports the observation by Blackemore and Palmer (1982) that a decrease in glial cells alone is unlikely to cause necrosis, and that vascular damage must play an important role in the damage of the CNS by irradiation.

Meninges

The lack of obvious lesions in the leptomeninges and the few changes found in most of the surface of the cortex – in contrast to the damage produced in the deeper layers of the cortex observed in our rats – is a phenomenon for which we do not have an explanation. Russel et al. (1949) reported similar findings in the irradiated brain of rabbits.

Necrosis

Investigations on the irradiated rat brain (Calvo et al. 1988) demonstrated the presence of white matter necrosis only at intervals of ⩾39 weeks after single doses of ⩾22.5 Gy. The fimbria of the hippocampus appeared to be the most radioresponsive. Necrosis of the white matter was preceded by changes in the vasculature and consisted of dilatation, enlargement of endothelial cell nuclei, thickening of the vessel wall, and hypertrophy of the adjacent astrocytes. These four parameters were highly correlated with each other and collectively appear to represent a tissue injury unit (TIU). Incidence and severity of damage to this gliovascular unit appear to increase with time after irradiation until necrosis develops. The latency associated with 50% incidence (LP_{50}) of the effect for the TIU was 11–13 weeks shorter than that for necrosis after single doses of 22.5 and 25 Gy.

Summary and Conclusions

1. The white matter of the brain of Spraque–Dawley rats, locally irradiated with X-rays at low single doses (20–25 Gy) showed morphological changes during the latent period preceding initiation of necrosis.
2. Morphological changes could be seen in the stroma and in the parenchymal components of the brain. Blood vessel changes preceded parenchymal changes.

3. Incidence and severity of lesions increased with time and dose.
4. Telangiectasia began to appear in the vessels of the white matter between the twelfth and fourteenth months after irradiation with a dose of 20 Gy, in the absence of necrosis.
5. Necrosis occurred within 9–12 months in the white matter after 22.5 or 25 Gy, and it developed in the fimbria earlier than in other areas of the brain.
6. The latency associated with 50% of rats developing necrosis in the fimbria (LP_{50}) was 48.7 ± 2.9 weeks after 22.5 Gy and 35.9 ± 2.6 weeks after 25 Gy.
7. Marked changes were seen in the vessels and their associated astrocytes during the latent period preceding necrosis. Such changes consisted of vessel dilatation, vessel wall thickening, enlargement of endothelial cell nuclei, and astrocyte hypertrophy. These changes have been referred to collectively as a tissue injury unit (TIU) and were accompanied by edema and perivascular infiltration of lymphocytes and monocytes.
8. The latency for the TIU preceded necrosis by 15.6 weeks after 22.5 Gy and by 11.1 weeks after 25 Gy.
9. Quantitative changes in the glial cells were also observed: astrocytes and oligodendrocytes increased in number at the margin of necrotic areas but disappeared from their center.
10. Necrosis appeared as small focal areas in tracts of white matter that were related to damaged vessels. The necrotic areas ended as pseudocysts after being dissolved by phagocytes.
11. The neurons in which the damaged tracts originated showed changes only in the immediate vicinity of damaged vessels.
12. The gray matter of the cortex showed morphological changes at a later time and after higher doses than those necessary to initiate white matter changes.

References

Archambeau JO, Ines A, Fajardo LF (1984) Response of the swine skin microcirculation to acute single exposures of X-rays: quantification of endothelial cell changes. Radiat Res 98:37–51

Arnold A, Bailey P (1954) Alterations in the glial cells following irradiation of the brain in primates. Arch Pathol 57:383

Blackemore WF (1971) The ultrastructure appearance of astrocytes following thermal lesions of the rat cortex. J Neurol Sci 12:319–332

Blakemore WF, Palmer AC (1982) Delayed infarction of spinal cord white matter following X-irradiation. J Pathol 137:273–280

Calvo W, Hopewell JW, Reinhold HS, van den Berg AP, Yeung TK (1987) Dose-dependent and time-dependent changes in the choroid plexus of the irradiated rat brain. Br J Radiol 60:1109–1117

Calvo W, Hopewell JW, Reinhold HS, Yeung TK (1988) Time- and dose-related changes in the white matter of the rat brain after single doses of X-rays. Br J Radiol 61:1043–1052

Caveness W, Tanaka A, Hess KH, Kemper TL, Tso MO, Zimmerman LE (1974) Delayed brain swelling and functional derangement after X-irradiation of the right visual cortex in *Macaca mulatta*. Radiat Res 57:104–120
Cervós-Navarro J (1964) Electronenmikroskopische Befunde an den Capillaren des Kaninchengehirns nach Einwirkung ionisierender Strahlen. Arch Psychiatr Nervenkr 205:204–214
Haymaker W, Ibrahim MZ, Miquel J, Call N, Riopelle A (1968) Delayed radiation effects in the brains of monkeys exposed to X- and gamma-rays. J Neuropathol Exp Neurol 27:50–79
Hopewell JW (1971) A quantitative study of the mitotic activity in the subependymal plate of adult rats. Cell Tissue Kinet 4:273–278
Hopewell JW (1983) Radiation effects on vascular tissue. In: Potten CS, Hendry JH (eds) Cytotoxic insult to tissue: effects on cell lineages. Churchill Livingstone, Edinburgh, pp 228–257
Hopewell JW, Wright EA (1970) The nature of latent cerebral irradiation damage and its modification by hypertension. Br J Radiol 43:161–167
Hopewell JW, Calvo W, Reinhold HS (1989) Radiation effects on blood vessels: role in late normal tissue damage. In: Steel GG, Adams GE, Horwich A (eds) The biological basis of radiotherapy, 2nd edn. Elsevier, Amsterdam
Hortega P del Rio, Penfield W (1927) Cerebral cicatrix: the reaction of neuroglia and microglia in brain wounds. Bull Johns Hopkins Hosp 41:278–303
Klatzo I (1967) Neuropathological aspects of brain edema. Neuropathol Exp Neurol 26:1–13
Leone J, Ochs S (1978) Anoxic block and recovery of axoplasmic transport and electrical excitability of nerve. J Neurobiol 9:229–245
McDonald LW, Hayes TL (1967) The role of capillaries in the pathogenesis of delayed radionecrosis of brain. Am J Pathol 50:745–764
Plotnikova ED, Levitman MK, Shaposhnikova VV, Koshevoj LV, Eidus LK (1988) Protection of microvasculature in rat brain against late radiation injury by gammaphos. Int J Radiat Oncol Biol Phys 15:1197–1201
Reinhold HS (1974) Structural changes in blood vessels. Curr Top Radiat Res Q 10:58–74
Reinhold HS, Hopewell JW (1980) Late changes in the architecture of blood vessels of the rat brain after irradiation. Br J Radiol 53:693–696
Reinhold HS, van Putten WL, Hopewell JW, van der Kogel AJ (1984) The late period in clinical radiation myelopathy. Int J Radiat Oncol Biol Pys 10:2385–2387
Reinhold HS, Calvo W, Hopewell JW, van den Berg AP (1990) Development of blood vessel-related radiation damage in the fimbria of the central nervous system. Int J Radiat Oncol Biol Phys 18:37–42
Remler M, Marcussen WH, Tiller-Borsich J (1986) The late effects of radiation on the blood brain barrier. Int J Radiat Oncol Biol Phys 12:1965–1969
Rubinstein LJ, Klatzo I, Miquel J (1962) Histochemical observations on oxidative enzyme activity of glial cells in a local brain injury. J Neuropathol Exp Neurol 21:116–137
Russel DS, Wilson CW, Tansley K (1949) Experimental radio-necrosis of the brain in rabbits. J Neurol Neurosurg Psychiatry 12:187–195
Yoshii Y, Phillips TL (1982) Late vascular effects of whole brain X-irradiation in the mouse. Acta Neurochir (wien) 64:87–102
Zeman W, Samorajski T (1971) Effects of irradiation on the nervous system. In: Berdjis CC (ed) Pathology of irradiation. Williams and Wilkins, Baltimore

Myelopathy and Hyperfractionated Accelerated Radiotherapy: A Radiobiological Interpretation

C.S. Wong[1], J. Van Dyk[2], and R.P. Hill[3]

[1] Department of Radiation Oncology, Princess Margaret Hospital, Toronto, Ontorio, Canada
[2] Department of Clinical Physics, Princess Margaret Hospital, Toronto, Ontario, Canada
[3] Research Division, Princess Margaret Hospital, Toronto, Ontario, Canada

Introduction

Where there is a rapid repopulation of tumor clonogens, a gain in local control should be realized by administering radiation treatments in a shorter overall time, thereby reducing the opportunity for proliferation of tumor cells during the treatment. Because of the differential effect of fractionation in early- versus late-responding normal tissues, decreased overall treatment time must be done in the context of keeping the fraction size small. The only feasible approach is to administer multiple fractions per day and use short interfraction intervals. Provided repair of sublethal radiation damage is largely complete within the interfraction interval, excessive late morbidity would not be expected. These radiobiological rationales of accelerated hyperfractionated radiotherapy thus suggest an altered fractionation scheme in which the overall treatment time is reduced, the dose per fraction is reduced, and multiple fractions are given per day.

The efficacy of accelerated hyperfractionated regimes on local tumor control and survival remains uncertain and mature data from well-designed prospective randomized trials are awaited. An unexpected late morbidity was the observations of radiation myelopathy. In the continuous hyperfractionated accelerated radiotherapy (CHART) regime at the Mount Vernon Hospital, Middlesex, England, there have been 4 cases of radiation myelopathy (Saunders et al. 1991). In a protocol of hyperfractionated accelerated radiotherapy for thyroid cancer at the Princess Margaret Hospital, Toronto, Canada, 2 patients were reported to have developed radiation myelopathy (Wong et al. 1991). All 6 patients developed radiation myelopathy at dose levels which were not expected to be associated with a significant risk to the spinal cord. In this article these cases will be analyzed in the context of the available clinical and radiobiological data, and a discussion of the possible radiobiological explanation for the myelopathy and the clinical implications will be presented.

Princess Margaret Hospital Experience

From January 1, 1975 to June 30, 1982, 32 patients underwent a protocol of accelerated hyperfractionated radiotherapy for anaplastic thyroid carcinomas. The clinical characteristics of these patients have been detailed previously (Wong et al. 1991). Most patients were given an initial single dose of 5 Gy using ^{60}Co or ^{137}Cs to prevent upper airway problems. This was followed by a protocol of accelerated hyperfractionated radiotherapy at a fraction size of 1 Gy, given 4 times a day to a total dose of 30–45 Gy. An interfraction interval of 3 h was chosen to allow patients to complete 4 fractions per day during the normal working hours of the radiotherapy clinics. Patients were not treated over weekends. Radiotherapy was given by ^{60}Co or 25 MV photons using anterior – posterior parallel-opposed fields. The volume irradiated encompassed the entire neck and upper mediastinum to the level of the carina. An anterior attenuator was routinely used for contour correction. A posterior spinal cord shield was introduced for most patients at 30–40 Gy. Fourteen patients received additional doxorubicin at 40 mg/m^2 intravenovsly every 3 weeks. There was a minimum follow-up of 3 years in all patients.

Only 7 of 32 patients achieved local control of 1 year or longer. The median survival was less than 6 months. The protocol was discontinued after 32 patients were treated. Early reactions, in particular in the skin and esophageal mucosa, were described as more intense than with conventional radiotherapy. No patients, however, failed to complete the protocol because of acute morbidity. All 6 patients who did not complete radiation therapy did so because of rapidly progressive local cancer or distant metastases.

An unexpected late morbidity was radiation myelopathy in 2 patients, neither of whom received doxorubicin. These 2 patients developed symptoms and signs of myelopathy at 8 and 13 months after spinal cord doses of 39.9 Gy and 48.3 Gy respectively. No errors were found when the radiotherapy records were reviewed.

Chart Regime

The CHART regime was initiated at the Mount Vernon Hospital in January 1985 and closed in March 1990 after the inclusion of 263 patients with mostly head and neck tumors or locally advanced non-small-cell carcinoma of the bronchus. A randomized multicenter trial is currently in progress in the United Kingdom and Europe comparing the CHART regime with conventional fractionation (Saunders et al. 1991). The initial 38 patients received a minimum tumor dose of 50.4 Gy in 36 treatments at a fraction size of 1.4 Gy over 12 days. An interfraction interval of 6 h was chosen. Because of acceptable acute morbidity, the total dose given to the subsequent patients was increased to 54 Gy using a fraction size of 1.5 Gy. The interfraction interval was kept at 6 h. Most patients received an initial dose of 42 Gy, followed by a volume reduction with the spinal cord excluded. The maximum allowable spinal cord dose was 44 Gy in the initial phase and a further 0.3–0.5 Gy in the boost fields.

Early reactions in the oral and pharyngeal mucosa were described as pronounced, but all healed eventually. Skin reactions were less severe than with conventional radiotherapy. There was no incidence of mucosal ulceration or bone necrosis when the experience was last updated. There was also a suggestion of better recovery of parotid function (Saunders et al. 1991).

An unexpected finding was the observation of 4 patients who developed radiation myelopathy. These patients presented at 6, 11, 12, and 24 months after total spinal cord doses of 46.0, 45.2, 48.3, and 46.6 Gy respectively (Saunders et al. 1991). All patients were treated for tumors of the head and neck. The permitted cord dose was reduced to a maximum of 40 Gy subsequent to the presentation of these cases. No further cases of radiation myelopathy had been observed when the experience was last updated (Saunders et al. 1991). There has not been an incidence of radiation myelopathy in the patients with bronchogenic carcinoma.

Discussion

All 6 patients developed radiation myelopathy at spinal cord doses which were considered to be well within spinal cord tolerance when these trials were commenced. When these cases were initially reported and analyzed (Dische and Saunders 1989; van der Kogel 1989; Wong et al. 1991a), there was no apparent explanation for the spinal cord damage seen. These cases of myelopathy therefore raise serious concern about the underlying radiobiological model upon which these altered fractionation schemes are based.

The first question to be addressed is: Did these patients have radiation myelopathy? The onset of neurological symptoms in these patients were consistent with the latent periods described for radiation myelopathy (Schultheiss et al. 1984). Their neurological symptoms and signs were consistent with the anatomical level of the spinal cord irradiated, and the clinical course was compatible with radiation injury. The diagnosis of radiation myelopathy is essentially a diagnosis of exclusion, as rarely is there histological confirmation. In these patients no other pathological process was apparent, thus the answer to the question above is affimative.

Clinical Spinal Cord Tolerance

The accepted spinal cord tolerance dose is generally considered to be 50 Gy given as 2 Gy daily fractions over 5 weeks (Schultheiss 1990). This estimate of the tolerance dose comes from extrapolation of data from retrospective series of patients, generally treated at much larger doses per fraction. Very few of these series gave the actual number of patients at risk, thus an incidence value is difficult to establish. In a series of 19 patients with radiation myelopathy reviewed by Reinhold et al. (1976), the lowest cord dose was 53.4 Gy in 26 fractions. In the series by Abbatucci et al. (1978) the lowest cord dose in patients with myelopathy was 51 Gy in 18 daily fractions. There was no incidence of myelopathy in 210 patients who received a lower cord dose with a follow-up of 2 years or longer. McCunniff and Liang (1989) reported only a single patient with radiation myelopathy out of 82 head and neck cancer patients followed for at least a year and in whom the cord dose exceeded 56 Gy in daily fraction sizes of 1.3–1.8 Gy. In a review of the incidence of myelopathy after irradiation of the cervical spinal cord for head and neck cancer at the University of Florida, Marcus and Million (1990) reported only 2 cases of radiation myelopathy out of a total of 1112 evaluable patients. These patients all had a minimum of 30 Gy to at least 2 cm of the cervical spinal cord, and had a minimum of 1 year of follow-up. The risk of myelopathy at each dose level was 0/124 at 30.0–39.9 Gy, 0/442 at 40.0–44.9 Gy, 2/471 at 45.0–49.9 Gy, and 0/75 at a dose of 50.0 Gy or greater. These results suggest that the risk of myelopathy following the spinal cord "tolerance" dose, i.e., 50 Gy in 2 Gy daily fractions, is indeed very small, probably less than 0.5%.

In the series from the Princess Margaret Hospital (Wong et al. 1991), 2 of 32 patients developed radiation myelopathy. Most patients, however, died within 6 months of treatment, with only 7 patients surviving a year or longer. In a recent literature review of more than 300 cases of radiation myelopathy, the median latent period was approximately 20 months (Schultheiss et al. 1984). Therefore, the actuarial risk of myelopathy for this protocol is much greater. In CHART, 4 cases of radiation myelopathy were observed in the 74 cases of head and neck carcinoma (Saunders et al. 1991). The actuarial 2-year survival for these patients was 63%. No myelopathy cases were observed in the patients treated for carcinoma of the bronchus. However, only 39 patients received a cord dose of 40 Gy or higher, and very few were long-term survivors (Saunders et al. 1991). Whilst it remains possible that the 4 cases in CHART and the 2 cases reported by Wong et al. (1991) were idiosyncratic responses, the actuarial incidences of radiation myelopathy in these protocols suggest otherwise.

In contrast to these results, only 1 case of myelopathy has been reported from the EORTC advanced head and neck trial (van der Bogaart et al. 1986). This patient received a cord dose of 56 Gy because of a calculation error. In this study, a dose of 48 Gy in 30 fractions was given 3 times a day with a 4-h interfraction interval over 10–12 days. Over 500 patients were treated and a maximum cord dose of 45 Gy was allowed. This conflicts with the CHART and Princess Margaret Hospital experience. However, it appears that a more conservative cord dose of a maximum of only 40 Gy was used (Dische 1991).

No apparent error was found in the treatment records of the CHART and Princess Margaret Hospital patients. It should be noted, however, that even though a review of all records suggested no dosimetric errors, technical errors can never be totally excluded. Both patients reported by Wong et al. (1991) were hypertensive. There is little evidence, however, to support the hypothesis that hypertension increases the susceptibility of spinal cord damage to irradiation. In rats, hypertension has been shown to shorten the latent period and also to lower the threshold of radiation damage to the cerebral hemispheres (Hopewell and Wright 1970). However, Reinhold et al. (1976) reported lower systolic blood pressure in their patients who developed radiation myelopathy. Dische et al. (1988) also found no association of radiation myelopathy with blood pressure. One of the myelopathy cases in CHART was described as having evidence from magnetic resonance imaging of cervical spondylosis (Dische and Saunders 1989). Whether this could predispose the patient to radiation myelopathy is conjectural. None of the other myelopathy patients in CHART appeared to have any unusual susceptibility for spinal cord damage.

In the accelerated hyperfractionation protocols, when compared with standard fractionated radiotherapy, three other parameters, in addition to the total dose, were altered: (1) the overall treatment time was reduced; (2) the interfraction interval was reduced; and (3) the fraction size was reduced. How might these changes alter the effect of radiation damage?

Influence of Overall Treatment Time

Could reducing the overall treatment time increase the risk of myelopathy? Human myelopathy data have been reasonably well described by isoeffect formulae with a small time component (Wara et al. 1975; Reinhold et al. 1976; Abbatucci et al. 1978). However, changes in overall treatment time in these retrospective series have been invariably related to changes in fractionation, such that the actual contribution of time could not be adequately assessed. In the rat spinal cord there was no evidence of a change in tolerance dose which could be attributed to time unless the treatment time exceeded 8 weeks (van der Kogel 1986; Wong et al. unpublished). These results suggest that a proliferative response probably does not occur for many weeks after the beginning of irradiation. This is consistent with the slow rate of turnover of target cells in the central nervous system. Extrapolation of these animal results would suggest that reducing the overall time from 5 or 6 weeks to 2 weeks will be unlikely to increase the risk of myelopathy.

Effect of Small Fraction Sizes

A significant thrust in the application of altered fractionation regimes in clinical radiotherapy is the apparent satisfactory description of biological and clinical data by the linear-quadratic (LQ) model. This model describes cell survival by the mathematical formula:

$$\text{Surviving fraction, } S = \exp - (\alpha d + \beta d^2)$$

Late-responding normal tissues have been shown to have small α/β values, whereas tumor cells and early-responding normal tissues have large α/β values. This suggests that reducing the size of the dose per fraction will result in differential sparing of late-responding normal tissues (Peters and Ang 1986). From the studies of normal tissues which have been reported so far, it can be concluded that the dose-fractionation response is described accurately by the LQ model over the radiation dose range from large single doses down to doses per fraction of about 2 Gy (Joiner 1989). Below 2 Gy per fraction the limited data from the literature have been controversial. For the rat spinal cord, initial analysis of data from Ang et al. (1985) and van der Schueren et al. (1988) suggested that the LQ model (α/β of 1.7 Gy) overestimated the isoeffect dose when treratments were below 2 Gy per fraction, i.e., the spinal cord would be seriously overdosed if the LQ model, based on data from large doses per fraction, were used to predict doses in clinical radiotherapy for small fraction sizes. These animal experiments of Ang et al. (1985) and van der Schueren et al. (1988) were done with irradiations given twice daily with a 4 h interval between the 2 daily fractions. In a subsequent reanalysis of the data (Thames et al. 1988) combined with data from experiments on repair kinetics (Ang et al. 1987), the pooled results could be fitted to the incomplete repair (IR) version of the LQ model (Thames 1985) assuming monoexponential repair kinetics and using a larger α/β value of 2.7 Gy and a repair half-time of 1.6 h.

In recent experiments by Wong et al. (1992), significant sparing at small fraction sizes has been observed in rat spinal cord. These experiments were done with irradiations given once daily. For fraction sizes ranging from 25.0 to 2.0 Gy per fraction, the data indicated consistency with the LQ model and gave an α/β value of 2.4 Gy. For fraction sizes ranging from 2 down to 1 Gy per fraction, the data, however, were inconsistent with the LQ model and gave a very small α/β value of 0.48 Gy. It was concluded that the LQ model based on data from large doses per fraction in fact underestimated and did not overestimate the sparing effect of small doses per fraction *provided sufficient time was allowed between each fraction for repair of sublethal damage*. These results also suggest that the IR model previously used in the reanalysis (Thames et al. 1988) of the data by Ang et al. (1985) and van der Schueren et al. (1988) might have underestimated the amount of incomplete repair between fractions with short intervals.

Effect of Short Interfraction Intervals

The IR model is an extension of the LQ model; and repair of sublethal damage is assumed to recover monoexponentially with time (Thames 1985).

Initial studies of repair kinetics in the rat spinal cord suggested a fairly good fit of the data to the IR model with a repair half-time of approximately 1.5 h (Ang et al. 1987). There also appeared to be no significant influence of fraction size (1.7–17.5 Gy) on the rate of repair (Ang et al. 1987). However, in recent experiments on repair kinetics in rat spinal cord using 2 Gy per fraction (Ang et al. 1990), significant recovery of sublethal damage was observed between 8 and 24 h, and the IR model with monoexponential repair kinetics could not satisfactorily describe the data. These animal results are therefore consistent with the data of Wong et al. (1992), and suggest that the previous reanalysis of the spinal cord data by Thames et al. (1988) using the IR model was invalid, and would have underestimated the amount of incomplete repair between fractions with short intervals in the experiments of Ang et al. (1985) and van der Schueren et al. (1988).

In an experiment by Lavey et al. (1991) in which the effect of hyperfractionation in mouse spinal cord was assessed, it is of interest that no increase in tolerance was observed when an irradiation scheme of twice-daily fractions of 1.2 Gy separated by 8 h was compared with a scheme of daily fractions of 2 Gy. Regardless of the models used to describe the data, experiments using short interfraction intervals suggested little further sparing of the rat or mouse spinal cord below 2 Gy per fraction. Data with irradiations given once daily, however, revealed significant sparing at small fraction sizes. The most likely explanation for the discrepancy is that the IR model with monoexponential repair kinetics does not adequately describes Elkind repair in the rat spinal cord, and that repair is incomplete even after an interfraction interval of 8 h. These results are therefore consistent with the presence of a slow component of the repair process.

In an analysis of the clinical myelopathy data following accelerated hyperfractionated radiotherapy by Wong et al. (1991), the IR model (α/β value of 2–4 Gy, monoexponential repair kinetics, half-times 1.5–3 h) was used to compare the spinal cord doses received by the patients who developed myelopathy with the accepted spinal cord tolerance dose, i.e., 50 Gy in 2 Gy daily fractions. Even allowing for lack of complete repair, when the doses were expressed in α damage units, these myelopathy cases received doses either below or only approaching what is generally accepted to be the tolerance dose for the spinal cord. It was concluded that there was no apparent radiobiological explanation for the observations if the radiobiological models were valid. The recent animal data from Wong et al. (1992) on small fraction sizes and Ang et al. (1990) on repair kinetics suggested that the most plausible explanation for the myelopathy was that the short interfraction intervals used in these accelerated regimes did not allow adequate time for repair.

To conclude, observations of six myelopathy cases in patients treated with accelerated hyperfractionated radiotherapy and recent animal data both suggest limitations of the LQ or the IR model and indicate that these models should be used with caution to predict spinal cord tolerance doses for altered fractionation regimes in clinical radiotherapy. The clinical observations also underscore the importance of obtaining radiobiological data in clinically relevant dose-fractionation schemes to confirm or refute predictions from biological models. The ultimate test of the validity of a biological model is, however, the clinical observations. At present, in clinical protocols of multiple daily fractions, it is essential to space the fractions with as long an interfraction interval as possible. In view of the devastating effect of radiation myelopathy, repair of sublethal damage in the spinal cord or central nervous system cannot be regarded to be complete even after an interfraction interval of 8 h.

Acknowledgments. This work was supported by a Terry Fox Program Project Grant from the National Cancer Institute (Canada).

References

Abbatucci JS, Delozier T, Quint R, Roussel A, Brune D (1978) Radiation myelopathy of the cervical spinal cord: time, dose and volume factors. Int J Radiat Oncol Biol Phys 4:239–248

Ang KK, van der Kogel AJ, van der Schueren E (1985) Lack of evidence for increased tolerance of rat spinal cord with decreasing fraction doses below 2 Gy. Int J Radiat Oncol Biol Phys 11:105–110

Ang KK, Thames HD, van der Kogel AJ, van der Schueren E (1987) Is the rate of repair of radiation-induced sublethal damage in rat spinal cord dependent on the size of dose per fraction? Int J Radiat Oncol Biol Phys 13:557–562

Ang KK, Jiang GL, Thames HD, Stephens LC (1990) Repair kinetics in rat spinal cord (abstract). In: Proceedings of the 38th annual meeting of the Radiation Research Society, New Orleans, p 113

Dische S (1991) Accelerated treatment and radiation myelitis. Radiother Oncol 20:1–2

Dische S, Saunders MI (1989) Continuous, hyperfractionated, accelerated radiotherapy (CHART): an interim report upon late morbidity. Radiother Oncol 6:65–72

Dische S, Warburton MF, Saunders MI (1988) Radiation myelitis and survival in the radiotherapy of lung cancer. Int J Radiat Oncol Biol Phys 15:75–81

Hopewell JW, Wright EA (1970) The nature of latent cerebral irradiation damage and its modification by hypertension. Br J Radiol 43:161–167

Joiner MC (1989) The dependence of radiation response on the dose per fraction. BIR Rep 19:20–26

Lavey RS, Johnstone AK, Tracy JT, Taylor JMG, McBride WH (1991) Effect of hyperfractionation on "spinal cord" tolerance. Int J Radiat Oncol Biol Phys 21S:164–165

Marcus RB, Million RR (1990) The incidence of myelitis after irradiation of the cervical spinal cord. Int J Radiat Oncol Biol Phys 17S:163

McCunniff AJ, Liang MJ (1989) Radiation tolerance of the cervical spinal cord. Int J Radiat Oncol Biol Phys 16:675–678

Peters LJ, Ang KK (1986) Unconventional fractionation schemes in radiotherapy. In: DeVita V, Hellman S, Rosenberg A (eds) Important advances in oncology. Lippincott, Philadelphia, pp 269–286

Reinhold HS, Kaalen JGAH, Unger-Gils K (1976) Radiation myelopathy of the thoracic spinal cord. Int J Radiat Oncol Biol Phys 1:651–657
Saunders MI, Dische S, Grosch EJ, Fermont DC, Ashford RFU, Maher EJ, Makepeace AR (1991) Experience with CHART. Int J Radiat Oncol Biol Phys 21:871–878
Schultheiss TE (1990) Spinal cord radiation "tolerance": doctrine versus data. Int J Radiat Oncol Biol Phys 19:219–221
Schultheiss TE, Higgins EM, El-Mahdi AM (1984) The latent period in clinical radiation myelopathy. Int J Radiat Oncol Biol Phys 10:1109–1115
Thames HD (1985) An "incomplete-repair" model for survival after fractionated and continuous irradiations. Int J Radiat Biol 47:319–339
Thames HD, Ang KK, Stewart FA, van der Schueren E (1988) Does incomplete repair explain the apparent failure of the basic LQ model to predict spinal cord and kidney responses to low doses per fraction? Int J Radiat Biol 54:13–19
Van de Bogaert W, van der Schueren E, Horiot JC (1986) (EORTC cooperative group of radiotherapy). Early results of the EORTC randomized clinical trial on multiple fractions per day (MFD) and misonidazole in advanced head and neck cancer. Int J Radiat Oncol Biol Phys 12:587–591
Van der Kogel AJ (1986) Radiation-induced damage in the central nervous system: an interpretation of target cell responses. Br J Cancer 53 [Suppl]:207–217
Van der Kogel AJ (1989) Continuous hyperfractionated, accelerated radiotherapy. Radiother Oncol 16:75–77
Van der Schueren E, Landuyt W, Ang KK, van der Kogel AJ (1988) From 2 Gy to 1 Gy per fraction: sparing effect in rat spinal cord? Int J Radiat Oncol Biol Phys 14:297–300
Wara WM, Phillips TL, Sheline GE, Schwarde JG (1975) Radiation tolerance of the spinal cord. Cancer 35:1558–1562
Wong CS, van Dyk J, Simpson WJ (1991) Myelopathy following hyperfractionated accelerated radiotherapy for anaplastic thyroid carcinoma. Radiother Oncol 20: 3–9
Wong CS, Minkin S, Hill RP (1992) Linear quadratic model underestimates sparing effect of small doses per fraction in rat spinal cord. Radiother Oncol 23:176–184

Irradiation-Induced Brain Dysfunction in Children

R. Korinthenberg

Abteilung Neuropädiatrie und Muskelerkrankungen, Universitätskinderklinik, W-7800 Freiburg, Fed. Rep. of Germany

Introduction

Radiotherapy of the brain and its surrounding tissues contributes significantly to the improvement in long-term event-free survival of children suffering from brain tumors or leukemia. With the prolonged life span the aspects of quality of life and treatment-related sequelae with possible damage to the central nervous system (CNS) are gaining greater importance.

In adults, cranial radiation of 54 Gy delivered in 30 fractions over 42 days is considered safe with respect to vascular damage and radiation necrosis (Marks et al. 1981). However, in the young child there is increased vulnerability due to the immaturity of the brain. The development of the child's brain, especially in infancy, is characterized by formation of dendrites and synapses, proliferation of glial cells, and myelination of the central pathways. This process is not completed before the end of the second decade of life (Volpe 1987). It is evident that these developmental events can be disturbed by ionizing radiation.

In the child, as in the adult, acute clinical side effects of cranial radiotherapy are rare and limited to signs of edema and increased intracranial pressure. These symptoms can easily be treated with corticosteroids. Acute electroencephalographic (EEG) changes are minimal. On another level of function, radiotherapy causes a disturbance of the blood–brain barrier. Studying patients with acute lymphoblastic or myeloblastic leukemia undergoing radiotherapy, we found a significant increase in the concentration of albumin, lactate dehydrogenase, and some neutral amino acids in the cerebrospinal fluid (CSF). These elevated CSF levels were apparently due to radiation-induced disturbance of passive and active transport mechanisms (Korinthenberg et al. 1990). Although there was no correlation with clinical symptoms or EEG changes, our observations may explain why cytotoxic drugs such as methotrexate are more toxic with concomitant radiotherapy than without.

Recent Results in Cancer Research, Vol. 130

Four to six weeks after completion of cranial radiotherapy, a syndrome of postirradiation somnolence occurs in about two thirds of patients with leukemia and some children with brain tumors (Boller et al. 1990; Freeman et al. 1973). The syndrome is characterized by apathy, loss of appetite, vomiting, and sometimes low-grade fever. The course is always self-limiting with resolution of symptoms within 2–3 weeks. The pathogenesis is unknown. A transient disturbance of myelin synthesis has been discussed (Freeman et al. 1973). During this period of somnolence, and for some weeks thereafter, the children exhibit abnormalities on the EEG with diffuse slowing of varying degree. These abnormalities must be distinguished from similar changes due to more severe complications such as CNS leukemia, intracranial infection, or bleeding (Korinthenberg and Igel 1990).

To monitor the function of the white matter and conductivity of the optic pathways during and after radiotherapy, serial testing of the visual evoked potentials (VEP) has been done. Russo et al. (1985) reported a significant increase of VEP latency in 10 of 11 patients 3–6 months after radiotherapy with 18 Gy. Verity et al. (1990) were unable to confirm this observation by serial testing up to 6 weeks after radiotherapy. It remains unclear whether the conflicting results are due to the different study designs with different length of observation or to differences in the chemotherapeutic regimen.

While the impact of these acute and subacute changes on long-term sequelae is unknown, reports on delayed and permanent morphological and functional abnormalities are of greater significance.

For many years, abnormalities on cranial computed tomography or magnetic resonance imaging have been reported in children treated with radiotherapy and chemotherapy. These abnormalities consist primarily of inner and outer brain atrophy, dystrophic calcifications of subcortical white matter and basal ganglia, and white matter hypodensity (Brecher et al. 1985; Parker et al. 1986). The incidence and etiology of these findings have long been disputed, because most investigations were performed in patients with neurological abnormalities. Thus, their true incidence has often been overestimated. Prospective studies of a larger number of unselected patients have helped to clarify the situation, although many questions remain because of different study designs and treatment modalities.

Ochs (1989) has reviewed and compiled the findings on more than 700 patients with acute lymphoblastic leukemia treated with different forms of CNS therapy, with and without radiotherapy (Table 1). Despite rather variable data it seems clear that calcifications and atrophy are at least partly due to radiotherapy, while white matter hypodensity is most likely caused by chemotherapy. The role of radiotherapy as a causative mechanism in brain calcifications is underlined by the fact that calcifications have also been observed in patients with brain tumors who received radiotherapy without additional chemotherapy (Pearson et al. 1983) (Fig. 1). However, to the author's knowledge, no reliable data have been published on the incidence of calcifications in children with brain tumors.

Table 1. Cranial computed tomographic changes after CNS prophylaxis in ALL (%) (adapted from Ochs 1989)

Method	*n*	Atrophy	Calcification	Hypodensity
With radiotherapy				
24 Gy cr, 5–8 itMTX, or 24 Gy csp	349	15.5	8.5	3.5
24 Gy cr, 35 itMTX	32	25.0	18.7	12.5
18 Gy cr, 5 itMTX	48	35.0	0.0	0.0
18 Gy cr, 18 itMTX	55	1.9	7.2	5.4
Without radiotherapy				
ivMTX (0.5 g/m^2), itMTX	104	3.8	0.0	<1.0
ivMTX (1 g/m^2), itMTX	52	1.9	0.0	19.2
it MTX	82	4.6	0.0	3.5

cr, cranial; csp, craniospinal radiotherapy; ivMTX, intravenous methotrexate; itMTX, intrathecal methotrexate

The microscopical findings in areas of radiation-induced calcifications consist predominantly of a mineralizing microangiopathy, which differs from the huge white matter calcifications seen in subacute necrotizing leukoencephalopathy due to CNS leukemia, radiotherapy, and high cumulative methotrexate doses (Bleyer 1981).

At the electrophysiological level, dystrophic calcifications are often accompanied by nonspecific pathological EEG findings, such as focal or diffuse dysrhythmia (Korinthenberg 1986). However, in the whole population of irradiated children, alterations in the EEG are an infrequent observation. We have performed a prospective study on a cohort of patients with acute lymphoblastic leukemia (ALL) surviving in first complete remission. All children had had treatment discontinued at least 2 years previously. Eleven patients with standard risk leukemia had been irradiated with 18 Gy, 13 patients with standard risk had received CNS treatment with intermediate-dose intravenous methotrexate without radiotherapy, and 15 patients with increased risk of recurrence had been irradiated with 24 Gy. On quantitative EEG spectral analysis we detected no abnormalities in the standard risk patients compared with age-matched controls and no difference between the irradiated and nonirradiated groups. Significant abnormalities were observed in the increased risk group after 24 Gy irradiation. These abnormalities correlated more with preexisting EEG changes at diagnosis (probably due to subclinical CNS infiltrations) than with radiotherapy (Korinthenberg and Igel 1990).

Testing the VEP in the long-term follow-up after leukemia treatment has once again produced conflicting results. Russo et al. (1985) found pathological changes in a third of 34 irradiated patients. Verity et al. (1990) reported a slight increase in the latencies of the flash VEP, but no changes

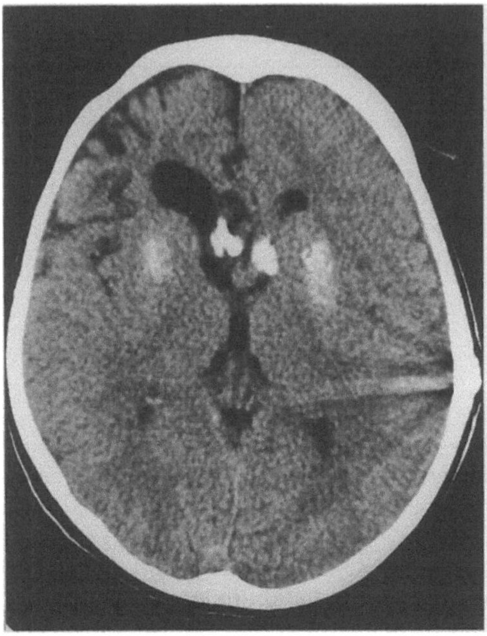

Fig. 1. Calcification of the basal ganglia in a child after radiotherapy of an incompletely resected craniopharyngioma

in pattern VEP in 23 patients. Latency in irradiated patients with medulloblastoma who had not received chemotherapy was normal. Thus, the authors conclude that the latency abnormalities might be due to chemotherapy rather than to radiotherapy. We have tested the pattern VEP in the abovementioned group of 39 patients with ALL, and did not find any abnormalities at all (Korinthenberg and Igel 1990).

For the child surviving in the long term, deficits in daily living skills or academic performance are of greater importance than the morphological or electrophysiological alterations discussed earlier. It is evident that in children with brain tumors neurological, neuropsychological, and psychiatric problems can persist after cessation of treatment. It is less well understood, however, which aspects of these deficits might be due to the tumor itself, to surgical treatment, or to radiotherapy.

During the last 15 years many studies have tried to address the role of radiotherapy in brain dysfunction. Various study designs have been applied. Cohorts of patients with different brain tumors have been compared with the normal population or with healthy siblings (Danoff et al. 1982; Holldack et al. 1985). This particular study design is hardly able to differentiate with respect to the pathogenesis of the existing damage. Cognitive deficits due to tumor site or surgery are hardly to be expected when comparing a cohort of patients with posterior fossa tumors with the normal population or siblings (Lebaron et al. 1988; Packer et al. 1987; Riva et al. 1991), although the effect of a raised intracranial pressure and the importance of the brainstem for attentional processes may not be negligible. Thus, studies comparing children with medulloblastomas treated with radiotherapy with children suffering from cerebellar astrocytomas treated with surgery alone (Hirsch et al. 1979; Zarbock et al. 1989) are more suitable for delineating the toxicity of cranial irradiation. Similarly, studies performing serial testing before and after radiotherapy may illustrate the adverse effects of radiotherapy (Bordeaux et al. 1988; Duffner et al. 1988; Ellenberg et al. 1987).

Reviewing the available literature, a significant decline in the IQ score is often found, even in children with only minor neurological sequelae. Twelve to sixty percent of children exhibit an IQ score below the normal range. The performance IQ is usually more affected than the verbal IQ (Duffner et al. 1988; Ellenberg et al. 1987; Lebaron et al. 1988; Riva et al. 1991). Academic achievement is very frequently altered, up to 70% of the children needing some kind of special education (Duffner et al. 1988; Lebaron et al. 1988) Neuropsychological testing reveals that poor school performance is due to deficits in attention, perception, fine motor coordination, and psychomotor speed (Duffner et al. 1988; Packer et al. 1987). Although the data are somewhat controversial, the site and extension of the tumor (Danoff et al. 1982; Riva et al. 1991), raised intracranial pressure (Packer et al. 1987), radiotherapy (especially in combination with young age) (Lebaron et al. 1988; Riva et al. 1991; Zarbock et al. 1989), and adjuvant chemotherapy (Duffner et al. 1988) significantly contributed to these abnormalities. The importance of radiotherapy can be delineated most conclusively from the prospective studies of Duffner et al. (1988), and Ellenberg et al. (1987; Table 2).

Due to the large number of surviving patients and to the primarily non-neurological character of the disease, a lot of interest has focused on neuropsychological and academic function in long-term survivors of ALL. As in brain tumors, study designs have usually relied on a comparison of the

Table 2. Significant predictors of IQ at the 1–4 year follow-up in children with brain tumors (adapted from Ellenberg et al. 1987)

Predictor variable	% of accounted variance (cumulative)	*p* value
IQ at 1 month post-diagnosis	0.62	<0.001
Age at diagnosis	0.70	<0.001
Radiation therapy	0.75	<0.001
Age at diagnosis + radiation therapy	0.80	<0.001
Tumor site	0.83	$0.1 > p > 0.05$

patients with a normal population (Appleton et al. 1990; Brouwers and Poplack 1990; Peckham et al. 1988; Schuler et al. 1990), with healthy siblings (Said et al. 1989; Schlieper et al. 1989) or with other cancer patients who received chemotherapy with or without local radiotherapy for solid tumors other than brain tumors (Harten et al. 1984; Waber et al. 1990). There is a smaller number of studies published comparing irradiated with nonirradiated leukemia patients (Mulhern et al. 1988; Rowland et al. 1984), or applying serial testing in one patient cohort (Chessells et al. 1990; Longeway et al. 1990; Rubenstein et al. 1990).

In 1988 Cousens et al. reviewed 31 neuropsychological studies in patients with ALL. Sixteen groups reported a significant decline in IQ score, 14 groups a non-significant decline, and only one group a higher IQ score in the patient population than in the control group. Twenty of the 31 studies were considered adequate for a meta-analysis. The analysis demonstrated a significant decline in IQ score of 10 points in irradiated patients versus controls. Differences were greater in comparison with healthy siblings than with other cancer patients, suggesting that chemotherapy alone has some negative influence on neuropsychological function also. Children of young age (under 4 years) at the time of radiotherapy suffered significantly more severe side effects than older children. Time elapsed since treatment correlated positively with loss of IQ, demonstrating that irradiation induced a retardation of the maturation of the CNS during childhood.

The small IQ loss of 10 points cannot alone adequately explain the problems of the affected children and possible therapeutic consequences. The poor performance in the standardized IQ tests and the school problems encountered in 30%–50% of patients with ALL are caused by a number of specific neuropsychological deficits. These were revealed by properly conducted studies. The deficits reported can extend to nearly all aspects of higher nervous function, namely perception, attention and concentration, memory function, and psychomotor coordination (Appleton et al. 1990; Brouwers and Poplack 1990; Harten et al. 1984; Peckham et al. 1988; Schuler et al. 1990). The pattern of these deficits is rather variable, depending on an individual vulnerability of the nervous system (Peckham et al. 1988; Schlieper et al. 1989). The resulting clinical syndrome is that of so-called minimal cerebral dysfunction, that can also be observed with different etiologies.

According to a large number of studies the major contributing factor to these neuropsychological problems is cranial radiotherapy, especially when administered at a young age (Harten et al. 1984; Rowland et al. 1984; Said et al. 1989; Schileper et al. 1989). Whether a reduction in dosage from 24 to 18 Gy is of great benefit has yet to be determined (Chessells et al. 1990). Another important factor is the concomitant administration of cytotoxic drugs, especially parenteral methotrexate (Chessells et al. 1990). Children suffering from CNS leukemia are at a very high risk for severe adverse effects due to the disturbance of the blood–brain barrier and – especially at relapse – high cumulative doses of radiotherapy and cytotoxic drugs (Longeway et al. 1990). Two studies demonstrated more severe problems in girls than in boys (Schlieper et al. 1989; Waber et al. 1990). Lastly, the socioeconomic status of the family has to be considered (Waber et al. 1990). The relationship between neuropsychological dysfunction and pathological cranial computed tomographic findings is still under debate, with an equal number of studies reporting either a strong correlation between the two (Brouwers and Poplack 1990; Chessells et al. 1990) or none at all (Harten et al. 1984; Schuler et al. 1990).

Whole-brain radiotherapy is an indispensable therapeutic measure for many children with ALL or brain tumors. An exact knowledge of the functional deficits following cranial radiation is of great importance not only for designing less toxic treatment strategies in the future, but also for planning early and adequate help for the individual child.

References

Appleton RE, Farrell K, Zaide J, Rogers P (1990) Decline in head growth and cognitive impairment in survivors of acute lymphoblastic leukaemia. Arch Dis Child 65:530–534

Bleyer WA (1981) Neurologic sequelae of methotrexate and ionizing radiation: a new classification. Cancer Treat Rep 65 [Suppl 1]:89–98

Boller O, Kraus E, Rautenberg M (1990) Das Apathie-Syndrom als Folge einer postoperativen Bestrahlung bei kindlichen Hirntumoren. Neurochirurgia 33 [Suppl 1]:33–35

Bordeaux JD, Dowell RE Jr, Copeland DR, Fletcher JM, Francis DJ, van Eys J (1988) A prospective study of neuropsychological sequelae in children with brain tumors. J Child Neurol 3:63–68

Brecher ML, Berger P, Freeman Al, Krischer J, Boyett J, Glicksman AS, Foreman E, Harris M, Jones B, Cohen M, Duffner PK, Rowland JH, Huang YP, Batnitzky S (1985) Computerized tomography scan findings in children with acute lymphocytic leukemia treated with three different methods of central nervous system prophylaxis. Cancer 56:2430–2433

Brouwers P, Poplack D (1990) Memory and learning sequelae in long-term survivors of acute lymphoblastic leukemia: association with attention deficits. Am J Pediatr Hematol Oncol 12:174–181

Chessells JM, Cox TCS, Kendall B, Cavanagh NPC, Jannoun L, Richards S (1990) Neurotoxicity in lymphoblastic leukemia: comparison of oral and intramuscular methotrexate and two doses of radiation. Arch Dis Child 65:416–422

Cousens P, Waters B, Said J, Stevens M (1988) Cognitive effects of cranial irradiation in leukemia: a survey and meta-analysis. J Child Psychol Psychiat 29:839–852

Danoff BF, Cowchock S, Marquette C, Mulgren L, Kramer S (1982) Assessment of the long-term effects of primary radiation therapy for brain tumors in children. Cancer 49:1580–1586

Duffner PK, Cohen ME, Parker MS (1988) Prospective intellectual testing in children with brain tumors. Ann Neurol 23:575–579

Ellenberg L, McComb JG, Siegel SE, Stowe S (1987) Factors affecting intellectual outcome in pediatric brain tumor patients. Neurosurgery 21:638–644

Freeman JE, Johnston PGB, Voke JM (1973) Somnolence after prophylactic cranial irradiation in children with acute lymphoblastic leukemia. Br Med J 4:523–525
Harten G, Stephani U, Henze G, Langermann HJ, Riehm H, Hanefeld F (1984) Slight impairment of psychomotor skills in children after treatment of acute lymphoblastic leukemia. Eur J Pediatr 142:189–197
Hirsch JF, Renier D, Czernichow P, Benveniste L, Pierre-Kahn A (1979) Medulloblastoma in childhood: survival and functional results. Acta Neurochir (wien) 48:1–15
Holldack J, Kalff R, Schindler H, Rappen U, Havers W (1985) Neurologische und psychosoziale Störungen bei Kindern mit Hirntumoren. Klin Padiatr 197:188–191
Korinthenberg R (1986) Leukämie und Nervensystem. Das Hirnstrombild im Erkrankungsund Behandlungsverlauf der akuten Leukämien des Kindesalters. Thieme, Stuttgart
Korinthenberg R, Igel B (1990) Prospective neurophysiological study in children treated for acute lymphoblastic leukaemia: serial EEG during treatment and long-term follow up with evoked potentials. Eur J Pediatr 15:127–131
Korinthenberg R, Ullrich K, Ritter J, Stephani U (1990) Electrolytes, amino acids and proteins in lumbar CSF during the treatment of acute leukemia in childhood. Acta Paediatr Scand 79:335–342
Lebaron S, Zeltzer PM, Zeltzer LK, Scott SE, Marlin AE (1988) Assessment of quality of survival in children with medulloblastoma and cerebellar astrocytoma. Cancer 62:1215–1222
Longeway K, Mulhern, R, Crisco J, Kun L, Lauer S, Casper J, Camitta B, Hoffman RG (1990) Treatment of meningeal relapse in childhood acute lymphoblastic leukemia. II. A prospective study of intellectual loss specific to CNS relapse and therapy. Am J Pediatr Hematol Oncol 12:45–50
Marks JE, Baglan RJ, Prassad SC, Blank WF (1981) Cerebral radionecrosis: incidence and risk in relation to dose, time, fractionation and volume. Int J Radiat Oncol Biol Phys 7:243–252
Mulhern RK, Wasserman AL, Fairclough D, Ochs J (1988) Memory function in disease-free survivors of childhood acute lymphocytic leukemia given CNS prophylaxis with or without 1800 cGy cranial irradiation. J Clin Oncol 6:315–320
Ochs JJ (1989) Neurotoxicity due to central nervous system therapy for childhood leukemia. Am J Pediatr Hematol Oncol 11:93–105
Packer PJ, Zimmerman RA, Bilaniuk LT (1986) Magnetic resonance imaging in the evaluation of treatment-related central nervous system damage. Cancer 58:635–640
Packer RJ, Sposto R, Atkins TE, Sutton LN, Bruce DA, Siegel KR, Rorke LB, Littman PA, Schut L (1987) Quality of life in children with primitive neuroectodermal tumors (medulloblastoma) of the posterior fossa. Pediatr Neurosci 13:169–175
Pearson ADJ, Campbell AN, McAllister VL, Pearson GL (1983) Intracranial calcification in survivors of childhood medulloblastoma. Arch Dis Child 58:133–136
Peckham VC, Meadows AT, Bartel N, Marrero O (1988) Educational late effects in long-term survivors of childhood acute lymphocytic leukemia. Pediatrics 81:127–133
Riva D, Milani N, Pantaleoni C, Ballerini E, Giorgi (1991) Combined treatment modality for medulloblastoma in childhood: effects on neuropsychological functioning. Neuropediatrics 22:36–42
Rowland JH, Glidewell OJ, Sibley RF, Holland JC, Tull R, Berman A, Brecher ML, Harris M, Glicksman AS, Forman E, Jones B, Cohen ME, Duffner PK, Freeman AI (1984) Effects of different forms of central nervous system

prophylaxis on neuropsychologic function in childhood leukemia. Clin Oncol 2:1327–1335
Rubenstein CL, Varni JW, Katz ER (1990) Cognitive functioning in long-term survivors of childhood leukemia: a prospective analysis. J Dev Behav Pediatr 11:301–305
Russo A, Tomarchio S, Pero G, Consoli G, Marina R, Rizzarai C, Schiliro G (1985) Abnormal visual-evoked potentials in leukemic children after cranial radiation. Med Pediatr Oncol 13:313–317
Said JA, Waters BGH, Cousens P, Stevens MM (1989) Neuropsychological sequelae of central nervous system prophylaxis in survivors of childhood acute lymphoblastic leukemia. J Consult Clin Psychol 57:251–256
Schlieper AE, Esseltine DW, Tarshis E (1989) Cognitive function in long survivors of childhood acute lymphoblastic leukemia. Pediatr Hematol Oncol 6:1–9
Schuler D, Bakos M, Borsi J, Gacsaly I, Kamanchey R, Kardos G, Koos R, Nagy Cs. Revesz T, Somlo P, Gebauer E (1990) Neuropsychologic and CT examinations in leukemic patients surviving 10 or more years. Med Pediatr Oncol 18:123–125
Verity CM, Morgan H, Mott M, Oakhill A (1990) Do visual evoked potentials detect neural damage in children treated for cancer? Dev Med Child Neurol 32:481–492
Volpe JJ (1987) Neurology of the newborn, 2nd edn. Saunders, Philadelphia
Waber DP, Urion DK, Tarbell NJ, Niemeyer C, Gelber R, Sallan SE (1990) Late effects of central nervous system treatment of acute lymphoblastic leukemia in childhood are sex-dependent. Dev Med Child Neurol 32:238–248
Zarbock G, Matthes-Martin S, Schulte FJ (1989) Lebensqualität und Restschadenssymptomatik bei Kleinhirntumoren im Kindes- und Jugendalter. Klin Padiatr 201:337–345

Central Nervous System Injury from Implanted Isotopes

C.B. Ostertag

Abteilung Stereotaktische Neurochirurgie, Neurochirurgische Universitätsklinik, W 7800 Freiburg, Fed. Rep. of Germany

Introduction

Stereotactic interstitial irradiation of brain tumors is a technique based on the principle of selectively irradiating a tumor while protecting the healthy surrounding brain (Hilaris 1975). Clinical follow-up studies indicate that it constitutes an effective adjuvant therapy for tumors of the central nervous system (Bernstein and Gutin 1981; Gutin and Leibel 1985; Ostertag 1991). However, interstitial irradiation also exerts toxic effects on the adjacent brain which constitute a limiting factor. Clinical experience with high-energy gamma emitters such as gold-198 (^{198}Au) and iridium-192 (^{192}Ir) has shown evidence that the injury is not so much inflicted by direct radiation, as it is in standard external beam radiotherapy, but is caused by secondary effects. The tissue response is characterized at the periphery of the complete radionecrosis by a zone of irregular and incomplete demyelination with reactive gliosis. A temporary, extensive, spatially restricted vasogenic cerebral edema which can result in demyelination has been demonstrated. In order to elucidate the tissue response to interstitial irradiation we studied sequentially the morphological and physiological effects caused by gamma emitters with different energies and different dose rates in an animal model, with particular emphasis on the process of vasogenic edema.

Experimental Dose Effects

Experimental dose effects on the brain (beagle) caused by the gamma emitters iodine-125 (^{125}I, half-life 60.2 days, 0.028–0.035 MeV), iridium-192 (^{192}I, half-life 74.2 days, 0.30–0.61 MeV) and gold-198 (^{198}Au, half-life 2.7 days, 0.41 MeV) were examined sequentially over 5–365 days. Permanent low-activity, low dose rate implants were compared over time with temporary high-activity, high dose rate implants, both delivering the same accumulated total radiation dose. Particular attention was paid to the morphological development, size, and composition of the radiation necrosis, as well as the changes in the blood–brain barrier. Single seeds of ^{125}I and ^{198}Au or wire pieces of ^{192}Ir were stereotactically implanted into the left frontal centrum semiovale of 6-month-old beagle dogs. The implants were either permanent (lost implants) or temporary removable implants, i.e., the radioactive source was held in the tip of a Teflon catheter. After observation periods between 5 and 365 days the animals were killed. The procedures for implantation, tissue perfusion, and histological and immunohistological staining are described elsewhere (Janzer et al. 1986; Ostertag and Weigel 1982; Ostertag et al. 1982, 1983, 1984a). The dosimetry for permanent low dose rate and for temporary high dose rate implants was calculated such that a 26000 (10000) cGy isodose was achieved at 5 (10) mm distance from the source. Isodose distribution and accumulated tissue dosage were calculated on the assumption of a point source of irradiation. For a detailed description of quantitative measurement of capillary transfer rates, i.e., quantitative autoradiographic and computer tomographic methods employed in the different experimental series, see Groothuis et al. (1987, 1991). Four animals served as controls, i.e., an inactive seed of ^{125}I or ^{198}Au was implanted into the left centrum semiovale using the same experimental procedures of physiological measurements and histopathology.

Sequential Histological Changes

Radionecroses were manifest as early as 10 days after implantation. Within 25 days a coagulation necrosis developed in the immediate vicinity of the radioactive source which later increased in size and became progessively mineralized (Fig. 1). Staining for serum proteins revealed the presence of perifocal edema, which extended into the white matter of the entire ipsilateral hemisphere. Vessels within the developing radionecrosis showed the typical hyaloid vessel wall degeneration. Vessels outside the radionecrosis, however, even within a distance of 1 mm, were inconspicuous. A reactive gliosis with a dense fibrillary network of astrocytes positive for glial fibrillary acidic protein (GFAP) was found around the radionecrosis in the surrounding white matter. GFAP-positive astrocytes were in later stages also found in the contralateral hemisphere as a reaction to vasogenic edema spreading via the corpus callosum. Demyelination was always restricted to the ipsilateral centrum semiovale without affecting the internal capsule or the contralateral hemisphere. However, the neurons next to the radionecrosis but not incorporated in it appeared to be morphologically intact, even at a distance of 0.2 mm.

A remarkable factor was the time course of lesion growth (Fig. 2). Whereas the size of the radiation lesion resulting from low dose rate permanent implants had not reached its maximum until after 70 days, the

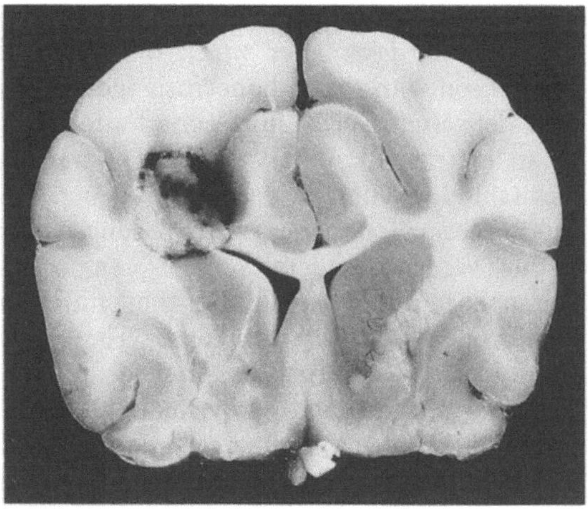

Fig. 1. Coronal brain section at the level of the implant (^{125}I seed temporary implant) after 25 days. A well-demarcated, partly calcified, partly hemorrhagic radionecrosis is demonstrated along with a pallor of the ipsilateral white matter and a midline shift, indicating vasogenic edema

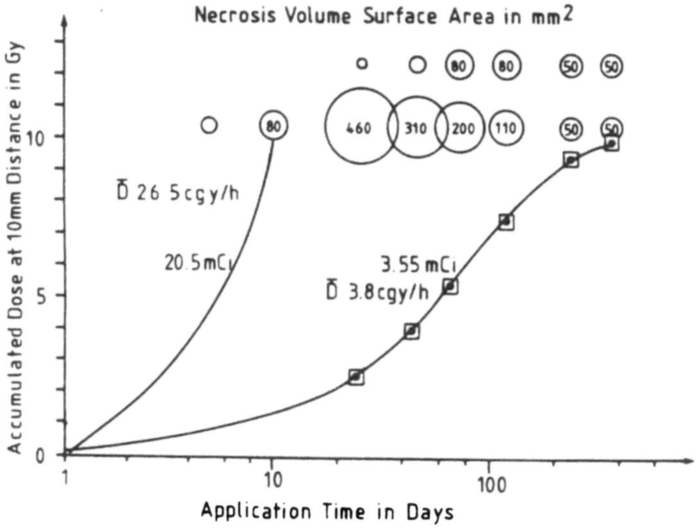

Fig. 2. The relationship between accumulated dose and the surface area of volumes of radionecrosis after ^{125}I implants over time (*upper line of circles*, permanent implants; *lower line of circles*, temporary implants)

radionecrosis after high dose rate temporary implants showed its maximum size after 25 days, after which the lesion decreased relatively quickly in comparison with the radionecrosis induced by permanent implants. A high dose delivered over a short period affected a larger volume, thus resulting in an increased capillary surface of impaired endothelial cells with the inevitable induction of vasogenic edema. Under low doses and long-term exposure small necroses were produced along with moderate, but long-lasting vasogenic edema. When temporary implants were used, lively macrophage activity set in after the emitter had been removed and the zone of necrotic tissue then decreased. The extent of the demyelination in the white matter was directly related to the intensity of the vasogenic edema. The glial reaction and demyelination clearly exceeded the physical penetration depth of the gamma radiation, at least that of ^{125}I gamma radiation, and were therefore considered secondary effects.

Sequential Changes in Capillary Permeability

All of the experimental animals showed nodular lesions (in the early stages) or ring-shaped lesions of the blood–brain barrier on standard computed tomography by the time the first examination was carried out. The measured values for the blood-to-tissue transfer rate K_1 were between 3.5 ml/100 g/min $\times 10^3$ after 70 days and 12.8 ml/100 g/min $\times 10^3$ after 12 days. The values for K_1 in normal brain tissue of dogs were between 0.1 and 0.3 ml/100 g/min $\times 10^3$. That is, the capillary permeability in a localized zone surrounding the implant was 10–40 times higher than that in normal brain tissue. The vascular volume also fell within the range of 0.4–2.0 ml/100 g and thus did not differ from normal brain tissue (1.3 ± 0.3 ml/100 g). Whereas after permanent interstitial irradiation the value of K_1 remained rather constant over a period of up to 1 year the value of K_1 after temporary irradiation had a peak after the maximum volume of radionecrosis had developed, and following that returned gradually to normal (Groothuis et al. 1987).

Discussion

The morphological analyses of brains treated with standard radiation therapy for cerebral gliomas have shown that radiation damage to the normal brain constitutes a risk when doses of 50–60 Gy in standard fractionation are exceeded (Bloom and Walsh 1975; Leibel and Sheline 1987). Radiosensitivity is enhanced when peritumoral edema is present (Burger et al. 1979). Delayed radionecrosis outside the treatment volume with widespread demyelination and vessel wall degeneration can be observed (Burger et al. 1979; Caveness 1980; Hall 1978). With respect to therapeutic principles, stereotactic interstitial irradiation for brain tumors has little in common with standard radiation therapy. Standard radiation therapy is based on a differential biological sensitivity of normal and neoplastic cells to radiation (therapeutic ratio). Interstitial irradiation, however, is not based principally on a differential sensitivity. Using interstitial irradiation therapy a high (i.e., necrotizing) radiation dose is delivered to a precisely defined tissue volume (i.e., tumor volume) without affecting surrounding normal brain. As with conventional radiotherapy, however, the risk of radiation-induced injury of the healthy tissue depends largely on the cumulative dose, the volume irradiated, and the dose rate.

Clinical follow-up examinations using computed tomography have demonstrated extensive, although temporary, edema surrounding the radionecrosis (Ostertag et al. 1979). However, computed tomographic or magnetic resonance findings alone can be misleading as the discrimination of white matter edema and tumor invasion might be difficult as shown by stereotactic biopsies (Daumas-Duport et al. 1984). Autopsy data on the response of the brain to interstitial irradiation are rare and inconsistent since most patients were treated with external beam radiation in addition to interstitial irradiation, thus demonstrating cumulative radiation toxicity (Davis et al. 1984; Kiessling et al. 1984; Szikla et al. 1979).

The effects of scattering and attenuation in tissue vary considerably for the three isotopes used in the experiment. The specific dose rate factor, i.e., the dose rate per unit activity, divided by the geometrical attenuation is not a constant with distance, particularly not for ^{125}I (Anderson et al. 1981; Hilaris 1975; Krishnaswamy 1978; Sondhaus 1981). We, like other students of the subject, found that the volume of the radionecrosis and the extent of the vasogenic edema can be highly influenced by the total dose and the application time (Fike and Cann 1984; Fike et al. 1985; Turowsky et al. 1986). Lower dose rates caused small radionecroses, which did not increase in size after 100 days. When the dose is delivered continuously, typical repair mechanisms of the cells such as reproduction, redistribution, and repair of sublethal damage are obstructed. The continuous low dose rate, however, was effective enough to inhibit macrophage activity, which is why the radionecrosis had not decreased after an observation period of at least 1 year. We also observed long-lasting edema as a side effect (Fike and Cann 1984). A high dose rate administered over a short time produced a larger necrosis accompanied by extensive vasogenic edema. However, after removal of the radiation source, repair processes such as macrophage activity were able to take effect and the lesion almost completely disappeared. The volume of radionecroses in normal brain tissue therefore depends on the total dose, the dose rate, and energy of the implanted radioactive source. In neoplastic tissue other factors such as neovascularization and susceptibility of tumor cells to radiation are contributing factors.

In a previous experiment we had studied the necrotizing effect of ^{125}I seeds in neoplastic tissue (Ostertag et al. 1984b). Brain tumors induced in dog by avian sarcoma virus (ASV) were chosen to serve as a primary model for human brain tumors. ASV tumors are autochthonous, i.e., their blood supply and growth are characteristic of a primary brain tumor. The model is extensively studied with respect to its biological and physiological characteristics (Bullard and Bigner 1980). The tumor type most often induced is an anaplastic glioma. The ^{125}I implants produced sharply delineated calcifying necroses with vital unaffected tumor outside the necroses. The necrotizing and calcifying effect was apparent as early as 18 days and complete after 90 days. The response of neoplastic tissue to interstitial irradiation in terms of the volume of necrosis was 3–5 times greater when compared with ^{125}I radionecroses in normal brain tissue. The necrobiotic characteristics, however, were apparently similar.

The temporary, spatially limited opening of the blood–brain barrier is considered a specific side effect of interstitial irradiation in the brain. The amount of blood-borne fluid that crosses the blood–brain barrier depends on the total surface area of the irradiated defective capillaries. Experimental and clinical results from blood-to-tissue transport studies are usually expressed in terms of a transfer constant K_1, which characterizes the unidirectional transfer across capillaries (Groothuis et al. 1987, 1991). Using [^{14}C]alpha-aminoisobutyric acid (AIB) autoradiography it could be shown that in comparison with normal brain the layer of irradiated brain tissue on the surface of a necrosis volume develops higher capillary permeability (up to 7.7 times higher) and maintains this over a period of several months in the case of low dose rate permanent interstitial irradiation (Groothuis et al. 1987). More recently quantitative computer tomographic methods as described by Groothuis et al. (1991) were used which allow sequential quantitative in vivo measurements of individual animals. The values for K_1 after temporary interstitial high dose rate irradiation exceeded those found after low dose rate permanent irradiation for all three gamma emitters. There was a positive correlation between the volume, i.e., capillary surface area, and the blood–tissue transfer rates. With ^{198}Au implants, whether permanent or temporary, the highest K_1 values were found. K_1 values for the ^{192}Ir temporary implant were slightly lower. The finding of increased capillary permeability, although restricted in both space and time, has far-reaching clinical implications. Under clinical conditions the time factor cannot be changed when permanent (lost) implants are used. With lost implants no corrections can be made. This also applies to overdoses, so that consequently overdosing is frequently observed in clinical situations. Moderate underdosing often requires reimplantation, or results in incomplete control of tumor growth. Larger tumors present a problem because of the risk of long-lasting, chronic vasogenic edema. The edema phase can be shortened by using temporary implants with a moderate dose rate in which case repair processes are free to take place after removal of the radioactive source from the brain. For the clinical application it was concluded that temporary ^{125}I implants with dose rates of 10 cGy/h might be the most favorable. The clinical results obtained so far demonstrate a positive tendency (Ostertag et al. 1984b). Toxic vasogenic edema formation no longer poses a serious problem since the introduction of temporary ^{125}I implants. The careful manipulation of dose rates and total tumor dose can help to minimize the toxic effects of interstitial irradiation.

Acknowledgments. The author gratefully acknowledges the support of P. Kleihues, Abt. Neuropathologie, Universität Zürich, and of M. Kiessling, Abt. Neuropathology, Universität Heidelberg. Thanks go to H.K. Leetz, Institut für Radiologische Physik der Universität des Saarlandes, Homburg/Saar, FRG, for providing the dosimetry calculations. The author is indebted to his collaborators P.C. Warnke and F.J. Hans, and to Mrs. A. Korst for technical assistance. The studies were supported by the Deutsche Forschungsgemeinschaft (OS 58/2-1 and OS 58/2-2).

References

Anderson LL, Hsin MK, Ing-Yuan D (1981) Clinical dosimetry with ^{125}I. In: George FW (ed) Modern interstitial and intracavitary radiation cancer management. Masson, New York

Bernstein M, Gutin PH (1981) Interstitial irradiation of brain tumors: a review. Neurosurgery 6:741–750

Bloom HJG, Walsh LS (1975) Tumors of the central nervous system. In: Bloom HJG, Lemerle J, Neidhardt MK (eds) Cancer in children: clinical management. Springer, Berlin Heidelberg New York

Bullard DE, Bigner DD (1980) Animal models and virus induction of tumors. In: Thomas DGT, Graham DI (eds) Brain tumors: scientific basis, clinical investigation and current therapy. Butterworth, London, pp 51–84

Burger PC, Mahaley MS, Dudka L, Vogel FS (1979) The morphologic effects of radiation administered therapeutically for intracranial gliomas. Cancer 44:1256–1272

Caveness WF (1980) Experimental observations: delayed necrosis in normal monkey brain. In: Gilbert HA, Kagan AR (eds) Radiation damage to the nervous system. Raven, New York, pp 1–38

Daumas-Duport C, Blond S, Vedrenne CL, Szikla G (1984) Radiolesion versus recurrence: bioptic Data in 39 gliomas after interstitial, or combined interstitial and external radiation treatment. In: Gybels J, Hitchcock ER, Ostertag C, Rossi GF, Siegfried J, Szikla G (eds) Advances in stereotactic and functional neurosurgery 6. Springer, Vienna New York, pp 291–299 (Acta Neurochirurgia, Supplementum 33)

Davis RL, Barger GR, Gutin PH, Philips TL (1984) Response of human malignant gliomas and CNS tissue to iodine brachytherapy: a study of seven autopsy cases. In: Gybels J, Hitchcock ER, Ostertag C, Rossi GF, Siegfried J, Szikla G (eds) Advances in stereotactic and functional neurosurgery 6. Springer, Vienna New York, pp 301–305 (Acta Neurochirurgia, Supplementum 33)

Fike JR, Cann ChE (1984) Contrast medium accumulation and washout in canine brain tumors and irradiated normal brain: a CT study of kinetics. Radiology 151:115–120

Fike JR, Cann CE, Phillips TL, Bernstein M, Gutin PH, Turowsky K, Weaver KA, Davis RL, Higgins RJ, DaSilva V (1985) Radiation brain damage induced by interstitial 125-I sources: a canine model evaluated by quantitative computed tomography. Neurosurgery 16:530–537
Groothuis DR, Wright DC, Ostertag CB (1987) The effect of I-125 interstitial radiotherapy on blood–brain barrier function in normal canine brain. J Neurosurg 67:895–902
Groothuis DR, Vriesendorp F, Kupfer B, Warnke PC, Lapin GD, Kuruvilla A, Vick NA, Mikhael MA, Patlak CS (1991) Quantitative measurements of capillary transport in human brain tumors by computed tomography. Ann Neurol 30:581–588
Gutin PH, Leibel SA (1985) Stereotactic interstitial irradiation of malignant brain tumors. Neurol Clin 3:883–893
Hall EJ (1978) Radiobiology for the radiologist. Harper and Row, Hagerstown
Hilaris BS (1975) Handbook of interstitial brachytherapy. Publishing Sciences Group, Acton
Janzer RC, Kleihues P, Ostertag CB (1986) Early and late effects on the normal dog brain of permanent interstitial iridium-192 irradiation. Acta Neuropathol 70:91–102
Kiessling M, Kleihues P, Gessaga E, Mundinger F, Ostertag ChB, Weigel K (1984) Morphology of intracranial tumours and adjacent brain structures following interstitial iodine-125 radiotherapy. In: Gybels J, Hitchcock ER, Ostertag C, Rossi GF, Siegfried J, Szikla G (eds) Advances in stereotactics and functional neurosurgery 6. Springer, Vienna New York, pp 281–289 (Acta Neurochirurgia, Supplementum 33)
Krishnaswamy V (1978) Dose distribution around an 125-I seed source in tissue. Radiology 126:489–491
Leibel SA, Sheline GE (1987) Radiation therapy for neoplasms of the brain. J Neurosurg 66:1–22
Ostertag CB (1992) Iodine-125 interstitial irradiation for cerebral gliomas. Acta Neurochir (Wien) 119:53–61
Ostertag ChB, Weigel K (1982) Three-dimensional CT scanning of the dog brain. J Comput Assist Tomogr 6(5):1036–1037
Ostertag CB, Weigel K, Birg W (1979) CT changes after long-term interstitial iridium-192 irradiation of cerebral gliomas. In: Szikla (ed) Stereotactic cerebral irradiation. Inserm symposium 12. Elsevier/North-Holland, Amsterdam
Ostertag ChB, Hossmann KA, von der Kerckhoff W (1982) Radiation effects of iridium-192 implants in the cat brain. Nucl Med 21:99–104
Ostertag ChB, Weigel K, Warnke P, Lombeck G, Kleihues P (1983) Sequential morphological changes in the dog brain after interstitial iodine-125 irradiation. Neurosurgery 13:523–528
Ostertag CB, Groothuis D, Kleihues P (1984a) Effects on tumour and brain: experimental data on early and late morphologic effects of permanently implanted gamma and beta sources (iridium-192, iodine-125 and yttrium-90) in the brain. In: Gybels J, Hitchcock ER, Ostertag C, Rossi GF, Siegfried J, Szikla G (eds) Advances in stereotactics and functional neurosurgery 6. Springer, Vienna New York, pp 271–280 (Acta Neurochirurgia, Supplementum 33)
Ostertag ChB, Warnke P, Kleihues P, Bigner D (1984b) Iodine-125 interstitial irradiation of virally induced dog brain tumors. Neurol Res 6:176–180
Sondhaus CA (1981) I-125: physical properties, photon dosimetry and effectiveness. In: George FW (ed) Modern interstitial and intracavitary radiation cancer management. Masson, New York
Szikla G, Betti O, Blond S (1979) Data on late reactions following stereotactic

irradiation of gliomas In: Szikla G (ed) Stereotactic cerebral irradiation. Inserm symposium 12. Elsevier/North-Holland, Amsterdam
Turowsky K, Fike JR, Cann CE, Higgins RJ, Davis RL, Gutin PH, Phillips TL, Weaver KA (1986) Normal brain iodine-125 radiation damage: effect of dose and irradiated volume in a canine model. Radiology 158:833–838

Long-Term Cerebral Side-Effects of Total Body Irradiation and Quality of Life

M. Peper[1], P. Schraube[1], B. Kimmig[1], C. Wagensommer[2], M. Wannenmacher[1], and R. Haas[3]

[1] University of Heidelberg, Department of Radiology, Im Neuenheimer Feld 400, W-6900 Heidelberg, Fed. Rep. of Germany
[2] University of Heidelberg, Department of Psychology, Hauptstr. 47–51, W-6900 Heidelberg, Fed. Rep. of Germany
[3] University of Heidelberg, Department of Internal Medicine V, Hospitalstr. 3, W-6900 Heidelberg, Fed. Rep. of Germany

Introduction

Total body irradiation (TBI) in preparation for bone marrow transplantation (BMT) is a routine treatment for malignant hematological disorders. With increasing survival rates the evaluation of long-term side effects and the patient's quality of life has become an important issue. However, long-term neurological and psychological side effects of BMT combined with TBI have not yet been evaluated in adults. In the following sections some introductory remarks on psychological assessment in research on radiotherapy will be made.

The Concept of "Quality of Life" in Radiation Oncology

The effects of radiation and chemotherapy can be evaluated in terms of their impact on the patient's quality of life (e.g., Holland et al. 1986; Aaronson and Beckmann 1987; von Kerekjarto et al. 1989). Unfortunately, no general definition of the concept "quality of life" exists. The operationalization of this term depends on the theoretical background of the researcher and the disease in question. In short, a definition of quality of life may include objective and subjective criteria of health. However, assessment of the long-term effects of cerebral radiotherapy should not be limited to the physiological level. Several different criteria of quality of life can be defined, depending on the method used. These methods can be classified according to the possibility of an intersubjective confirmation of the results.

First, oncological, neurological, and neuroradiological methods can be applied to describe the biological status after radiotherapy. Second, behavior samples may be taken by means of a neuropsychological assessment. This approach is appreciated by workers in neuropsychological toxicology, who have developed methods for a finer-grained analysis of behavioral

Recent Results in Cancer Research, Vol. 130

impairment (e.g., Hartman 1988). Neuropsychological deficits may involve disturbances in memory, attention, visuomotor coordination, and visuoperceptual speed (Lezak 1983). Third, behavior ratings may be performed by family members of the patient or the hospital staff. Finally, self-reported data on present or past psychosocial stress, and emotional or physical complaints, as well as inventory ratings on individual differences in illness behavior, can be assessed (e.g., King et al. 1985). In particular, affective symptoms such as irritability, depression, and psychophysiological disorders have frequently been reported as concomitants of neurotoxic exposure (Hartman 1988). These issues are addressed by psychological oncology. A summary of determinants which might influence the quality of life after irradiation of the brain is given in Table 1.

Determinants of Quality of Life in Patients after Irradiation of the Brain

Neurological and Radiological Determinants

Long-term neurological and neuroradiological side effects of the treatment of childhood acute lymphoblastic leukemia have been well documented (e.g., Eiser 1978; Kretzschmar et al. 1980; Brouwers et al. 1985). A considerable rate of morphological changes could be observed with increasing survival time. According to Poplack and Brouwers (1985), five different effects of delayed central nervous system (CNS) toxicity can be described in childhood leukemia: subacute leukoencephalopathy, mineralizing microangiopathy, subacute necrotizing leukomyelopathy, multiple focal necroses and generalized cortical atrophy.

Table 1. Determinants of quality of life after total body irradiation and bone marrow transplantation

- Dose, fraction, and localization of irradiation
- Chemotherapy, drugs, and medication

- Nervous system pathology (e.g., previous focal pathology or radiation-induced pathology)
- Non-neurological medical problems

- Behavioral and neuropsychological symptoms of neurotoxicity

- Cognitive and functional status in everyday life

- Subjective cognitive problems (e.g., concentration and memory problems)
- Subjective emotional problems (e.g., anxiety, depression, fatigue, irritability)
- Psychosocial determinants (e.g., coping behavior, social support)

Necrotizing leukoencephalopathy is the most prominent long-term side effect and may prevail in patients with a high total dose of brain irradiation and previous intrathecal methotrexate (MTX) instillation. This process is characterized by a multiple demyelination. Side effects may range from minor neurological and neuropsychological dysfunction to progressive dementia (Bleyer 1981). Degenerative mineralizing microangiopathy may disrupt arteries and may lead to a degeneration of the gray matter. Cortical atrophy is the most common concomitant of elective irradiation of the brain. Multiple focal necrosis may cause a loss of cortical tissue and general cortical atrophy.

Neuropsychological Determinants

Neuropsychological side effects have been studied extensively in children (Eiser 1978; Meadows et al. 1981; Brouwers et al. 1985; Ochs et al. 1991). However, neuropsychological determinants of quality of life have not been well investigated in adults. Patients with elective prophylactic brain irradiation for small cell lung cancer or hematological disorders (acute lymphoblastic leukemia/acute myeloblastic leukemia (ALL/AML) and non-Hodgkin's lymphoma (NHL)) have been evaluated for neuropsychological long-term effects. The extent of the neuropsychological impairment in patients after high-dose irradiation is obviously associated with the total dose and the dose of a single fraction. A correlation of atrophy indices and behavioral deterioration yields significant results in this group (Laukkanen et al. 1988).

We know of only one study investigating treatment side effects in adult survivors of systemic hematological disorders. Tucker et al. (1989) investigated 24 patients who received CNS prophylaxis including intrathecal MTX instillation and whole brain irradiation (24 Gy) with conventional fractions. Neurological symptoms and moderate brain atrophy with enlargement of sulci were found. This was more pronounced in patients older than 30 years at the time of treatment. However, severe memory and concentration difficulties could not be found. In general, neuropsychological deficits in patients treated with high-dose radiotherapy of the brain can be observed in motor functions, visuomotor coordination, short-term memory, concentration, and general speed (Johnson et al. 1985; Lee et al. 1986; Laukkanen et al. 1988).

Subjective and Psychosocial Determinants

Laukkanen et al. (1988) reported slight depression in a few patients and increased anxiety in more than one half of their patients. In the Tucker et al. study (1989), less than one fifth of the patients described the following complaints: forgetfulness, poor concentration, unsteadiness, poor hearing, anxiety, headaches, pins and needles. However, in these early studies of radiation toxicity a detailed assessment of emotional symptoms or psychosocial determinants was not performed.

It is the aim of the present study to assess *subjective indicators* of quality of life (self-ratings on physical, cognitive, and emotional complaints) in patients who received TBI conditioning for BMT. These subjective indicators were also related to behavior-observation data of relatives and to more objectively defined neuropsychological and oncological variables. Detailed information on neurobehavioral and neuroradiological results will be presented elsewhere (Peper et al. 1993).

Materials and Methods

Subjects

Between 1984 and 1991 125 patients with malignant hematological disorders were treated with TBI conditioning for BMT. Transplantations were carried out at the Department of Internal Medicine V, University of Heidelberg, Germany (for details see Körbling et al. 1989).

The "pre-TBI group" included 14 patients (6 male, 8 female) with a mean age of 35.5 years (range 16–49 years) who were examined prior to the termination of radiotherapy and prior to BMT. All surviving patients of the abovementioned population were asked to participate ("post-TBI group"). Nineteen patients refused. Out of this sample, 20 patients (14 male, 6 female) with a mean age of 38.0 years (range 17–52 years) participated voluntarily. Mean observation (survival) time after TBI was 30.5 months with a range of 9–67 months. As a control group, 11 patients with chronic renal dysfunction were examined who had received no previous chemo- or radiotherapy and had no history of neurological disease. This group was chosen in order to determine the specificity of changes in quality of life. Due to the chronicity of the disease, psychosocial and neuropsychological problems can be expected in this group, too. These patients were matched to the TBI groups with respect to age, sex, and education.

Medical and demographic data are summarized in Table 2. Diagnostic categories were not evenly distributed in both groups. The frequency of leukemia was greater in the post-TBI group (AML/ALL, $n = 17$; NHL, $n = 3$). All three groups were comparable with respect to age and premorbid intelligence. There is a greater proportion of patients with university degrees in the post-TBI group.

Previous Treatment

The time interval between the beginning of previous chemotherapy and radiotherapy varied between 6 months and 4 years. Chemotherapy protocols

Table 2. Personal and medical data

	Controls	Pre-TBI	Post-TBI
n	11	14	20
Age (years)[a]	35.5 (13)	35.5 (11)	38.0 (10)
Sex (male/female)	7/4	6/8	14/6
Estimated premorbid IQ[a,b]	95.7 (8)	95.8 (7)	97.5 (7)
Education (years)[a]	8.5 (1)	9.9 (2)	10.2 (2)
Survival time (months)[a]	NA	NA	30.5 (17)
Leukemia		(43%)	(85%)
AML		5	13
ALL		1	4
Lymphoma		(57%)	(15%)
CC-CB lymphoma		6	2
T cell lymphoma		1	
Immunoblastoma			1
Burkitt lymphoma		1	

NA, not applicable
[a] Means (and standard deviations) are given
[b] According to Wilson et al. (1979), Kessler et al. (1988)

were heterogeneous and included two or three cycles in most cases. More than 80% of both patient groups were within the first or second remission period. Exposure to chemotherapy was identified by the number of remissions. One patient in the post-TBI group had received a previous brain irradiation (24 Gy) and 2 patients had had a previous brain irradiation combined with MTX instillation.

Exposure

All patients received a hyperfractionated and accelerated treatment scheme: 14.4 Gy in 12 fractions within a period of 4 days. They received high-dose cyclophosphamide between TBI and BMT (cf. Körbling et al. 1989).

Procedure

All TBI patients underwent a general neurological, oncological, and neuroradiological examination. A neuropsychological examination comprised procedures to evaluate cognitive functions. Several questionnaires were administered for patients to register their complaints. Subjective cognitive and emotional problems were also assessed in an interview. A German questionnaire of general health complaints (Beschwerdenliste: von Zerssen 1975) and an attention inventory (Zimmermann and Poser 1993) with a three-factorial structure including distractability, fatigue, and initiative were used. An adjective checklist (Eigenschaftswörterliste-K: Janke and Debus 1978) with five factors including well-being, deactivation, emotional irritation, extraversion, and anxiety/depressed feelings was used to assess mood changes. The two primary factors "positive" and "negative mood" were derived from these scales.

In an attempt to validate findings, a behavioral rating was performed by family members according to Kessler et al. 1988. This questionnaire includes rating scales on cognitive functions (attention, memory, orientation, communication) and noncognitive functions (emotional instability, mood and depression, activation level, etc.).

Statistical Methods

Mann–Whitney Tests and Spearman rank correlations were computed due to distribution and scale attributes.

Results

Physical and Neurological Examination

All patients were in good general condition. No evidence of neurological deficits was found except a slight reduction in reflexes in 2 patients of the pre-TBI group and 3 patients of the post-TBI group. No patient had severe brain atrophy. However, a small subgroup of patients had moderate atrophy. Several atrophy indices derived from cranial computed tomography (CT) showed a slight increase in the post-TBI group.

Psychological Results

Subjective Complaints

Subjective complaints were independent of sociodemographic data and diagnosis. Information on personal problems was assessed in an interview and by means of a health complaint inventory. During radiotherapy all patients reported increased fatigue and concentration difficulties. Several patients experienced memory difficulties or emotional problems. Most frequent noncognitive complaints were fatigue and rapid exhaustion. Four patients did not report any difficulties. In the post-TBI group only 3 patients did *not* complain about emotional or functional problems. Memory and concentration difficulties were the most frequently reported cognitive complaints. Two patients mentioned difficulties in word retrieval and thinking. In contrast, controls mainly reported on impairments in performance and endurance. A more general reduction of physical fitness was described, but no cognitive complaints. Self-reported complaints are summarized in Table 3.

Health complaints were reported by all groups. These problems were more frequently described by the female subgroups (percentile 75). Gender differences were evident within the pre-TBI group ($p = 0.06$). In the attention questionnaire there was a trend for post-TBI patients to report increased distractability and slowing of mental processes compared with controls ($p = 0.07$). However, there were no significant differences when means of all groups were compared with a normative sample provided by

Table 3. Self-reported complaints (% of patients)

	Pre-TBI	Post-TBI	Controls
Cognitive complaints			
Concentration	100	75	0
Memory impairment	71	70	0
Thought disturbances	0	15	0
Word retrieval	14	10	0
Emotional complaints			
Inner tension	29	40	18
Depressive thoughts	29	30	0
Emotional instability	0	20	0
Anxiety	29	20	0
Irritability	14	20	0
Depressive feelings	14	15	0
Psychophysiological complaints			
Joint ache	29	35	27
Cold feet	29	35	18
Feeling cold	0	35	18
Rapid heart rate	14	35	27
Feelings of numbness	29	30	18
Hot flushes	14	30	18
Headaches	14	15	18
Constipation	0	15	0
Rapid exhaustion	43	40	36
Fatigue	100	35	18
Extra need for sleep	14	35	0
Sleep disorders	0	15	36
Loss of energy	29	20	18
Reduced fitness	0	15	18

the test authors (<0.1 SD). Positive mood descriptions were less frequent in the pre-TBI group compared with controls ($p = 0.02$) or the post-TBI group ($p = 0.08$). Negative emotions were not significantly increased. Deactivation was described more frequently by women than by men in the post-TBI group ($p = 0.03$).

Finally, behavior observation data were analyzed, but only minor cognitive problems could be observed by relatives within all groups. However, noncognitive problems such as emotional instability were observed more frequently in the post-TBI group than in the control group ($p = 0.01$). Questionnaire data are summarized in Table 4.

Correlation Analyses

Self-reported data were not significantly correlated with behavior observation data or CT atrophy indices. However, in the post-TBI group the ventricular index (CT) was correlated with the cognitive observation score ($r_S = -0.56$; $p < 0.05$) and with the noncognitive observation score ($r_S = -0.83$; $p < 0.001$). The validity of the cognitive observation score is supported by its correlation with neuropsychological measures such as "logical memory" from the Wechsler Memory Scale-R ($r_S = -0.73$;

Table 4. Summary of questionnaire data[a]

	Controls	Pre-TBI	Post-TBI
Health complaints[b]	61.7 (20)	72.6 (16)	65.0 (31)
Attention questionnaire[c]			
Distractability	59.6 (3)	58.0 (3)	53.8 (8)
Fatigue	36.8 (2)	35.0 (4)	34.8 (5)
Initiative	27.1 (3)	26.8 (2)	25.6 (4)
Mood adjective checklist			
Well-being	39.3 (10)	21.3 (22)	39.3 (24)
Deactivation	14.0 (6)	20.6 (14)	14.2 (10)
Extraversion	5.8 (5)	5.7 (10)	4.6 (6)
Emotional irritability	10.5 (5)	17.4 (10)	16.2 (10)
Anxiety/depressed feeling	21.2 (11)	21.0 (9)	18.4 (16)
Behavior observation scores[c,d]			
Cognitive functions	107.1 (4)	107.4 (5)	106.7 (4)
Noncognitive functions	171.6 (4)	166.4 (8)	162.6 (9)

[a] Means (and SD) are given; for an explanation of inventories see text
[b] Gender norms (T-score); health complaint questionnaire (von Zerssen 1975)
[c] A higher raw score indicates fewer complaints
[d] Behavior rating was performed by family members

$p < 0.05$). Logical memory was also correlated with the ventricular index. In the pre-TBI group no such correlations could be found.

The correlation of observation time with emotion (positive mood: $r_S = -0.46$; $p < 0.09$; negative mood: $r_S = 0.51$; $p < 0.06$) approaches significance in the post-TBI group. A similar association was found for the number of remissions.

Discussion

Quality of life can be regarded as a multidimensional concept (von Kerekjarto et al. 1989). According to Aaronson (1986) several important dimensions of this concept can be identified: symptoms of the disease, side effects of the treatment, functional status, psychological distress, and social interactions. The aim of the present study was to investigate subjective indicators of these dimensions in patients with chronic hematological disorders treated with total body irradiation and bone marrow transplantation.

Primary complaints, as described by our patients, may be summarized as follows: Severe cognitive dysfunction was experienced by none of the groups. Subjective memory problems and concentration difficulties were comparable in both groups. Emotional symptoms such as inner tension or emotional instability were also experienced by both groups. However, post-TBI patients more frequently described distractability and slowing of mental functions. This trend could not be confirmed by a behavior rating performed by relatives. Significant others are probably more sensitive to noncognitive behavioral changes: emotional instability was observed more frequently after TBI compared with controls.

TBI and BMT can be regarded as having a major impact upon the physical and social integrity of the individual. It is not surprising that this treatment coincides with considerable general complaints and reduced well-being. Women in particular reported reduced well-being and elevated health complaints. However, emotional problems (emotional instability and, in women, deactivation and a reduction in positive mood) persisted years after therapy; the extent of emotional problems even seems to increase with survival time. For example, the duration of the disease was correlated with mood, but not with neuropsychological or CT variables. Neuser (1989) found that patients even feel better in the preparatory and conditioning phase prior to BMT when compared with subsequent weeks.

Emotional symptoms frequently occur in the course of dementing diseases. For example, depression has been described as a significant precursor of the full syndrome of Alzheimer's dementia (Reding et al. 1985). It is characterized by social withdrawal, pervasive sadness, irritability, hopelessness, and psychomotor retardation (Sunderland et al. 1988). Similar emotional symptoms have been described as sequelae of chronic exposure to neurotoxic substances (Hartman 1988).

In psychological oncology, emotional symptoms are usually attributed to the individual coping behavior of the patient. However, at least in Alzheimer's dementia, neuropathological changes of emotion-related structures such as the medial temporal cortex seem to precede the general cortical atrophy seen in later stages. Given that cerebral radiotherapy leads to mild forms of dementia, emotional changes can also be interpreted as early neurotoxic sequelae which might be due to alterations of specific subcortical or allocortical structures (e.g., basal ganglia, thalamus, amygdala). The weak association of general atrophy and emotional variables found in our follow-up group does not rule out the possibility of a specific subcortical damage.

Patients with leukemia and lymphomas have different protocols of chemotherapy. Thus, differential effects on quality of life may be expected. Nonparametrical tests, however, did not show any difference between the diagnostic groups.

It has been pointed out above that quality of life can be defined on different methodological levels. Medical methods are generally accepted for the objective evaluation of long-term effects of brain irradiation. From a psycho-oncological perspective, neurological, neuroradiological, and neuropsychological sequelae can be interpreted as inversely defined determinants of quality of life. However, absence of cerebral atrophy does not prove that behavioral or emotional functions are intact (e.g., Bigler et al. 1985; Bigler 1988). Even if a neuropsychological assessment yields only a minimal cognitive impairment (cf. Tucker et al. 1989) it is uncertain how subjective emotional, motivational, and psychosocial consequences will influence the patient's quality of life. Emotional problems seem to be perceived more accurately than cognitive difficulties by the patient.

In our study a marked decline in quality of life on a subjective level could not be confirmed. However, there was considerable variability within the post-TBI patients. One of our patients who was treated with radiotherapy combined with MTX instillation showed the most distinct long-term effects on objective and subjective indices of quality of life. He developed moderate brain atrophy and described memory and concentration problems. On the neuropsychological level, a subclinical impairment of attentional performance and mnestic processing could be found. Radiogenic impairment of the blood–brain barrier and an increase in intracerebral concentration of MTX have been discussed as a possible mechanism of this increased neurotoxicity (Stephani et al. 1983; Griffin et al. 1977).

Since the association of objective and subjective determinants is usually not very strong (cf. von Kerekjarto et al. 1989) and the predictive value of neurological or neuropsychological indicators for everyday behavior is limited, we suggest that the assessment of subjective indicators of quality of life should be an essential addition to radiological treatment evaluation methods.

Acknowledgments. We are grateful to Prof. Dr. Huber and Dr. Twittenhof for providing control patients.

References

Aaronson NK, Beckman J (1987) The quality of life of cancer patients. Raven, New York

Aaronson NK (1986) Methodological issues in psychosocial oncology with special reference to clinical trials. In: Ventafridda V, van Dam FSAM, Yancik R, Tamburini M (eds) Assessment of quality of life and cancer treatment. Excerpta Medica, Amsterdam, pp 29–41

Bigler ED (1988) Neuropsychological and computed tomographic identification in dementia. In: Whitaker HA (ed) Neuropsychological studies of nonfocal brain damage. Springer, Berlin Heidelberg New York, pp 61–85

Bigler ED, Hubler DW, Cullum CM, Turkheimer E (1985) Intellectual and memory impairment: CT volume correlations. J Nerv Ment Dis 173:347–352

Bleyer WA (1981) Neurologic sequelae of methotrexate and ionising radiation: a new classification. Cancer Treat Rep 65 [Suppl]:89–98

Brouwers P, Riccardi R, Fedio P, Poplack DG (1985) Long-term neuropsychologic sequelae of childhood leukaemia: correlation with CT brain scan abnormalities. J Pediatr 106:723–728

Eiser C (1978) Intellectual abilities among survivors of childhood leukaemia as a function of CNS irradiation. Arch Dis Child 53:391–395

Griffin TW, Rasey JS, Bleyer WA (1977) The effect of photon irradiation on blood–brain barrier permeability to methotrexate in mice. Cancer 40:1109–1111

Hartman DE (1988) Neuropsychological toxicology. Pergamon, Oxford

Holland JC, Silberfarb P, Tross S, Cella D (1986) Psychosocial research in cancer: the cancer and leukaemia group B (CALGB) experience. In: Ventafridda V, van Dam FSAM, Yancik R, Tamburini M (eds) Assessment of quality of life and cancer treatment. Excerpta Medica, Amsterdam, pp 89–101

Janke W, Debus G (1978) Die Eigenschaftswörterliste EWL. Hogrefe, Göttingen

Johnson BE, Becker J, Gott WB et al. (1985) Neurologic, neuropsychologic and computed cranial tomography scan abnormalities in 2- to 10-year survivors of small cell lung cancer. J Clin Oncol 3:1659–1667

Kerekjarto M von, Schulz KH, Kramer C, Fittschen B, Schug S (1989) Grundlegende Aspekte zum Konzept der Lebensqualität. In: Verres R, Hasenbring M (eds) Jahrbuch der psychosozialen Onkologie. Springer, Berlin Heidelberg New York, pp 18–29 (Handbuch der Medizinischen Psychologie, vol 3)

Kessler J, Denzler P, Markowitsch HJ (1988) Demenz-Test. Beltz, Weinheim

King KB, Nail LM, Kreamer K, Strohl RA, Johnson JE (1985) Patients' descriptions of the experience of receiving radiation therapy. Oncol Nurs Forum 12(4):55–61

Körbling M, Hunstein W, Fliedner T, Cayeux S, Dörken B, Fehrentz D, Haas R, Ho AD, Keilholz U, Knauf W, König A, Mende U, Pezzutto A, von Reumont J, Wolf GK, Wannenmacher M, zum Winkel K, Rother K (1989) Disease-free survival after autologous bone marrow transplantation in patients with acute myelogenous leukemia. Blood 74:1898–1904

Kretzschmar K, Gutjahr P, Kutzner J (1980) CT studies before and after CNS treatment for acute lymphoblastic leukaemia and malignant non-Hodgkin's lymphoma in childhood. Neuroradiology 20:173–180

Laukkanen E, Klonoff H, Allan B, Graeb D, Murray N (1988) The role of prophylactic brain irradiation in limited stage small cell lung cancer: clinical, neuropsychologic, and CT sequelae. Int J Radiat Oncol Biol Phys 14:1109–1117
Lee JS, Umsawasdi T, Lee YY et al. (1986) Neurotoxicity in longterm survivors of small cell lung cancer. Int J Radiat Oncol Biol Phys 12:313–321
Lezak MD (1983) Neuropsychological assessment. Oxford University Press, Oxford
Meadows AT, Massari JD, Fergusson J, Gordon J, Littman PH, Moss K (1981) Declines in IQ scores and cognitive dysfunctions in children with acute lymphocytic leukaemia treated with cranial irradiation. Lancet 1:1015–1018
Neuser J (1989) Psychische Belastung unter Knochenmarkstransplantation: hat soziale Unterstützung Pufferwirkung? In: Verres R, Hasenbring M (eds) Jahrbuch der psychosozialen Onkologie. Springer, Berlin Heidelberg New York, pp 151–160 (Handbuch der Medizinischen Psychologie, vol 3)
Ochs J, Mulhern R, Fairclough D, Parvey L, Whitaker J, Ch'ien L, Mauer A, Simone J (1991) Comparison of neuropsychologic functioning and clinical indicators of neurotoxicity in long-term survivors of childhood leukaemia given cranial radiation or parenteral methotrexate: a prospective study. J Clin Oncol 9:145–151
Peper M, Schraube P, Kimmig B, Wannenmacher M, Haas R (1993) Neuropsychological side-effects of total body irradiation (to be published)
Poplack DG, Brouwers P (1985) Adverse sequelae of central nervous system therapy. Clin Oncol 4:263–285
Rubin PH, Wasserman TH (1988) The late effects of toxicity scoring. J Radiat Oncol Biol Phys 14:29–38
Stephani U, Rating D, Korinthenberg R, Siemes H, Riehm H, Hanefeld F (1983) Radiation-related disturbance of blood/brain barrier during therapy of acute lymphoblastic leukaemia. Lancet 4:1036–1037
Tucker J, Prior PF, Green CR, Ede GMV, Stevenson JF, Gawler J, Jamal GA, Charlesworth M, Thakkar CM, Patel P, Lister TA (1989) Minimal neuropsychological sequelae following prophylactic treatment of the central nervous system in adult leukaemia and lymphoma. Br J Cancer 60:775–780
Von Zerssen D (1975) Die Beschwerdenliste. Beltz, Weinheim
Wilson RS, Rosenbaum G, Brown G (1979) The problem of premorbid intelligence in neuropsychological assessment. J Clin Neuropsychol 1:49–93
Zimmermann P, Poser U (1993) Ein Fragebogen erlebter Defizite der Aufmerksamkeit. Z Neuropsychol (to be published)

Eye Sequelae Following External Irradiation

M. Hempel and W. Hinkelbein

Department of Radiotherapy, University Hospital, W-7800 Freiburg, Fed. Rep. of Germany

Introduction

The first studies of the effects of ionizing radiation on the eye were by Chalupecky in 1897. Since then many studies have been published but nevertheless not all the risks to the eyes of radiotherapy are known in detail.

Well-known are the early reactions to irradiation such as conjunctivitis and keratoconjunctivitis. Special attention has been directed recently to radiation retinopathy (RR) and radiation neuropathy of the optic nerve (RON), while the well-known late effect of radiation-induced cataract has become less feared with the development of modern surgical or optical treatment.

The published data on the total dose causing RR or RON and the latent period of these severe complications differ over a wide range. Recent results with eye-preserving therapy in maxillary sinus carcinomas (42–66 Gy) showed a blindness rate of 33% ipsilateral and 10% bilateral (Jiang et al. 1991). Prospective studies with continuing ocular examinations are needed for the early identification of microangiopathy of the retina and optic nerve, and the frequency and extent of vision loss and complete blindness.

Acute Reactions

Conjunctivitis

Conjunctival hyperemia is often seen during the course of radiotherapy, while doses of approximately 50 Gy lead to real conjunctival damage with drying and scarring. Usually conjunctivities is transient and can be treated well by local steroids and antibiotics, if associated with infection. Severe, irreversible damage such as contracture is seen with doses of more than 60 Gy; symblepharon is seen after 80–100 Gy. The side effect of permanent

Recent Results in Cancer Research, Vol. 130

epilation of the eyelashes is seen with doses of 30 Gy or more (Merriam et al. 1972).

Keratitis and Corneal Ulceration

Transient punctate keratitis may develop during radiotherapy with doses of 30–50 Gy in 4–5 weeks (Merriam et al. 1972). Ulceration and perforation may occur after doses exceeding 60 Gy and may lead to loss of sight in the eye within months after therapy. Corneal damage can also be produced by a dry eye following atrophy of lacrimal glands in the dose range of 50–60 Gy (Merriam et al. 1972; Parsons et al. 1983). Similar doses may lead to obliteration of the lacrimal ducts. Therefore, in planning radiotherapy treatments shielding of the lateral part of the upper lid is recommended.

Late Reactions

Cataract

The degree of opacity varies from no visual impairment to complete loss of vision and is dose dependent. Cataract appears from within 6 months to many years (on average 2–3 years) after radiotherapy. Single doses producing opacities vary from 2 to 10 Gy. Doses inducing progressive cataracts with fractionated radiotherapy range from 10 to 15 Gy (Deeg 1984; Merriam and Focht 1962; Schipper et al. 1985).

The lenses of children are more radiosensitive than those of adults. In children who completed treatment for acute lymphoblastic leukemia, including cranial irradiation, one third showed posterior subcapsular lens opacities – though without optical significance (Elliot et al. 1985).

Cataract as a frequent and severe complication can be treated adequately by extraction of the lens and visual rehabilitation using contact lenses or lens implants.

Retinopathy

Radiation retinopathy (RR) is characterized by microaneurysms, "cotton-wool spots", hemorrhages, leakage of vessels with exudates, progressive occlusion of small vessels with ischemia and edema, and chronic changes including vitreous hemorrhage, retinal detachments, and optic nerve atrophy. Vascular changes in the retina begin at 30 Gy (Duke-Elder 1972). RR generally occurs 6 months to 3 years (range 1 month to 15 years) after radiotherapy. The clinical severity differs from little impairment to complete loss of vision.

The frequency, extent, and latency period of RR depend on total dose, size of fraction, and dose rate, all of which are dependent on the radiation field arrangement and beam energy. The threshold dose for RR seems to be 30–35 Gy (Merriam et al. 1972), but the lowest retinal dose described was 11 Gy (Elsas et al. 1988). There are many conflicting estimates of the frequency of RR (Table 1), but the true risk of visual impairment is not known with confidence. Daily fractions should not exceed 2 Gy. Combination with chemotherapy or diabetic and hypertensive disease are important cofactors in potentiating RR and shortening its latency period (Brown et al. 1981; Chan and Shukovsky 1976; Dhir et al. 1982; Hayreh 1970). No RR has been described after doses applied to children for acute lymphoblastic leukemia and cranial prophylactic irradiation (12–18–24 Gy) despite the enclosure of the whole of the posterior part of the eye in the irradiation field (Weaver et al. 1986).

No promising treatment exists for progressive severe retinal damage causing deterioration of vision and blindness. Some patients may benefit from photocoagulation treatment (Kinyoun et al. 1988).

Optic Neuropathy

Radiation optic neuropathy (RON) may cause unilateral or bilateral loss of vision ranging from mild to severe. There are two types of RON: (1) injury at the distal end of the nerve on or around the disk, and (2) more proximal injury with retrobulbar neuropathy or damage to the chiasma. The observed pathological changes are initial damage to capillaries and arterioles and later to the larger arteries, with subsequent damage to the fasciculus opticus.

The latency period varies from several months to many years. The development of RON is dose dependent. The smallest dose recorded as producing RON is 36 Gy, but mostly RON occurs with doses exceeding 50–60 Gy (Alberti 1991; Brown et al. 1981). Reducing the fraction size reduces the frequency of RON. Fraction sizes of 1.65–1.9 Gy and total doses of 60–73 Gy produce RON only in 8% of patients (Parsons et al. 1983). Combination with chemotherapy increases the incidence; some authors even found RON in patients who had had prophylactic cranial irradiation for acute lymphoblastic leukemia (Fishman et al. 1976; Margileth et al. 1977).

As in the case of RR there is as yet no effective treatment for visual loss after RON.

Summary

The early reactions of the eye to radiation are conjunctivitis and, with higher doses, corneal damage. The inflammatory reactions are transient and

Table 1. Frequency of radiation retinopathy (RR)

Reference	No. of patients evaluated	Dose (Gy)	% RR	% blindness	Latency period (yr)	Remarks
Perrers-Taylor	119	15–21				
et al. (1965)		27–31	20	0	2–4	
Shukovsky and Fletcher (1972)	15	55–74	46 (+RON)	22	2–3.5	Ethmoidal and upper nasal cavity
Chan and Shukovsky (1976)	22	60		10		Paranasal sinus
Schipper et al. (1985)	54	45	4.5	0	2	Retinoblastoma, 3 fractions/week
Thompson et al. (1983)	10	60–70	70	50	1–10	Posterior nasal space carcinomas
De Schryver et al. (1971)	30	15–35	60	0		Nasopharyngeal carcinoma
Karim et al. (1990)	45	52–100	16 (+RON)	2	1–3.3	Upper nasal cavity ethmoidal region external + brachytherapy boost
Brown et al. (1982)	33	25–55	100 (+RON)	20		Study on RR and RON
Parsons et al. (1988)	48	60–76		33 (+RON)	0.5–5, 8 bilateral	Nasal cavity and paranasal sinus
Nakissa et al. (1983)	30	34–75	25 (+RON)	7		Paranasal sinus

RON, neuropathy of the optic nerve

remit within a few weeks after the end of radiotherapy. Doses above 60 Gy can produce corneal ulcerations with the risk of perforation and loss of the eye.

The most frequent late reaction of the eye is cataract of the lens. The tolerance dose (about 5 Gy) is extremely low and the latent period varies from 6 months to 3 years. The lens in children has a much lower tolerance. The increasing potential for optical support and ophthalmic surgery over recent decades has reduced the fear of this complication.

The most severe late complications are retinopathy (RR) and neuropathy of the optic nerve (RON), both of which are caused by radiation-induced microangiopathy. Visual loss is very frequent and complete blindness is seen with high doses in the range of 50–60 Gy. The latent period of these injuries varies widely from 1 month to 15 years, but they usually occur within 3 years of treatment. Conflicting frequencies are reported in the literature. Beyond 30 Gy, usually no RR is seen. However, the lowest recorded dose producing RR is 11 Gy. In the high dose range of 60–70 Gy RR and RON are found in 10%–100% of patients. There is a great need for prospective trials to estimate the true risk to patients with nasopharyngeal, maxillo-ethmoidal, and orbital tumors, pituitary adenomas, and tumors of the salivary glands.

To minimize complications of radiotherapy to the eyes daily fractions should be reduced to 1.7–1.8 Gy. Whenever possible there should be sparing of the orbita and bulbus, especially the lateral two thirds, and a reduction of the dose to the chiasma is necessary. The greatest hazard is contralateral blindness, which must be avoided at all costs.

References

Alberti W (1991) Effects of radiation on the eye and ocular adnexa. In: Scherer E, Streffer C, Trott KR (eds) Radiopathology of organs and tissues. Springer, Berlin Heidelberg New York, pp 269–282

Brown GC, Shields JA, Sanborn G, Augsburger JJ, Savino PJ, Schatz NJ (1982) Radiation retinopathy. Ophthalmology 89:1494–1501

Brown GC, Shields JA, Sanborn G, Augsburger JJ, Savino PJ, Schatz NJ (1982) Radiation optic neuropathy. Ophthalmology 89:1489–1493

Chalupecky H (1897) Über die Wirkung der Röntgenstrahlen auf das Auge und die Haut. Zentralbl Augenheilkd 21:234–267

Chan RG, Shukovsky LJ (1976) Effects of radiation on the eye. Radiology 120:673–675

Deeg HJ (1984) Bone marrow transplantation: a review of delayed complications. Br J Haematol 57:185–208

De Schryver A, Wachtmeister L, Brayd I (1971) Ophthalmologic observations on long-term survivors after radiotherapy for nasopharyngeal tumors. Acta Radiol 10:193–209

Dhir SP, Joshi AV, Banerjee AK (1982) Radiation retinopathy in diabetes mellitus. Acta Radiol Oncol 21:111–113

Duke-Elder S (1972) System of ophthalmology, vol 14, part 2: injuries, nonmechanical injuries. Mosby, St Louis, pp 985–999

Elliot AJ, Oakhill A, Goodman S (1985) Cataracts in childhood leukemia. Br J Ophthalmol 69:459–461
Elsas T, Thorud E, Jetne V, Conradi IS (1988) Retinopathy after low dose irradiation for an intracranial tumor of the frontal lobe. Acta Ophthalmol (Copenh) 66:65–68
Fishman ML, Bean SC, Cogan DG (1976) Optic atrophy following prophylactic chemotherapy and cranial irradiation for acute lymphocytic leukemia. Am J Ophthalmol 82:571–576
Hayreh SS (1970) Post-radiation therapy: a fluorescence fundus angiographic study. Br J Ophthalmol 54:705–714
Jiang GL, Kian Ang K, Peters LJ, Wendt CD, Oswald MJ, Goepfert H (1991) Maxillary sinus carcinomas: natural history and results of postoperative radiotherapy. Radiother Oncol 21:193–200
Karim ABMF, Kralendonk JH, Njo KH, Tabak JM, Elsenaar WH, van Balen AThM (1990) Ethmoid and upper nasal cavity carcinoma: treatment, results and complications. Radiother Oncol 19:109–120
Kinyoun JL, Chittum ME, Wells CG (1988) Photocoagulation treatment of radiation retinopathy. Am J Ophthalmol 105:470–478
Margileth DA, Poplack DG, Pizzo PA, Leventhal BG (1977) Blindness during remission in two patients with acute lymphoblastic leukemia. Cancer 39:58
Merriam GR, Focht EF (1962) A clinical and experimental study of the effect of single and divided doses of radiation on cataract production. Trans Am Ophthalmol Soc 60:35–52
Merriam GR, Szechter A, Focht EF (1972) The effects of ionizing radiations on the eye. Front Radiation Ther Onc 6:346–385
Nakissa N, Rubin P, Strohl R, Keys H (1983) Ocular and orbital complications following radiation therapy of paranasal sinus malignancies and review of literature. Cancer 51:980–986
Parsons JT, Fitzgerald CR, Hood GI, Ellingwood KE, Bova FJ, Million RR (1983) The effects of irradiation on the eye and optic nerve. Int J Radiat Oncol Biol Phys 9:609–612
Parsons JT, Mendenhall WM, Mancuso AA, Cassisi NJ, Million RR (1988) Malignant tumors of the nasal cavity and ethmoid and sphenoid sinuses. Int J Radiat Oncol Biol Phys 14:11–22
Perres-Taylor M, Binkley D, Reynolds T (1965) Choroidoretinal damage as a complication of radiotherapy. Acta Radiol 3:431–440
Schipper J, Tan KEWP, van Peperizeel HA (1985) Treatment of retinoblastoma by precision megavoltage radiation therapy. Radiother Oncol 3:117–132
Shukovsky LJ, Fletcher GH (1972) Retinal and optic nerve complications in a high dose irradiation technique of ethmoid sinus and nasal cavity. Radiology 104:629–634
Thompson GM, Migdal CS, Whittle RJM (1983) Radiation retinopathy following treatment of posterior nasal space carcinoma. Br J Opthalmol 67:609–614
Weaver RG Jr, Chauvenet AR, Smith TJ, Schwartz AC (1986) Ophthalmic evaluation of long-term survivors of childhood acute lymphoblastic leukemia. Cancer 58:963–968

V. Particular Problems in Pediatric Radiotherapy

Late Side Effects of Pediatric Radiotherapy

R. Pötter

Klinik und Poliklinik für Strahlentherapie – Radioonkologie Westfälische, Wilhelms-Universität Münster, W-4400 Münster, Fed. Rep. of Germany

Introduction

During the last two decades the place of radiotherapy in the combination treatment of pediatric malignancies has changed considerably, mainly because of the high chemosensitivity of most pediatric tumors. The essential role of radiotherapy for local tumor control has been widely clarified for Hodgkin's disease, central nervous system (CNS) leukemia, soft tissue sarcoma, Ewing's sarcoma, retinoblastoma, and nephroblastoma (stage II N+, III) and is being clarified for the majority of CNS malignancies. Local radiotherapy is no longer commonly used within multimodal treatment of standard risk acute lymphoblastic leukemia (ALL), non-Hodgkin's lymphoma (NHL), prognostic favorable and operable nephroblastoma, operable osteosarcoma, extracranial germ cell tumors, histiocytosis X, and localized, chemoresponsive neuroblastoma. Late side effects of multimodal treatment will be observed with increasing frequencies due to the high cure rates – more than two thirds of all children with cancer survive (Table 1) – and the resulting long follow-up periods.

During the last decade treatment strategies have been increasingly tailored to the individual risk of disease and to the probability of late side effects expected from any of the applied treatment modalities: radiotherapy, chemotherapy, surgery. In particular this applies to Hodgkin's disease, nephroblastoma, subgroups of leukemia, neuroblastoma, soft tissue sarcoma, and Ewing's sarcoma.

Late side effects in pediatric radiotherapy are dependent on several parameters: total dose and single dose in the treatment volume and irradiation volume, the size of these volumes, the overall treatment time, the growth potential and repair capacity of the tissue involved, and the age of the child. The term "age of the child" reflects differences in radiosensitivity dependent on different periods of proliferation, differentiation, and maturation of the tissue involved. Radiosensitivity is regarded as highest at the

Recent Results in Cancer Research, Vol. 130

Table 1. Five-year survival rates in childhood malignancies (n = 9342) after treatment in the German cooperative clinical multicenter trials (GPO/DAL) (modified from Haaf et al. 1990)

Diagnosis	*n*	5-year survival rate (%)
Hodgkin's disease	498	94
Histiocytosis X	270	89
Germ cell tumors	274	85
Nephroblastoma	572	83
ALL	2896	77
Non-Hodgkin's-lymphoma	593	75
Osteosarcoma	287	65
Rhabdomyosarcoma	404	59
Ewing's sarcoma	222	59
CNS tumors	1195	52
Neuroblastoma	733	52
Acute leukemia without ALL	485	45
All malignancies	9342	69

time of onset of proliferative activity in a certain organ or tissue, for instance during infancy or adolescence in bone and soft tissue (Rubin et al. 1982). The clinical expression of a certain radiation-induced effect, on the other hand, becomes most evident during these periods of active proliferation irrespective of the time of induction.

As malignancies in childhood are nearly all treated with multimodal strategies, the side effects from drugs and surgical interventions have to be considered separately as well as in their interaction with radiotherapy. For side effects after combination with chemotherapy the following parameters have to be considered: the type of drug(s) and the interaction with normal tissue, the organ/tissue at specific risk from a certain drug, the cumulative dose, the method of drug administration, and the timing of drug administration relative to irradiation (before/after radiotherapy, simultaneous with radiotherapy). Regarding acute and late toxicity the most important known drugs are alkylating agents (gonads, bladder, kidney, induction of second malignancies), doxorubicin (heart, mucosa of the gastrointestinal tract, skin), actinomycin D (liver, skin), methotrexate (CNS), platin (ear, kidney), and bleomycin (lung). For side effects after combination with surgery the surgical procedure itself must be taken into account as well as the possible lasting or late effects following the surgical intervention. This is especially important for surgery in sarcoma and brain tumors.

Side effects from therapeutic X-rays in children have been studied for decades, mostly in small numbers of children for the endpoints of bone and soft tissue growth. Little attention has been paid to dose distribution within a given volume of a certain tissue investigated (Willich et al. 1990). Nevertheless, for assessing the effect of irradiation the crucial factors are the radiation dose and the irradiated volume in the tissue of interest. It is not necessarily meaningful to take the tumor dose (reference dose) as representative of the tissue dose and correlate this construct with an observed effect in this tissue. The questionable validity and reliability of such a procedure are evident. When reporting late effects from radiotherapy the minimal requirement is to state the mean applied total and single radiation dose in the tissue and the distribution of dose within the volume of the tissue investigated and the overall treatment time (Probert and Parker 1975). This is to be done for every single patient and correlated with the effect investigated (Pötter et al. this volume). Furthermore the minimum and maximum dose in the tissue based on calculated dose distributions, the beam quality, and the treatment technique (e.g., number of radiation fields, use of shielding blocks) including documentation (X-ray films, CT scans) must be indicated. The widely accepted ICRU recommendations for reporting dose in radiotherapy also represent a reliable basis for reporting side effects from radiotherapy (ICRU 1978).

This article will address only certain types of side effects, with special emphasis on a critical review from the radiotherapeutic point of view. As, except in immature organs during infancy and early childhood, a specific radiovulnerability has not been reported, organs such as lung, heart, kidney, bladder, liver, digestive tract, lymphatic system, bone marrow, eye, ear, salivary gland, and skin are not dealt with. Furthermore only sparse data exist for these organs with regard to late effects from pediatric radiotherapy.

Growth of Bone and Soft Tissue

Due to the different types of bone growth there are different patterns of irradiation effects: in tubular bones epiphyseal injury leads to an arrest of chondrogenesis with a resultant shortening of bone length, metaphyseal injury to deficiencies in absorption of bone and cartilage, and diaphyseal injury to an alteration of periosteal activity and impairment of bone modeling and bone thickness. The effects of irradicition on enchondral ossification in pelvic bones, vertebrae, ribs, and viscerocranium depend on the degree of injury to the different ossification and epiphyseal centers. The clinical picture from the irradiation effects on desmal ossification seems to be not very prounonced in the skull, whereas it may be significant in the clavicle. In addition to the direct irradiation effect on the parenchymatous cells in bone the dose-dependent damage of microvasculature contributes much to the development of late effects (Hopewell, this volume).

The most sensitive periods for the induction of bone and soft tissue effects are periods of rapid proliferation during the growth spurts in early childhood and adolescence. The amount of growth reduction is dependent on the growth potential and the degree of amplification of the (region of) X-ray-treated bone to be expected before adult target height and target shape are reached (Gonzalez Gonzalez and Breur 1982; Rubin et al. 1982; Fig. 1). In soft tissue the amount of growth reduction has to be calculated in a similar way, although based on different pathological mechanisms from connective tissue and muscle. In assessing the clinical effect the relative importance of bone and soft tissue effects have to be taken into account.

The age dependency of radiation effects on bone and soft tissue is sufficiently explained by this model without claiming a specific radiosensitivity. Several reports in the literature on vertebral growth in long-term survivors

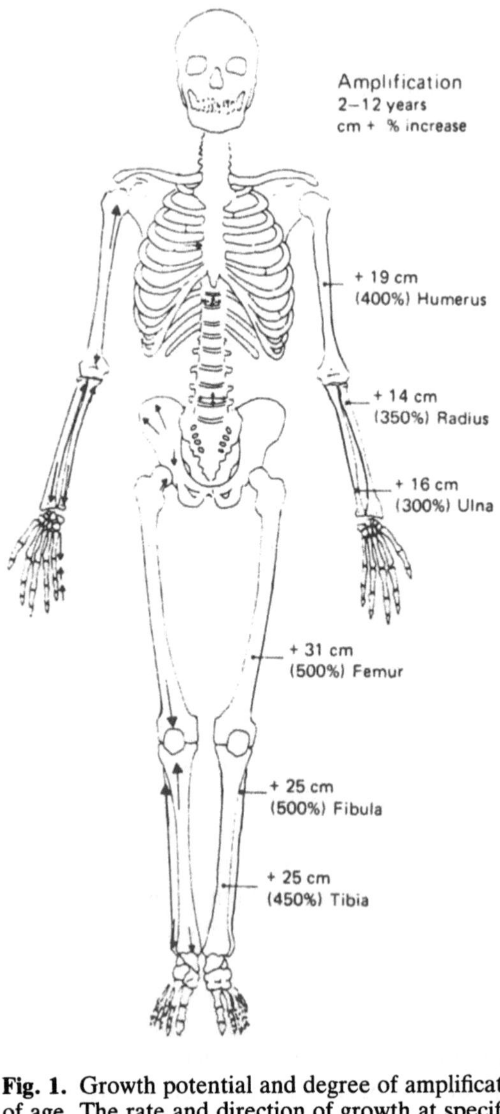

Fig. 1. Growth potential and degree of amplification of bone between 2 and 12 years of age. The rate and direction of growth at specific skeletal sites are indicated by the length and thickness of arrows. (Modified from Rubin et al. 1982)

after spinal irradiation in Hodgkin's disease, nephroblastoma, leukemia, and medulloblastoma support this model (Neuhauser et al. 1952; Probert and Parker 1975; Willich et al. 1990). No specification of radiation dose is given in some of these reports (see above). The side effect – reduction of sitting height – is described as much more severe after irradiation in early childhood.

Dose dependency of the degree of effect has also been described in detail. Sitting height, for example, is reduced less (within 1 standard deviation from the mean in older children, up to 2 standard deviations from the mean in young children) after doses up to 25 Gy compared with those of more than 35 Gy (Probert and Parker 1975). Shortening and scoliosis of the spine, soft tissue hypoplasia in one flank, and iliac hypoplasia have been reported after radiotherapy with 30–47 Gy in nephroblastoma that included these tissues within the treatment volume (Lemerle et al. 1989; Willich et al. 1990). Long-term follow-up studies after low-dose radiotherapy (10–30 Gy) which is nowadays commonly used in the treatment of Hodgkin's disease, leukemia, and nephroblastoma (stage II N+, III) will clarify the degree of effect after low-dose radiotherapy combined with multidrug chemotherapy. Earlier data (e.g., Neuhauser et al. 1952) and clinical experience suggest that late effects on growth to be expected after low-dose radiotherapy will probably be small.

The late effects of high-dose radiotherapy (40–60 Gy) in tubular bones (nowadays mostly Ewing's and soft tissue sarcoma), joints, and soft tissues of the extremities are very severe after treatment of young children, with significant functional impairments; they are much less after treatment of adolescents (Gonzalez Gonzalez and Breur 1982; Neff 1985; Lemerle et al. 1989; Pötter et al., this volume). Significant effects such as pathological fracture and severe fibrosis have been described by Tefft et al. (1976) after combination therapy with simultaneous chemotherapy. Nevertheless, more systematic analysis in larger numbers of patients for a given site is needed to clarify this issue, which will become possible because of the increasing cure rates achieved during the last decade (Table 1).

A systematic analysis is needed for assessing the late effects after high-dose radiotherapy of the pelvic region, the trunk, and the head and neck region. The reports published so far indicate several functional and cosmetic impairments after high-dose radiotherapy for Hodgkin's disease (Fig. 2) and especially for sarcoma in the head and neck: muscle atrophy, subcutaneous fibrosis, craniofacial deformity, dental problems, and temporomandibular joint fibrosis (Heyn 1985; Fromm et al. 1986). Again it has to emphasized that radiation dose and its volume distribution in the tissue of interest have to be correlated with the effect being investigated (see above); this is of particular importance because of the wide variety of different radiation techniques in sarcoma radiotherapy.

In assessing late effects after a combination of surgery and radiotherapy the late effects due to the surgical intervention must be carefully considered, especially in sarcoma compare Figs. 1 and 2; (Pötter et al., this volume).

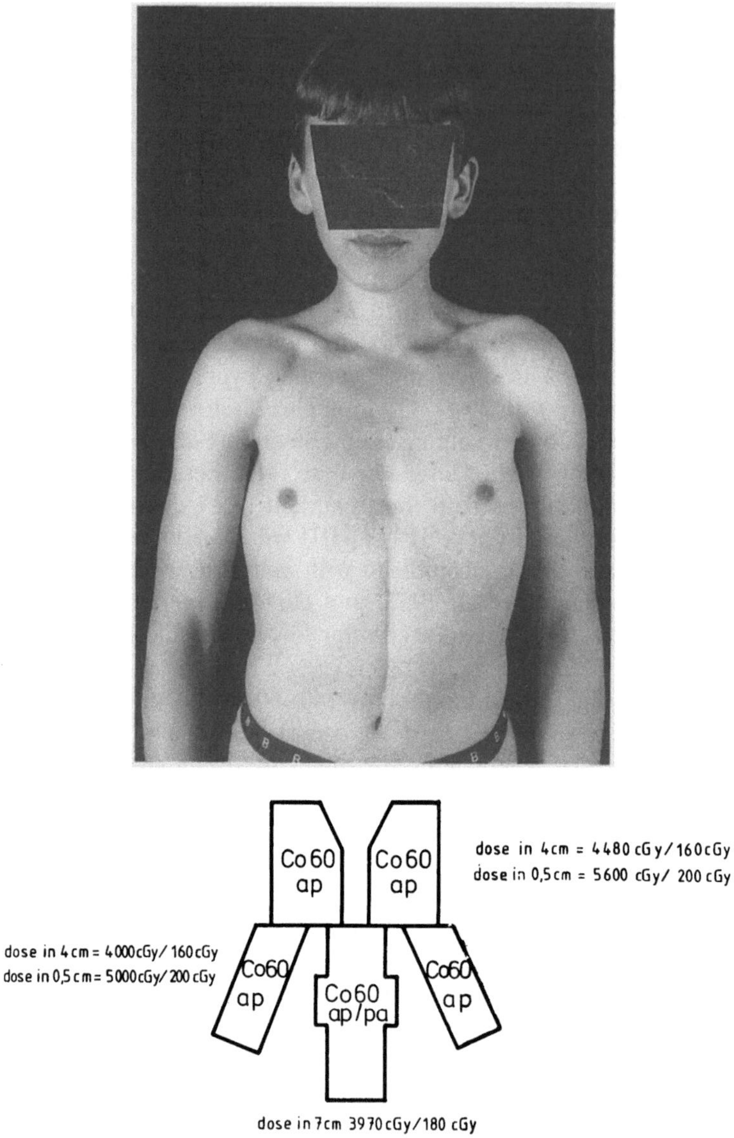

Fig. 2a,b. Soft tissue hypoplasia in the supra/infraclavicular axillary region and the neck, and clavicle hypoplasia in a boy 19 years old (**a**) who had been irradiated for Hodgkin's disease at the age of 8 years (**b**). The boy had been treated by anteroposterior (ap) ^{60}Co portals and opposed anteroposterior/posteroanterior (pa) portals in the mediastinum. The reference dose, the maximum dose total dose, and the dose per fraction are indicated in the diagram. To understand the distribution of soft tissue hypoplasia it is necessary to know the maximum total dose in the soft tissues, which is up to 55 Gy. Note that the protracted application of radiotherapy, lasting more than 6 months, did not avoid the remarkable hypoplasia

Endocrine Function

Hypothalamic–Pituitary Axis

The site of radiation-induced injury is most likely to be the hypothalamic region where the releasing hormones are produced (Blacklay et al. 1986; Lannering and Albertsson-Wiland 1987). The pituitary gland itself seems to be of minor importance.

Radiation-induced growth hormone deficiency has been investigated in children after radiotherapy for brain and nasopharyngeal tumors and after prophylactic irradiation of the brain in leukemia and medulloblastoma. The measurable impairment becomes evident within months or years after radiotherapy. For growth hormone deficiency the clinical endpoint is height and height velocity; the biochemical endpoint is spontaneous and stimulated growth hormone (GH) secretion (stimulation e.g., by insulin or arginine provocation tests).

After radiotherapy of brain and nasopharyngeal tumors with doses from 35 to 55 Gy to the hypothalamic–pituitary axis significant impairment of height and height velocity as well as of spontaneous and stimulated growth hormone secretion has been observed (Shalet 1985). Growth curves are likely to fall below the 10th percentile within a few years after treatment.

After radiotherapy for prophylactic treatment in leukemia with doses from 18 to 24 Gy radiation-induced effects are difficult to detect. In a large longitudinal national study on 107 long-term survivors from leukemia treated according to the BFM/DAL protocols in Germany from 1970 to 1979 no significant differences could be found in standing height when comparing the adult height achieved with the target height: mean values for boys were 179 cm, for girls 165 cm. A minor height loss (about 3 cm) was noted compared with the height of siblings (Brämswig et al. 1990b). Nevertheless, according to several reports in the literature there seems to be an impairment of stimulated growth hormone secretion (Shalet 1985) indicative of a rather modest radiation injury in this region which does not lead to a measurable clinical effect with regard to height. Loss of target height was more probable after 2 Gy per fraction than after low doses per fraction (1.2 Gy) when the same total dose (24 Gy) had been applied for cranial radiotherapy in leukemia (Brämswig et al. 1989).

Chemotherapy contributes only temporarily to growth retardation. When therapy is finished, growth is accelerated and the children usually catch up with their peers.

The clinical monitoring of growth-hormone-induced growth retardation is important as it can successfully be treated by replacement of growth hormone (Shalet 1989).

The risk of radiation injury to the other hypothalamic–pituitary axes has not been well stated yet. After doses above 35 Gy reduction of TSH secretion is to be expected within a few years in 30%–50% of children

(Pomarede et al. 1983). The risk for alteration of gonadotropin secretion is reported to be about 20%–40% after radiotherapy with doses above 35 Gy (Rappaport et al. 1982). Impairment of ACTH secretion seems to be very rare even after very high radiation doses (Lemerle et al. 1989). Diabetes insipidus has been reported due to tumor growth (craniopharyngioma, germinoma, histiocytosis X) or after surgical intervention.

Dose and treatment volume of radiotherapy are not specified in detail in the majority of the cited reports. As for brain radiotherapy a wide range of different indications exist; the indications for which a radiation dose above 30–35 Gy in the hypothalamic–pituitary region is justified are to be clarified and documented. Doses of 30–35 Gy seem to define the range above which clinically evident side effects from the different hypothalamic–pituitary axes become increasingly probable. From the biological behavior of the tumors to be irradiated and from the treatment planning and techniques nowadays available, the radiation dose to this region should only exceed 35 Gy if the tumor grows within this region or very close to it (e.g., craniopharyngioma, suprasellar germinoma, glioma of the optic chiasma, brain stem glioma, histiocytosis X). It seems questionable to include this region within a treatment volume (above 35 Gy) for reasons such as "sufficient safety margin" in cerebral gliomas or medulloblastoma (Fig. 3), or for standard prophylactic treatment in, for example, parameningeal sarcoma or nasopharyngeal cancer.

Gonads: Ovary

Due to the reproductive and endocrine function of the ovary, disturbances in ovarian function become clinically manifest in young girls at the start of puberty as impairment in the development of secondary sexual characteristics and libido, amenorrhea, and infertility. Measurable biochemical parameters are estradiol, FSH, and LH.

The place of radiation injury is assumed to be the follicle, leading to a loss of steroidogenesis and the oocyte with a resultant loss of fertility. There is a fixed population of oocytes in a girl at birth for which there is no possibility of regeneration: the number of oocytes thus decreases continuously with age. Consequently, the vulnerability of ovarian function, which is dependent on the number of oocytes, increases with age.

Little has been reported with regard to dose–effect relationships in ovarian function. In a large retrospective study on long-term surviving girls, the majority of whom had been treated for nephroblastoma and lymphoma, Stillman et al. (1981) found a close correlation between the location of the ovary in relation to the radiation field and the probability of ovarian failure: ovarian failure did not develop (0/34) if at least one ovary was completely outside the radiation field (estimated scattered mean ovarian tissue dose 54 cGy), it occurred rarely (5/35) if an ovary was at the edge of the treat-

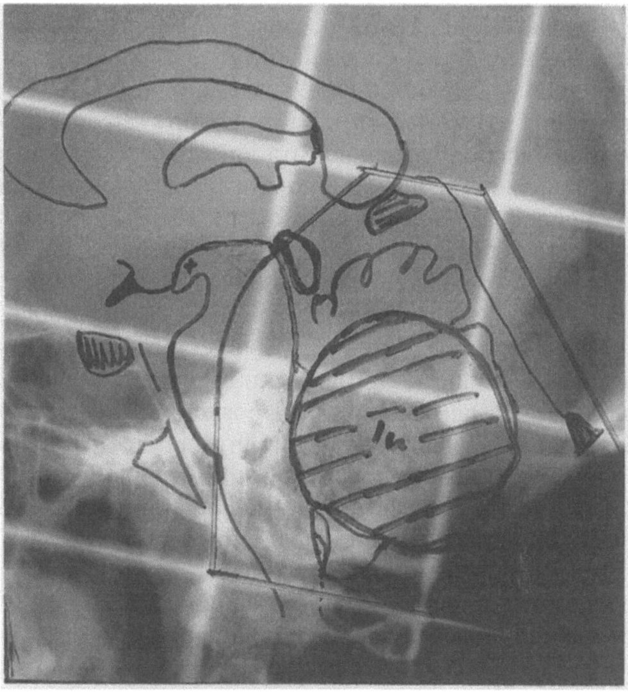

Fig. 3. Radiation portal of a medulloblastoma patient with sparing of the hypothalamic–pituitary region from the high-dose boost volume which has to encompass the region with primary tumor spread. Normal anatomy and tumor extension prior to surgery are superimposed on the midsagittal MRI scan before surgery. The *cross* indicates the corpora mamillaria, the most posterior area producing hypothalamic releasing hormones

ment field (estimated mean ovarian tissue dose 290 cGy), and it occurred often (17/25) if both ovaries were within the treatment field (estimated mean ovarian tissue dose 3200 cGy). It has to be taken into account that this analysis was based on radiotherapy field diagrams, that a number of patients had been treated with orthovoltage radiotherapy, and that the procedure of (retrospective) ovarian location was not clearly indicated.

A recent analysis reporting the Stanford experience in pelvic radiotherapy for girls with Hodgkin's disease underlined the importance of location of the ovaries following oophoropexy (Sy Orton et al. 1990): in all girls with ovarian failure following pelvic radiotherapy the position of the ovaries after oophoropexy made adequate shielding impossible. In 21 girls there was only one ovarian failure after ovarian tissue doses between 90 and 484 cGy which had been achieved by adequate shielding (Sy Orton et al. 1990). Normal pregnancies following oophoropexy and radiotherapy were observed.

On the basis of these data fractionated ovarian tissue doses up to 500 cGy do not seem to impair ovarian function. Doses reported in the literature up to more than 2000 cGy should be taken with great caution, because they might be based on assumed rather than adequately calculated ovarian tissue doses. Donaldson (1989) gives a dose of 2200 cGy for the right ovary in a young girl treated for left iliac Ewing's sarcoma (55 Gy) who maintained ovarian function; in her illustration of the radiation portals (CT, isodose distribution X-ray film) the normal topographic position of the ovary is, in my opinion, beyond the edge of the portal laterocaudal in the true pelvis (compare Fig. 4). If this assumption is true the applied radiation dose to the right ovary would have been far below 10% of the reference dose (≪550 cGy) and thus well within the tolerance dose reported above.

When reporting ovarian tissue tolerance doses the way of assessing the ovarian dose, including the location procedure itself, has to be valid and reproducible, particularly as the position of the ovary in a young girl is not fixed but only assumed to be within a certain anatomical region.

In the case of pelvic radiotherapy adequate location and shielding of the ovary directly prior and during radiotherapy is the most critical factor and has to be performed in a highly individualized way which can nowadays be based on magnetic resonance imaging or ultrasound studies (Fig. 4). In many cases, sometimes with the support of a surgical intervention, it will be possible to reduce the applied radiation dose to such an extent that it will be within the assumed tolerance levels.

After pelvic radiotherapy biochemical monitoring (estradiol, FSH, LH) is mandatory, particularly in the prepubertal phase as in the case of impairment hormone replacement is necessary in order to avoid disturbances in pubertal maturation and sexual development.

Gonads: Testis

As the reproductive and endocrine function of the testes are located in the germinal epithelium and in the interstitial cells of Leydig, the radiosensitivity of these different cell populations will be described.

An impairment of testicular function becomes clinically manifest at the start of puberty with the development of pubertal maturation, growth, gonadal function, libido (endocrine function), and fertility (reproductive function). Measurable endpoints are secretion of testosterone (HCG test) and LH (LHRH test) for endocrine function, and a spermiogram (testicular biopsy) and FSH test for reproductive function.

Only very few data are available by which the radiation dose that will damage the germinal epithelium can be determined. In the frequently cited work of Shalet on testicular function (Shalet et al. 1978) the testicular dose was calculated retrospectively in 10 men who had had abdominal radiotherapy for nephroblastoma many years before. Based on these findings a calculated radiation dose in the range 270–980 cGy led to an elevated FSH and a decreased sperm cell count in 7/10 men. The tolerance dose for an

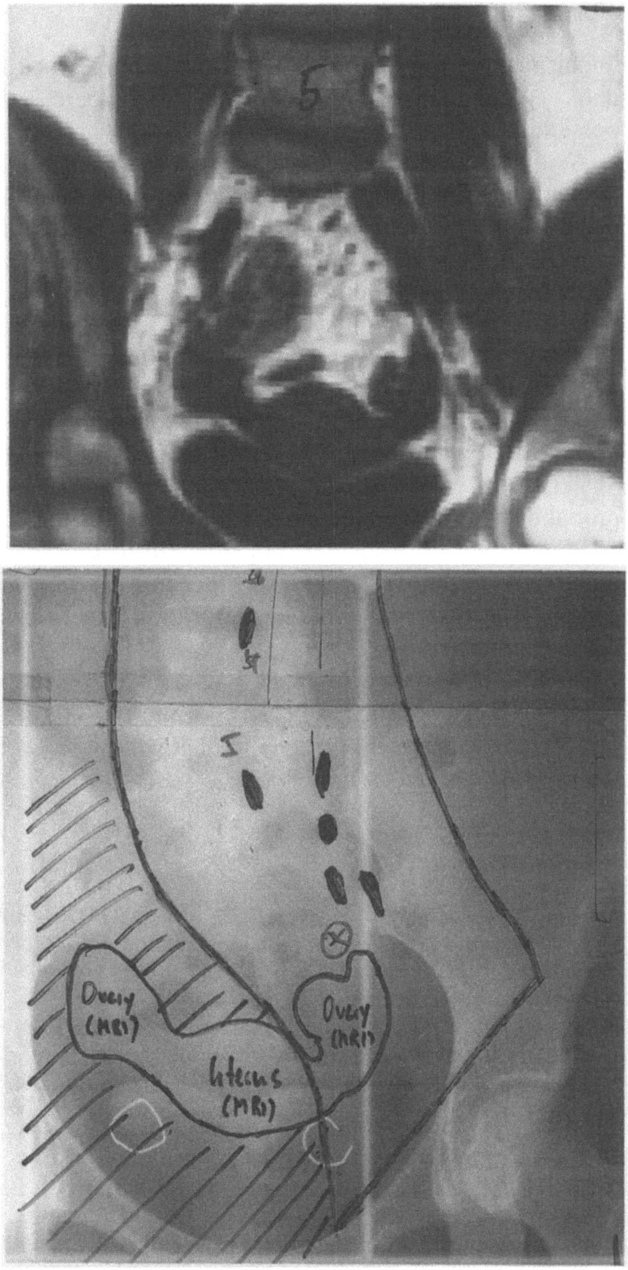

a

b

Fig. 4a,b. Coronal MRI scan (**a**) and radiation portal (**b**) in pelvic and abdominal recurrence of Hodgkin's disease in a 16-year-old girl. Delineation of the ovaries by superimposition of the MRI scan made adequate shielding of the right ovary for involved field radiotherapy (25 Gy) possible (>2 cm beyond the edge of the shielding block, which was 12 cm thick in the pelvis to avoid radiation transmission (*hatched line*)). The scattered right ovarian tissue dose was <10% of the reference dose (<2.5 Gy). Localization by ultrasound was not successful because of too much fatty tissue. One year later there was no indication of ovarian failure impairment of spermatogenesis in boys cannot be derived from these sparse data. A spontaneous normalization of a decreased sperm cell count is possible.

A valid and reliable tolerance dose assessment will have to be based upon in vivo measurements of the scattered radiation dose from abdominal, pelvic, and lower extremity radiotherapy in children and adolescents, which in turn will have to be correlated with functional measurement when these patients reach adulthood.

Leydig cell failure may occur when the testes are directly irradiated. Testes in children have been irradiated for leukemia relapse with doses between 12 and 24 Gy. Below 15 Gy the probability of testicular impairment is low, whereas testicular failure was reported in almost all children who had been treated with doses of 24 Gy (Brämswig, personal communication 1991; Shalet et al. 1985; Sklar et al. 1990). There is some evidence that the probability of damage increases with the age of the child at treatment.

Monitoring of testicular function (testosterone, LH) at the start of puberty is necessary because in the case of impairment disturbances in gonadal function and pubertal maturation can be avoided by testosterone replacement therapy.

Total dose and type of applied alkylating agent must always be stated in reporting gonadal function because of the well-known induction of gonadal injury, particularly in boys (spermatogenesis and Leydig cell function) (Brämswig et al. 1990a).

References

Blacklay A, Grossmann A, Ross RJM, Savage MO, Davies PSW, Plowman PN, Coy DH, Besser GM (1986) Cranial irradiation for cerebral and nasopharyngeal tumours in children: evidence for the production of a hypothalamic defect in growth hormone release. J Endocrinol 108:25–29

Brämswig JH, Wegele M, von Lengerke HJ, Müller R-P, Schellong G (1989) The effect of the number of fractions of cranial irradiation on growth in children with acute lymphoblastic leukaemia. Acta Paediatr Scand 78:296–302

Brämswig JH, Heimes U, Heiermann E, Schlegel W, Nieschlag E, Schellong G (1990a) The effects of different cumulative doses of chemotherapy on testicular function. Cancer 65:1298–1302

Brämswig JH, Zielinski G, Schellong G (1990b) Adult height, target height and siblings' adult height in 107 patients treated for acute lymphoblastic leukemia (ALL): comparison of the effects of 4 different chemotherapeutic regimens and different doses of cranial Irradiation (abstract). Suppl Hormone Research 32

Donaldson SS (1989) Pediatric patients: tolerance levels and effects of treatment. Front Radiat Ther Oncol 23:390–407

Fromm M, Littman P, Raney RB, Nelson L, Handler S, Diamond G, Stanley C (1986) Late effects after treatment of twenty children with soft tissue sarcomas of the head and neck: experience at a single institution with a review of the literature. Cancer 57:2070–2076

Gonzalez D, Breur K (1983) Clinical data from irradiated growing long bones in children. Int J Radiat Oncol Biol Phys 9:841–846

Haaf HG, Kaatsch P, Michaelis J (1990) Jahresbericht 1989 des Kinderkrebsregisters Mainz. IMSD, University of Mainz
Heyn RM (1985) Late effects of therapy in rhabdomyosarcoma. Clin Oncol 4:287–299
ICRU (1978) Report 29. Dose specification for reporting external beam therapy with photons and electrons. International committee on radiation units and measurements, Woodmont Avenue 7910, Washington, DC 20014
Lannering B, Albertsson-Wiland K (1987) Growth hormone release in children after cranial irradiation. Horm Res 27:13–22
Lemerle J, Dubousset J, Brauner R, Oberlin O, Habrand J, Thibaud E, Aubier F (1989) Séquelles chez les enfans guéris. In: Lemerle J (ed) Cancers de l'enfant. Flammarion, Paris, pp 173–217
Neff JR (1985) Late orthopaedic effects in Ewing's sarcoma. Clin Oncol 4(2):299–320
Neuhauser EBD, Wittenborg NH, Berman ČZ, Cohen J (1952) Irradiation effects on the growing spine. Radiology 59:637–650
Pomarede R, Brauner R, Rappaport R, Czernichow P (1983) Les séquelles thyroidienne des radiotherapies pour cancer de la tete et du cou chez l'enfant. Lemerle J (ed) Actualités carcinologiques de l'Institut Gustave Roussy. Masson, Paris, pp 211–221
Probert JC, Parker BR (1975) The effects of radiation therapy on bone growth. Radiology 114:155–162
Rappaport R, Brauner R, Czernichow P (1982) Effect of hypothalamic and pituitary irradiation on pubertal development in children with cranial tumors. J Clin Endocrinol Metab 54:1164–1168
Rubin P, van Houtte P, Constine L (1982) Radiation sensitivity and organ tolerances in pediatric oncology: a new hypothesis. Front Radiat Ther Oncol 16:62–82
Shalet SM (1985) The effects of cancer treatment on growth and sexual development. Clin Onol 4(2):223–238
Shalet SM (1989) Endocrine consequences of treatment of malignant disease. Arch Dis Child 64:1635–1641
Shalet SM, Beardwell CG, Jacobs HS, Pearson D (1978) Testicular funtion following irradiation of the human prepubertal testis. Clin Endocrinol 9:483–490
Shalet SM, Horner A, Ahmed SR, Morris-Jones PH (1985) Leydig cell damage after testicular irradiation for lymphoblastic leukaemia. Med Pediatr Oncol 13:65–68
Sklar CA, Robison LL Nesbit ME, Sather HN, Meadows AT, Ortega JA, Kim TH, Hammond GD (1990) Effects of radiation on testicular function in long-term survivors of childhood acute lymphoblastic leukemia: a report from the Children's Cancer Study Group. J Clin Oncol 8:1981–1987
Stillman RJ, Schinfeld JS, Schiff I, Gelber RD, Greenberger J, Larson M, Jaffe N, Frederick PL (1981) Ovarian failure in long-term survivors of childhood malignancy. Am J Obstet Gynecol 139:62–66
Sy Orton TT, Shostak CA, Donaldson SS (1990) Gonadal status and reproductive function following treatment for Hodgkin's disease in childhood: the Stanford experience. Int J Radiat Oncol Biol Phys 19:873–880
Tefft M, Lattin PB, Jereb B, Cham W, Ghavimi F, Rosen G, Exelby P, Marcove R, Murphy ML, D'Angio GJ (1976) Acute and late effects on normal tissues following combined chemo- and radiotherapy for childhood rhabdomyosarcoma and Ewing's sarcoma. Cancer 37:1201–1213
Willich E, Kuttig H, Pfeil G, Scheibel P (1990) Wirbelsäulenveränderungen nach Bestrahlung wegen Wilmstumor im Kleinkindesalter. Retrospektive interdisziplinäre Langzeitstudie an 82 Kindern. Strahlenther Onkol 166:815–821

Side-Effects After Combination Therapy for Ewing's Sarcoma

R. Pötter[1], C. Kuhnen[1], J. Ritter[2], B. Rath[2], P. Wuismann[3], M. von Eiff[4], H.-J. von Lengerke[5], J.H. Brämswig[2], and S. Paulus[3]

[1] Klinik für Strahlentherapie – Radioonkologie – Westfälische Wilhelms-Universität Münster, W-4400 Münster, Fed. Rep. of Germany
[2] Kinderklinik, Westfälische Wilhelms-Universität Münster, W-4400 Münster, Fed. Rep. of Germany
[3] Klinik für Orthopädie, Westfälische Wilhelms-Universität Münster, W-4400 Münster, Fed. Rep. of Germany
[4] Medizinische Klinik (Abteilung A), Westfälische Wilhelms-Universität Münster, W-4400 Münster, Fed. Rep. of Germany
[5] Institut für Klinische Radiologie, Westfälische Wilhelms-Universität Münster, W-4400 Münster, Fed. Rep. of Germany

Introduction

The late effects of combined therapy in Ewing's sarcoma, especially the effects of local therapy, are detected more clearly now as a result of a significant improvement in survival (about 65% 2-year survival rate: Jürgens et al. 1988). Because of the radiosensitivity of this tumor, radiotherapy has long been established as the local treatment, followed quite often by severe side effects: high doses (55–70 Gy) to the entire bone ("whole-bone" technique because of microscopic spread of tumor cells throughout the medullary cavity) caused significant atrophy in soft tissues as well as bone shortening and pathological fractures (Lewis et al. 1977; Neff 1985). In recent years better results have been reported after surgical therapy and after a combination of surgical and radiological local therapy (40–45 Gy) compared with high-dose radiotherapy (60 Gy) alone (Wilkens et al. 1986; Winkelmann and Jürgens 1989).

Possible late effects of the combined local therapy will be influenced by several factors:

1. The anatomical site and extension of the tumor.
2. The type of surgery.
3. The treatment volume and total dose of radiotherapy.
4. The age of the patient during therapy; this is important for those patients who are not fully grown at the time of treatment.

The conventional target volume for radiotherapy in Ewing's sarcoma includes the entire bone and the surrounding tissue at risk. Because of technical difficulties in making the target volume coincide with the treatment volume, treatment volumes are often larger than target volumes. This can

Recent Results in Cancer Research, Vol. 130

result in extended volumes of soft tissue and bone being irradiated. The late effects after radiation of large volumes are more significant, especially in growing tissues. Many authors today recommend discontinuing this method of whole-bone irradiation because of the great efficacy of chemotherapy (Hayes et al. 1989).

Material and Methods

Between 1975 and 1990, 47 patients with Ewing's sarcoma or malignant peripheral neuroectodermal tumor (Askin's tumor) were treated in the Department of Radiotherapy and Radiooncology of the University of Münster, FRG. All patients received radiotherapy to the primary tumor; the doses ranged between 36 and 62.4 Gray. The site and volume of the tumor as well as target volume, treatment volume, total dose, and the clinical result were reviewed for 20 cases to evaluate the effectiveness of radiotherapy. Target volume was defined according to the CESS recommendations (German Cooperative Ewing's Sarcoma Study 1981/86).

Twenty-two of 47 patients (47%) were alive on 1 January 1991; the median time of observation was 46.5 months. Follow-up examinations were possible in 17 patients to evaluate the late effects of combined therapy. Eleven patients presented with a tumor of the extremities (scapula included), 4 with a tumor of the thorax, and 2 with a tumor of the pelvis. Median age during therapy was 15.5 years (range 7–25 years). The median time after radiotherapy was 29 months.

The following functional and cosmetic results were examined:

1. Skin (atrophy, pigmentation, fibrosis, sensitivity).
2. Soft tissues (especially atrophy).
3. Limb shortening.
4. Function and mobility of irradiated or involved joints.

Radiological follow-ups helped to detect roentgenological changes and abnormalities in bony structure. Examination of special organs included pulmonary function, renal function (^{99m}Tc MAG3 scintigraphy), liver function (^{99m}Tc Jodida scintigraphy). Gonadal function (LH, FSH, androgens, estrogens) was reviewed in 11 patients (older than 12 years at the time of examination).

Local Control

Continuous local control was achieved in 36/47 patients (77%). No relationship between radiation dose and local control could be detected.

The relation between tumor, target, and treatment volumes varied between 1/2/2 and 1/12/42: no increase in local failure rate could be observed when only small margins were chosen (close correlation between tumor and treatment volume up to 1/2/2) compared with extensive margins (correlations down to 1/12/42). After irradiation of extremity tumors, no local failure occurred within the nonirradiated area of bone in cases where the whole bone had not been entirely included inside the radiation portal.

Side Effects

Extremities

The results were categorized according to the scheme of Jentzsch et al. (1981): minimal late effects (e.g., limb shortening up to 1.5 cm), significant late effects (e.g., limb shortening up to 2.5 cm), and severe late effects (complications severe enough to warrant an amputation).

Minimal Late Effects

Minimal late effects occurred in 4 patients. Atrophy of the extremity was the main local feature; atrophy of the thigh was up to 16%. Limitations of joint mobility could be fully compensated. The functional outcome after amputation of the lower leg and a prosthetic device was especially positive.

Significant Late Effects

Significant late effects occurred in 5 patients. Atrophy of the thigh was measured up to 17%, atrophy of the lower limb up to 23% (Fig. 1); maximal limb length shortening was 3 cm. A major functional restriction was due to palsy of the peroneus muscle after resection of the proximal fibula in 2 patients.

Severe Late Effects

Severe late effects occurred in 2 patients. In 1 patient (Ewing's sarcoma of the proximal ulna), high-dose radiotherapy (62.4 Gy) caused multiple pathological fractures and subsequent osteomyelitis which was finally responsible for an arthrodesis of the elbow. This patient suffered from severe atrophy and total functional loss of the entire lower arm. In the case of a Ewing's sarcoma of the proximal fibula amputation of the forefoot became necessary following postoperative complications.

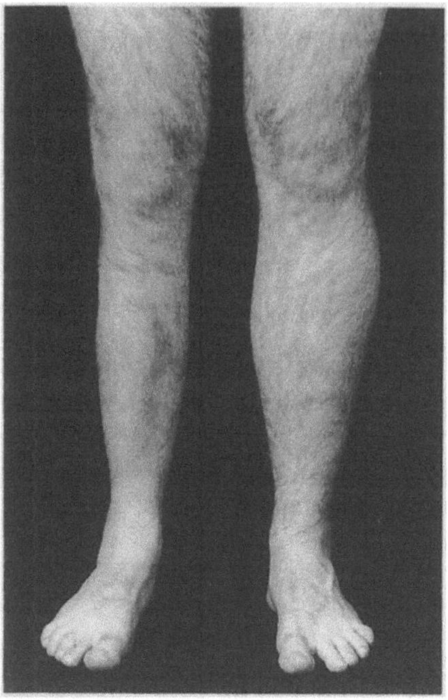

Fig. 1. Lower extremities of a 20-years-old man who had been treated at 14 years for a sarcoma of the right proximal fibula. Preoperative chemotherapy (Vincristine, Actinomycin D, Cyclophosphamide, Adriamycin, VACA) with good response was followed by wide resection of the proximal fibula. Postoperative radiotherapy with 36 Gy was given to the whole region of the fibula including the ankle joint together with VACA. Significant late effects 6 years after local therapy were palsy of the peroneus muscle (after surgery), soft tissue atrophy (23%) within the whole calf (not restricted to the radiation treatment volume) probably partly due to palsy-induced inactivity, valgus deformity of the ankle due to reduced growth of the lateral malleolus (within the radiation field), and 2.5 cm shortening of the right leg. There was pain in the leg only on exertion; otherwise there were no clinical symptoms

Post-therapeutic Valgus Deformity of the Ankle

Three patients presented with a valgus deformity of the articulatio talocruralis (up to 20°) after local therapy for a tumor of the fibula. In 2 of the 3 patients the deformity is mainly due to asymmetrical bone growth arrest following radiotherapy (36 Gy): the treatment field included the lateral part of the distal tibial growth plate whereas the medial part was excluded. The roentgenological appearance was of a continuously developing deformity over approximately 5 years (66 and 69 months).

In 1 patient with a tumor of the proximal fibula the distal third of the lower leg was not irradiated; the treatment volume was therefore significantly diminished. This patient developed a valgus deformity of the knee joint; the resulting abnormal relative positions of tibia, fibula, and talus caused the valgus of the ankle.

In all 3 patients radiogrophs revealed a thickened lateral corticalis tibiae compared with the medial side.

Thorax

Thoracic Wall

Following electron radiotherapy (45–60 Gy) significant pigmentation, multiple telangiectasis, and hair loss of the skin could be noticed on the anterior chest wall. One girl (aged 15.5 years during therapy) suffered severe soft tissue hypoplasia after surgery and high-dose radiotherapy, and hypoplasia of the irradiated breast (36 months after irradiation).

Scoliosis

Two patients, both with a similar tumor site in the right hemithorax (10th to 12th rib), developed a clinically significant scoliosis following combined local resection and radiotherapy (angle of scoliosis according to Cobb 19° and 22°, predominantly of the lumbar spine). The scoliosis could be detected roentgenologically just after the end of irradiation therapy in both cases; the convexity of scoliosis was directed to the side of the resected and irradiated hemithorax (convexity to the right with tumor of the right thorax: Fig. 2).

A so-called en bloc resection of the chest wall including several ribs preceded local radiotherapy in both patients. The convexity of scoliosis to the side of resection cannot be interpreted as a radiation-induced side effect (inadequate time lag and wrong side) but can be explained by a sudden muscular predominance of the contralateral side caused by the surgical resection: the loss of homolateral intercostal and autochthonic muscles of the ribs and back.

Pulmonary Function

Two patients (tumor of the right hemithorax, 10th to 12th rib) presented with severe pulmonary restrictive disease; pulmonary function showed a reduction in vital capacity (VC) to about 50% of the predicted normal value. The tumor site was locally resected (en bloc chest wall resection) and irradiated (45 Gy). This restrictive disease persisted without significant changes during longer periods of time (up to 40 months postoperatively). The reduction in VC occurred as early as 3 months after radiotherapy in the one patient (49%) and 6 months after radiotherapy in the other (43%). The

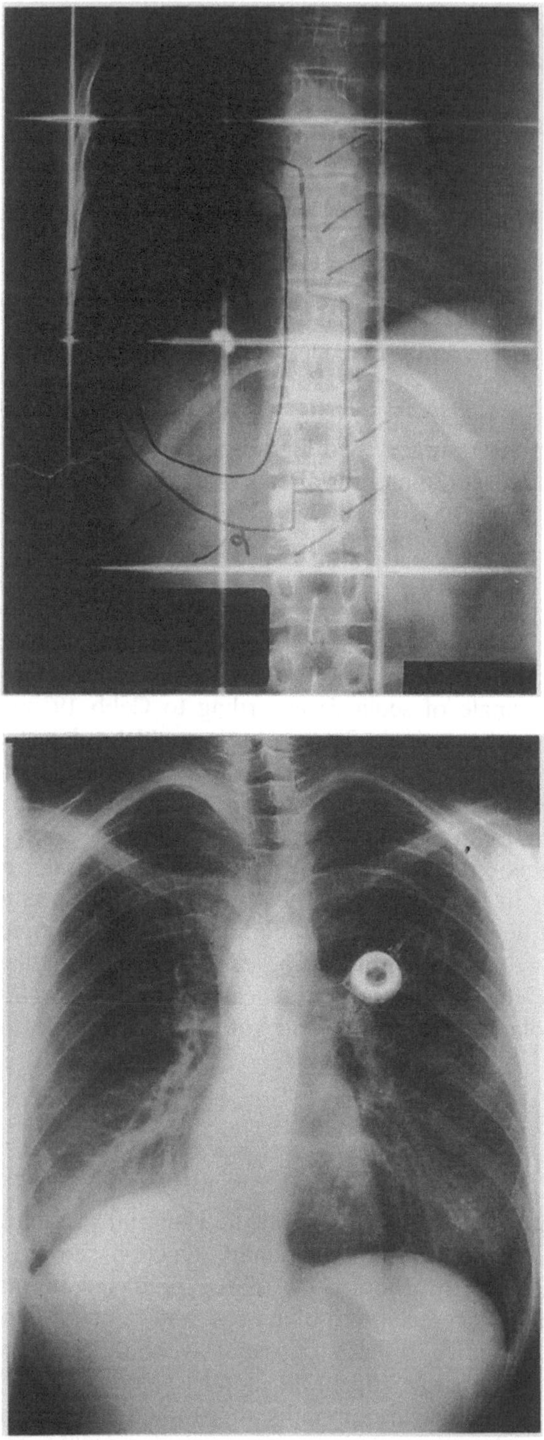

a

b

irradiated lung volume was rather small in both patients (<30% of the right lung; compare Fig. 2).

Pelvis

Only 2 patients with Ewing's sarcoma of the pelvis were examined. The late effects of combined treatment were dependent on the anatomical site of the tumor: the patient with a Ewing's sarcoma of the os ilium suffered from a severe restriction of hip and knee flexion following extensive pelvic resection; this should be evaluated as a very poor result according to Enneking's criteria (Thomas et al. 1987). The patient with a Ewing's sarcoma of the os pubis presented with only little functional loss of the lower extremity after resection of the os pubis.

Gonadal Injury

Elevated levels of FSH were measured in 4 of 7 male patients, indicating damage to spermatogenesis. LH was slightly elevated in 1 case. Two patients received radiotherapy to regions distant from the gonads (upper chest wall, below the knee joint); the testicular radiation dose could be estimated as less than 45 cGy (<1%), hence the influence of irradiation on gonadal injury was excluded in these cases. However, all patients had been treated with cytotoxic drugs, the cumulative doses of the alkylating agents (ifosfamide) being about 60000–70000 mg/m^2, which is known to be able to induce testicular damage.

Fig. 2. a Simulation film with radiation field (anteroposterior/posteroanterior) before second-look surgery in a 17-year-old girl with a tumor of the right lower chest wall (Askin's tumor) with destruction of ribs and infiltration of an intervertebral foramen. Local therapy consisted of primary marginal resection (including parts of the 12th rib) with intralesional resection at the intervertebral foramen. Postoperatively she received VAIA chemotherapy and radiotherapy (32 Gy). The radiation portal included parts of the thoracolumbar vertebral bodies. Second-look surgery involved resection of the 11th and 12th rib, soft tissue of the thoracic wall, and one nerve root. A postoperative radiation boost up to 45 Gy was given with sparing of the spinal cord together with chemotherapy (VAIA). **b** X-ray film 2 months after boost radiotherapy indicating a marked scoliosis of the thoracolumbar spine which is most probably a consequence of surgical resection and not induced by radiotherapy (convexity is on the right side and it occurred 2 months after radiotherapy). Right paramediastinal pneumonitis is related to the radiation portal. A Port-O-Cath for the application of chemotherapy can be seen

Secondary Malignancies

One acute nonlymphoblastic leukemia occurred 1 year after multimodal treatment according to CESS 86 for an Askin tumor in a 13-year-old girl (Vincristine, Actinomycin D, Iphosphamide, Adriamycin, VAIA, local radiotherapy (45 Gy), marginal resection). This secondary malignancy has to be interpreted as an adverse side effect, most probably from high-dose chemotherapy and in particular the high cumulative dose of alkylating agents.

Conclusion

Compared with the late side effects described in former reports following radiotherapy as the main local treatment (Lewis et al. 1977), the patients in this series generally presented with minor morbididty after combination local therapy.

References

Hayes FA, Thompson EI, Meyer WH, Kun L, Parham D, Rao B, Kumar M, Hancock M, Parvey L, Magill L, Hust HO (1989) Therapy for localized Ewing's sarcoma of bone. J Clin Oncol 7:208–213

Jentzsch K, Binder H, Cramer H, Glaubiger DL, Kessler RM, Bull C, Pomeroy TC, Gerber NL (1981) Leg function after radiotherapy for Ewing's sarcoma. Cancer 47:1267–1278

Jürgens H, Bier V, Dunst J, Harms D, Jobke A, Kotz R, Kühl J, Müller-Weihrich St, Ritter J, Salzer-Kuntschik M, Sauer R, Sternschulte W, Treuner J, Voute PA, Weinel P, Winkelmann W, Winkler K, Göbel U (1988) Die GPO cooperativen Ewing-Sarkom Studien CESS 81/86: Bericht nach 6 1/2 Jahren. Klin Padiatr 200:243–252

Lewis RJ, Marcove RC, Rosen G (1977) Ewing's sarcoma: functional effects of radiation therapy. J Bone Joint Surg [Am] 59:325–331

Neff (1985) Late orthopaedic effects in Ewing's sarcoma. Clin Oncol 4(2):299–317

Thomas IH, Cole WG, Waters KG, Menelaus MB (1987) Function after partial pelvic resection for Ewing's sarcoma. J Bone Joint Surg [Br] 69:271–275

Wilkins RM, Pritchard DJ, Burgert EO, Unni KK (1986) Ewing's sarcoma of bone: experience with 140 patients. Cancer 58:2551–2555

Winkelmann W, Jürgens H (1989) Lokalkontrolle bein Ewing-Sarkom. Vergleichende Ergebnisse nach intraläsionaler, marginaler bzw. Tumorrseketion im Gesunden. Z Orthop 127:424–426

Subclinical Impairment of Renal Function After Radiotherapy for Hodgkin's Disease in Children

R. Pötter[1], F. Roes[1], G. Schellong[2], P. Bartenstein[3], J.H. Brämswig[2], H.-J. von Lengerke[4], B. Rath[2], R. Mohring[1], and R. Rossi[2]

[1] Klinik für Strahlentherapie–Radioonkologie – Westfälische Wilhelms-Universität Münster, W-4400 Münster, Fed. Rep. of Germany
[2] Kinderklinik, Westfälische Wilhelms-Universität Münster, W-4400 Münster, Fed. Rep. of Germany
[3] Klinik für Nuklearmedizin, Westfälische Wilhelms-Universität Münster, W-4400 Münster, Fed. Rep. of Germany
[4] Institut für Klinische Radiologie, Westfälische Wilhelms-Universität Münster, W-4400 Münster, Fed. Rep. of Germany

Introduction

According to the results of the German multicenter trials in Hodgkin's disease in children (HD 82), projected 5-year event-free survival rates are 90% (stage IIIB/IV), 96% (stage IIB/IIIA), and 99% (stage I/IIA) (Schellong et al. 1989). Because of this favorable prognosis after stage-adjusted combined chemotherapy and radiotherapy (all stages) the avoidance of long-term treatment-related morbidity has become of great importance.

In Hodgkin's disease the frequent sites of subdiaphragmatic involvement are the paraaortic region including the splenic pedicle (124/156 patients (79%) stage III/IV HD 78/82: Kassner 1991) and the spleen (50/174 (with histological proof of involvement) patients (29%) all stages HD 82: Schellong et al. 1986)). The place for radiotherapy in these sites is increasing as a result of the abandonment of splenectomy, making the assessment of long-term radiation-related morbidity necessary. The role of splenectomy was questioned because of septic deaths occurring only in children after this procedure (n = 12, 1.9%) (Studienprotokoll DAL-HD 90, Schellong et al. 1990).

In radiotherapy of subdiaphragmatic Hodgkin's disease (excluding the pelvis) the most critical organ is the kidney because of its known radiovulnerability and its position near to the target volume. Little is known about the tolerance dose of the kidney in children, in particular if it is only partly irradiated (Mitus et al. 1969).

During the three German multicenter trials, in which more than 600 children were enrolled (HD 78, HD 82, HD 85/87), the protocols for radiotherapy changed as regards the radiation dose and treatment volume. In these protocols the radiation dose in the involved region has been reduced continuously from 36 Gy to 20/25 Gy (Schellong et al. 1989). In parallel with the change from Betatrons and ^{60}Co treatment machines to linear accelerators during this period in Germany, treatment techniques

Recent Results in Cancer Research, Vol. 130

for the radiotherapy of subdiaphragmatic Hodgkin's disease (including the splenic pedicle and the spleen) changed from multiple single fields (Abbatucci et al. 1976) to two opposing large fields with individual kidney shielding (Wannenmacher et al. 1978).

Aim of the Study

In order to introduce low-dose radiotherapy as a routine treatment for the spleen instead of splenectomy in subdiaphragmatic Hodgkin's disease within a treatment protocol a study was performed at one center in which different radiation doses and treatment techniques had been used. The aim was to evaluate the radiation-related long-term renal morbidity in the treatment for Hodgkin's disease in children, by investigating renal function after therapy (compare Le Bourgeois et al. 1979). These findings were correlated with the radiation dose within the kidney, which was retrospectively estimated by individual dose calculations taking into account the different prescribed radiation doses in the target and the different treatment techniques.

Material and Methods

Twenty children with Hodgkin's disease were irradiated for subdiaphragmatic disease at the University of Münster from 1979 to 1988 according to the cooperative multicenter German DAL protocols (HD 78, HD 82, HD 85/87). The mean age at diagnosis was 10 years, at investigation for renal function 17 years. All children had undergone staging laparotomy, and 18 had had a splenectomy. Renal function was studied in 17 children by ^{99m}Tc MAG3 scintigraphy (Bubeck et al. 1987), creatinine tests, sonography, and urinalysis 1–11 years (mean 6 years) after the end of therapy.

According to the multicenter protocols the stage-adjusted prescribed target doses for the paraaortic field and the splenic pedicle varied from 18 to 40 Gy. No specific treatment technique and no maximum dose for the kidneys (tolerance dose) were given in the national cooperative treatment protocols. The mean dose per fraction was 1.8 Gy (1.2–2.1 Gy) (Table 1). The mean treatment time was 3 weeks (2–9 weeks depending on total dose and duration of break) (Table 1). The rotational technique for the paraaortic field using photons (×18 MV, Betatron) was applied in combination with two fields for the splenic pedicle using ^{60}Co gamma-rays in 10 patients. The reference point for the rotational fields was the isocenter, for the two splenic pedicle fields a depth representing the assumed distance between the splenic pedicle and the entrance point on the skin. Dose correction taking into account the overlapping isodose curves from the different fields was carried out beginning with patient no. 4 (Table 1).

Opposed anteroposterior/posteroanterior (ap/pa) fields using ^{60}Co gamma-rays – in part with individual shielding of the kidney ($n = 3$) – were used in 5 patients. Opposed ap/pa fields with individual shielding of the kidney using photons (×10 MeV, linear accelerator) were applied in 5 patients. The reference point was half the diameter along the central beam.

For both kidneys the delivered total dose and the dose distribution were estimated retrospectively in every patient by computed dose calculation (Treatment Planning System) based on computed tomography, taking into account the different beam quality (×10 MeV, ×18 MeV, ^{60}Co), the field sizes, the field arrangements, and the prescribed total doses (Table 1, Fig. 1). Dose distribution from the computed plot was superimposed on the axial computed tomogram (Fig. 1), and from phantom measurements on the simulation film.

Results

A wide variation of applied radiation dose including a large inhomogeneity in dose distribution was found in the upper part of the left kidney as well as in the other parts of both kidneys. This was dependent in a rather complex way on prescribed total dose and treatment technique (Table 1, Fig. 1).

Clinically, renal dysfunction was not observed. Creatinine levels, urinalysis (1 exception), sonography (3 exceptions), and blood pressure were normal.

In the first 3 children the applied dose at the upper half of the left kidney (50–60 Gy) lies much above the prescribed target dose (36–40 Gy) due to the inhomogeneity of dose within the irradiated volume (Fig. 1). In these patients scintigraphy showed no uptake within the upper half of the left kidney (Fig. 3). Three sonograms revealed an increased echogenicity at the upper pole suggestive of fibrosis. A slight decrease in local clearance within the upper half of the left kidney was observed after doses from 30 to 40 Gy (Figs. 2 and 3). In one patient urinalysis revealed a glucosuria. No clearcut regional difference in the left kidney could be found within a wide range of lower doses from 12 to 30 Gy at the upper pole of the left kidney (Fig. 3).

Looking independently at the clearance of the right kidney no decrease can be seen after doses from 5 to 30 Gy. Comparing renal clearance of the two kidneys a difference in favor of the right kidney was only evident in patients with a distinct difference in local clearance within the left kidney.

The overall clearance is about 1 standard deviation below the average total clearance in patients treated with a dose above 30 Gy at the upper left pole and a dose in both kidneys between 15 and 30 Gy (rotational technique, ^{60}Co). Overall clearance is not decreased in patients treated with doses below 15 Gy in both kidneys independent of the dose at the upper part of the left kidney and has a value around the average (379 cm^3/min/1.73 m^2).

Table 1. Characteristics of radiotherapy in children ($n = 18$) treated for subdiaphragmatic Hodgkin's disease with different doses and treatment techniques during a 10-year period

Patient no.	Age at therapy	Radiation	Portal (cm)	Target dose (Gy)	Applied dose (Gy) to kidney				Dose per fraction	Treatment time (weeks)
					Upper left integral dose (range)		Right integral dose (range)			
1	9	× 18 Me V ^{60}Co	I 6 × 14 II 7 × 7 III 6 × 7	36	50.5	(45–54)	15	(4–26)	1.8	4 (15)
2	12	× 18 Me V ^{60}Co	I 6 × 14 II 8 × 8 III 8 × 8	40	56.5	(52–61)	16.5	(6–27)	1.8	5 (11)
3	13	× 18 Me V ^{60}Co	I 6 × 14 II 8 × 8 III 6 × 8	36	48	(45–51)	15	(6–24)	1.8	4 (9)
4	9	× 18 Me V ^{60}Co	I 6 × 9 II 6 × 6 III 5 × 6	36	38	(31–45)	14	(4–24)	1.8	4 (6)
5	15	× 18 Me V ^{60}Co	I 6 × 14 II 8 × 10 III 6 × 10	30	33	(28–38)	12	(4–20)	1.8	4 (6)
6	12	× 18 Me V ^{60}Co	I 6 × 14 II 7 × 8 III 6 × 8	25	22.5	(16–29)	12	(4–20)	1.8	3
7	6	× 18 Co ^{60} Me V	I 6 × 9 II 6 × 7 III 4 × 5	36	30	(20–40)	16	(4–28)	1.4	6 (9)
8	5	× 18 Me V ^{60}Co	I 6 × 14 II 5 × 8 III 5 × 8	20	21	(16–26)	9.5	(3–16)	1.4	3 (5)

9	14	× 18 Me V ^{60}Co	I 6 × 14 II 9 × 9 III 6 × 9	20	19	(12–26)	9.5	(3–16)	1.8	3
10	14	× 18 Me V ^{60}Co	I 6 × 14 II 6 × 8 III 6 × 10	25	20	(14–26)	11	(3–19)	2.1	3
11	10	^{60}Co	I 6 × 14 II 6 × 14	38	30		23	(15–30)	1.5	6
12	9	^{60}Co	I 7 × 14 II 7 × 13	18	12.5	(10–15)	7	(3–10)	1.2	3
13	5	^{60}Co		36						
14	10	^{60}Co	I 14 × 14 II 14× 14	25	14		14		1.5	3.5
15	9	^{60}Co	I 19 × 19 II 19 × 19	30	30		6		1.5	4
rec.[a]		× 10 Me V	I 23 × 24 II 23 × 24	15	15		7	(2–10)	1.5	2
16	6	^{60}Co	I 24 × 32 II 24 × 32	30	30		6		2.0	3
17	13	× 10 Me V	I 19 × 23 II 19 × 23	20	20		3		1.5	3
18[a]	15	× 10 Me V	I 23 × 27 II 23 × 27	20	20		3		1.5	3

Radiation quality, portal size, dose per fraction, and treatment time are given. In the comparison of prescribed doses in the target area and applied integral doses in different kidney regions the range describes the minimum and maxiumum estimated dose. In the column "Treatment time" the figures in parentheses indicate the overall treatment time if there was a break between two courses of radiotherapy. rec., relapse

[a] The liver hilus lymph nodes and the upper part of the right kidney were irradiated in combination with the splenic pedicle and the upper part of the right kidney

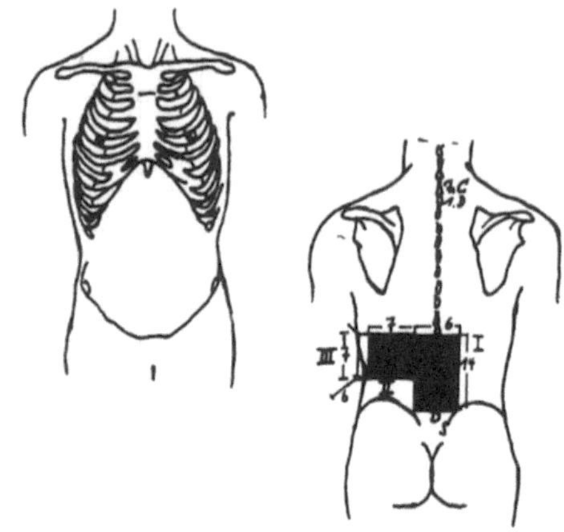

Fig. 1a,b. Calculated dose distribution for a complex field arrangement superimposed on an axial computed tomogram of the upper abdominal region in a 10-year-old girl (**b**). In the complex field arrangement the dose distribution for the rotational photon field and the dorsal and lateral ^{60}Co fields (**a**) are calculated separately. For estimating the resulting total dose in the target as well as in the kidney the overlapping isodose curves have to be summed for defined areas, resulting in an integral dose (Table 1, patients 1–6)

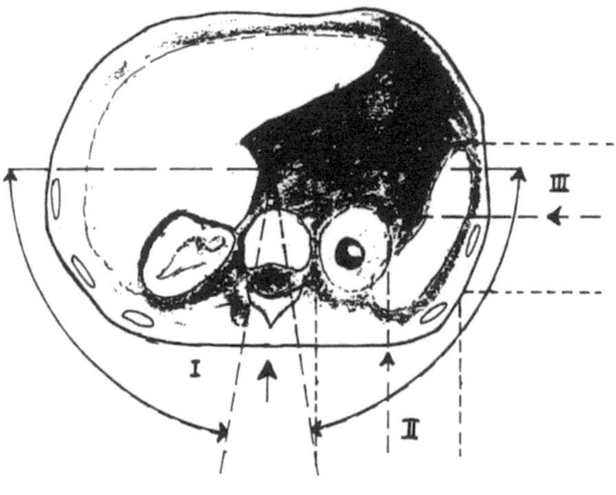

a

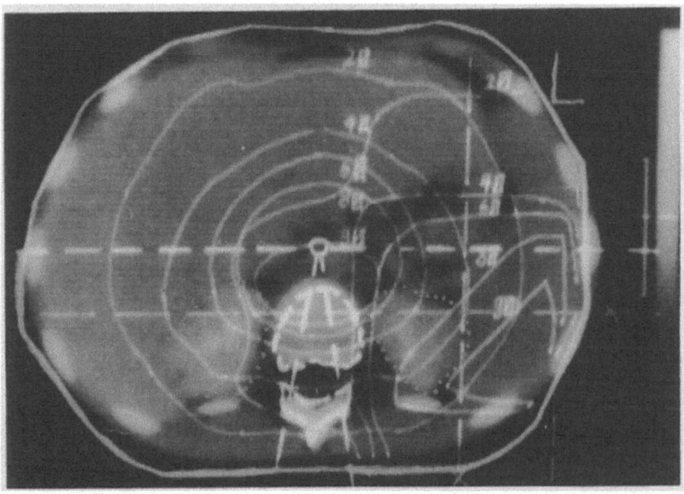

b

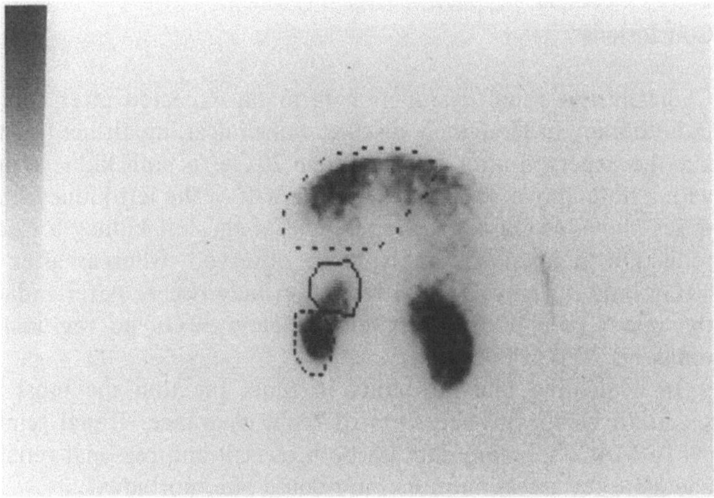

Fig. 2. Nephrography and scintigraphy (^{99m}Tc MAG3): There is a decrease in uptake in the upper half of left kidney, a difference in uptake between left and right kidney, and a decrease in overall uptake for both kidneys (not visible)

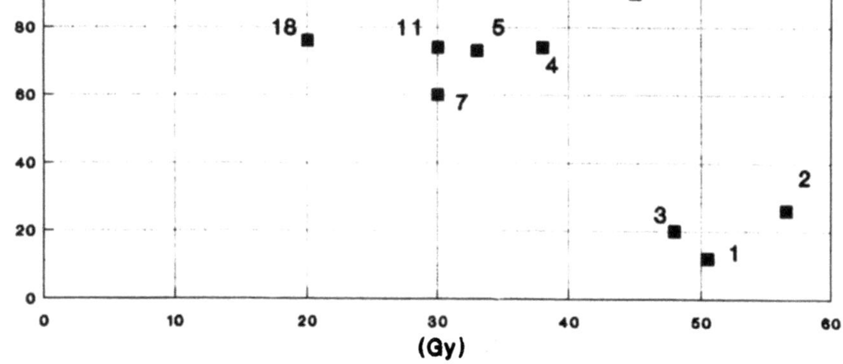

Fig. 3. Renal clearance and radiation dose. There is correlation between integrated dose and measured clearance (^{99m}Tc MAG3) at the upper part of the left kidney

Conclusions

Clinically, no renal dysfunction is to be expected after subdiaphragmatic radiotherapy in Hodgkin's disease. Subclinical impairment of renal function may be expected after a dose above 20 Gy to both kidneys in combination with a dose above 30 Gy in the upper half of the left kidney. After radiation doses above 45 Gy at the upper pole of the left kidney a clearcut regional reduction in uptake is likely to be observed, whereas after doses of 30–40 Gy only a slight regional reduction may occur. After radiation doses to the upper pole of the left kidney below 30 Gy no regional reduction in uptake is seen in this area.

In evaluating late morbidity in renal function the most sensitive tool seems to be the investigation of renal clearance. Renal scintigraphy (e.g. ^{99m}Tc MAG3), giving data on both overall and regional renal clearance, is adequate for assessing radiation-related late morbidity.

Over a long time period changes in treatment planning and delivery may lead to differences in dose distribution within the target volume and within radiosensitive organs. In order to be able to compare the radiation effects found in one-center and multicenter trials a standard prescription of radiation dose and treatment technique, as well as a standard way of reporting such data, is advisable both for the target and for radiosensitive organs. For evaluating late morbidity in a given tissue the applied radiation dose in that tissue with regard to the treatment technique and dosimetry in every individual patient has to be checked.

References

Abbatucci JS, Quint R, Bloquel J, Roussel A, Urbatjel M (1976) Techniken der Kurativen Telekobalttherapie. Enke, Stuttgart

Bubeck B, Brandau W, Eisenhut M, Weidenhammer K, Georgi P (1987) The tubular extraction rate (TER) of Tc-99MAG3: a new quantitative parameter of renal function. Nucl Compact 18:260–267

Kassner I (1991) "Involved-Field"- oder Extended-Field"-Radiotherapie im Rahmen einer kombinierten Behandlungsstrategie bei Kindern mit Morbus Hodgkin. Eine Analyse bei insgesamt 373 Patienten der kooperativen Therapiestudien DAL-HD-78 und DAL-HD-82. Dissertationsschrift, University of Münster

Le Bourgeois JP, Meignan M, Parmentier C, Tubiana M (1979) Renal consequences of irradiation of the spleen in lymphoma patients. Br J Radiol 52:56–60

Mitus A, Tefft M, Fellers FX (1969) Long term follow-up of Renal functions of 108 children who underwent nephrectomy for malignant disease. Pediatrics 44:912–921

Schellong G, Brämswig JH, Ludwig R, Gerein V, Jobke A, Jürgens H, Kabisch H, Stollmann B, Weinel P, Gadner H, Schwarze EW, Wannenmacher M (1986) Kombinierte Behandlungsstrategie bei über 200 Kindern mit Morbus Hodgkin: abgestufte Chemotherapie, Involved-Field-Bestrahlung mit erniedrigten Dosen und selektive Splenektomie. Ein Bericht der kooperativen Therapiestudie DAL-HD 82. Klin Pädiat 198:137–146

Schellong G, Hörnig I, Schwarze EW, Wannenmacher M (1989) Risk factor adapted treatment of Hodgkin's lymphoma in childhood: strategies and results of three consecutive multicenter studies in the Federal Republic of Germany. In: Diehl V, Pfreundschuh M, Löffler M (eds) New aspects in the diagnosis and treatment of Hodgkin's disease. Springer, Berlin Heidelberg New York, pp 205–213 (Recent results in cancer research, vol 117)
Schellong G, Pötter R, Hörnig-Tremz J, füi die DAL HD90-Studiengruppe (1990) Kooperative Therapiestudie DAL HD-90 zur Behandlung des Morbus Hodkin bei Kindern und Jugendlichen (Studienprotokoll). Studienleitung G. Schellong, Münster
Wannenmacher M, Slanina J, Kuphal K, Bruggmoser G (1978) Gegenwärtiger Stand der Großfeldtechnik unter Megavoltbedingungen bei der Strahlentherapie der Hodgkin'schen Erkrankung: Grundlagen, Durchführung, Nebenwirkungen. Radiologe 18:371–387

VI. Second Malignancies

Incidence of Secondary Malignancies in Patients with Hodgkin's Disease: Preliminary Results

J. Slanina, K. Henne, G. Schäffer, N. Hodapp, G. Moog, and H. Frommhold

Department of Radiotherapy, Radiological Clinic, University of Freiburg, Hugstetter Str. 55, W-7800 Freiburg i. Br., Fed. Rep. of Germany

Introduction

The term secondary malignancy relates simply to the sequence of occurrence of malignancies in an individual patient, and it is not possible to derive a causality from this temporal sequence. Also, although there is no doubt that ionizing radiation and/or chemotherapy may induce malignancies, there are a number of other factors which may also cause malignant tumors. For the treating physician it is not only of interest to know the frequency of occurrence of secondary malignancies. He also has to follow any clues to the cause of secondary malignancies, because prophylactic steps can only be taken with knowledge of the causality.

Material and Methods

Reported here are the preliminary results of a current investigation. Patients with Hodgkin's disease were observed with respect to secondary malignancies occurring during the follow-up period. To date we have evaluated the data on 996 evaluable patients out of a total of 1088 patients with surnames A to M, treated in Freiburg between 1940 and 1991.

As regards observation time there is a difference between the overall observation time and the observation time for secondary malignancies, because it is easier to get information about straightforward survival than about the status of health. As shown in Fig. 1, the median overall observation time is approximately 5.2 years and the median observation time for secondary malignancies approximately 3.6 years.

The patient characteristics of age, sex, initial staging, first treatment period, first treatment modality, and treatment modality until the incidence of a secondary malignancy are listed in Table 1. For comparison, some data from the International Database on Hodgkin's Disease (IDHD) (Henry-

Recent Results in Cancer Research, Vol. 130

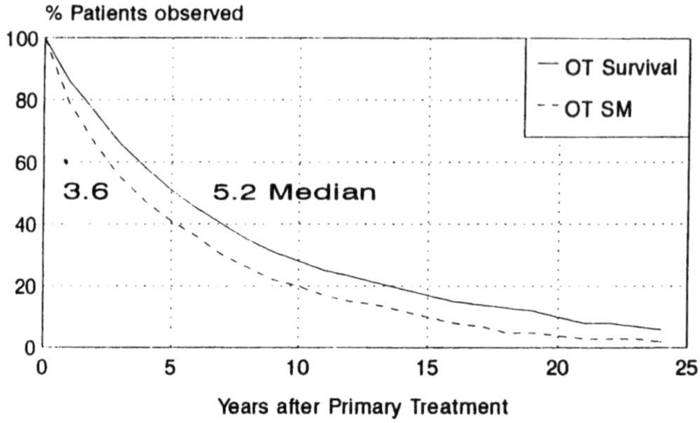

Fig. 1. Observation time (OT) of secondary malignancies (SM) versus observation time of survival. Freiburg 1940–1991, patients with surnames A–M, n = 996

Table 1. Initial patient characteristics and treatment

	Freiburg	Paris[a]	Milan[b]
n (total)	996	14.225	764
Sex ratio (M:F)	1.15:1	1.54:1	–
Age (average)	33.7	34.5	–
Stage			
I	21%	21%	–
II	43%	43%	–
III	29%	23%	–
IV	7%	13%	–
First treatment in			
1940–1960	22%	0%	0%
1961–1970	26%	7%	100% (1965–1976)
1971–1980	24%	57%	
1981–1991	28%	36%	0%
Primary treatment modality			
Radiation therapy alone	54%	42%	–
Chemotherapy alone	7%	24%	–
Combined modality	38%	32%	–
Not treated	1%	2%	–
Treatment modality until secondary malignancy			
Radiation therapy alone	37%	–	52%
Chemotherapy alone	1%	–	10%
Combined modality	62%	–	38%
Not treated	0%	–	0%

[a] Henry-Amar and Somers (1990)
[b] Valagussa et al. (1980)

Amar and Somers 1990) and from a Milan patient group (Valagussa et al. 1980) are included.

Results

Of the total group of 996 patients, 33 (3.3%) suffered from secondary malignancies. Calculated by the life-table method the cumulative risk of a secondary malignancy occurring within 5, 10, 15, and 20 years of primary treatment was 1%, 3%, 8%, and 19% respectively (Table 2). There is a remarkable peak incidence at 15–19 years after therapy that is clearly illustrated in Fig. 2. In this diagram the incidence of secondary malignancies is plotted as a percentage of patients at risk in the observed interval. Most of the secondary malignancies occur after a latency period of 15 years and the peak occurrence is between 16 and 20 years.

Table 2. Incidence of secondary malignancies as a function of time since initial therapy

Time at risk (yr)	Secondary malignancies	
	n	%[a]
0–4	8	1
5–9	5	3
10–14	7	8
15–19	9	19
–20	4	–
	33	

[a] Cumulative risk

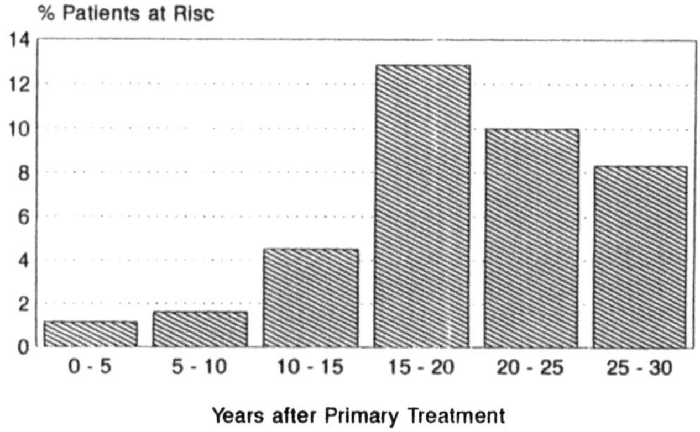

Fig. 2. Incidence of secondary malignancies plotted as a percentage of patients at risk. Freiburg 1940–1991, surnames A–M, $n = 996$

The details of the 33 secondary malignancies are listed in Table 3. A surprising finding is the fact that there is no case of secondary leukemia to be found in this series.

Treatment was divided into primary treatment and treatment until occurrence of a secondary malignancy. The treatment modalities were categorized as radiation therapy alone, chemotherapy alone, radiation therapy + MOPP (mustine, vincristine, procarbazine, prednisone) or similar drug combinations, radiation therapy + ABVD (doxorubicin, bleomycin, vinblastine) or similar drug combinations, radiation therapy + MOPP + ABVD, and radiation therapy + any other chemotherapy without MOPP or ABVD. Table 4a shows the incidence of secondary malignancies with respect to different treatment modalities at primary therapy. Table 4b shows the same with respect to different treatment modalities for the whole treatment until occurrence of a secondary malignancy.

The number of patients dying from secondary malignancies, the overall number of deaths, and the total number of patients are listed in Table 5 for both the Freiburg patient group and the IDHD group (Henry-Amar and Somers 1990). The percentage of secondary malignancies causing death in the two groups differs by a factor of 3.5.

A further question of interest is whether there is a correlation between radiation dose and incidence of secondary malignancies. Table 6 shows that secondary malignancies are located not only in the centre of the irradiation field but also at the margin of the field or outside the directly irradiated volume. Therefore, the radiation dose exposure in the areas of secondary malignancies varies over a wide range (Table 7).

Discussion

Typical examples of increased cancer incidence after exposure to ionizing radiation are leukemias in atomic bomb survivors (Bizzozero et al. 1966)

Table 3. Types of secondary malignancy

Breast Cancer	6
Lung cancer	4
Colorectal cancer	4
Non-Hodgkin's lymphoma	3
Soft tissue sarcoma	3
Brain tumor	3
Stomach cancer	2
Seminoma	2
Basal cell carcinoma	2
Pleural mesothelioma	1
Osteosarcoma	1
Cervix carcinoma	1
Urinary bladder carcinoma	1
	33

Table 4. Rates of incidence of secondary malignancies with respect to different treatment modalities

	n	Years after treatment (median)	% incidence within			
			3 years	5 years	10 years	20 years
(*a*) *Primary treatment*						
RT	530	5.0	1.3 (371)	1.6 (264)	3.9 (140)	19.0 (28)
CT	70	4.0	2.0 (48)	– (27)	– (10)	– (2)
RT + MOPP	102	5.0	1.8 (71)	– (55)	14.1 (25)	– (1)
RT + ABVD	36	2.5	0 (13)	0 (5)	0 (1)	– (0)
RT + MOPP + ABVD	38	5.0	0 (27)	0 (19)	– (0)	– (0)
RT + other	210	3.5	0 (122)	0 (92)	0 (41)	9.4 (17)
(*b*) *Treatment until occurence of secondary malignancy* (*overall*)						
RT	368	3.6	2.0 (235)	3.0 (180)	3.0 (103)	24.0 (18)
CT	11	1.3	17.0 (4)	– (1)	– (1)	0 (0)
RT + MOPP	169	5.3	0 (127)	1.0 (100)	4.0 (47)	28 (7)
RT + ABVD	50	2.1	0 (26)	0 (14)	0 (3)	0 (1)
RT + MOPP + ABVD	86	3.9	0 (64)	0 (43)	14.0 (6)	43 (2)
RT + other	312	3.0	0 (202)	0 (134)	0 (59)	8 (19)

Numbers in brackets denote patient numbers available for analysis CT, chemotherapy; RT, radiotherapy; MOPP and ABVD, see text

Table 5. Deaths caused by secondary malignancies

Series	Patients (*n*)	Total deaths (*n*)	Deaths from secondary malignancy	
			n	%
Paris[a]	14225	4139	413	10
Freiburg	996	576	16	2.8

[a] Henry-Amar and Somers (1990)

Table 6. Location of secondary malignancies with respect to the irradiation field

	n	%
Centre	9	27
Margin	11	33.5
Outside	12	36.5
Not irradiated	1	3

Table 7. Irradiation dose exposure of the areas of secondary malignancies

Dose (Gy)	No. of secondary malignancies
0.0	1
0.05	1
0.1	2
0.2	2
0.4	1
0.5	1
0.9	2
2	1
7	1
8	2
15	5
20	4
25	1
35	1
40	2
42	2
44	3
45	1

and thyroid cancers in children irradiated for benign conditions (Swelstad et al. 1977). However, in the reports of secondary malignancies in patients treated for cancer, the causative effect of the treatment is more difficult to establish (Colemann 1982; Hellbardt et al. 1990; Penn 1982; Seydel 1975). A multifactorial etiology has been postulated comprising impaired cellular immunity, especially in patients with advanced Hodgkin's disease, immunosuppressive effects of intensive treatment, and direct cellular effects of irradiation and chemotherapy (Canellos et al. 1975; Casciato and Scott 1979; Sieber and Adamson 1975; Valagussa et al. 1980). Cancer patients may be predisposed to develop secondary malignancies independent of the treatment (Colemann 1982) and there are no characteristic histopathological features in radiation-induced and/or chemotherapy-induced tumors (Boice 1981). Moreover, there is no "control group" without treatment in which one could evaluate the incidence of secondary malignancies (Arseneau et al. 1977).

The same applies also to the Freiburg patient group. Compared with the IDHD group (Henry-Amar and Somers 1990) it differs with respect to the male/female ratio, the year of primary treatment, and the percentage of patients receiving primary chemotherapy alone (Table 1). The fraction of deaths related to secondary malignancies for the Freiburg group is 2.8% (Table 5). This is markedly less than the 10% for the IDHD group (Henry-Amar and Somers 1990). One reason for this could be that there is no complete follow-up for the Freiburg group. The mean value for the lack of observation time for surviving patients who withdrew from the study is about 2.5 years. For the whole group of 996 patients there is a lack of about 1 year for a mean observation period of about 8 years.

The cumulative risk of secondary malignancy in the Freiburg group 10 years after primary treatment is about 3%. This is again less than the 7.3% for the Milan group of patients with Hodgkin's disease (Valagussa et al. 1980) or the 7% for a group of patients with seminoma reported by Hellbardt and coworkers (1990) who underwent radiation therapy with rather small extent and dose. In the last group the cumulative risk of secondary malignancy 15 and 20 years respectively after primary treatment is 16%; in the Freiburg patient group it is 8% and 19% respectively (Table 2).

It is remarkable that in the Freiburg group no incidence of second leukemia has been observed (Table 3) – a finding contrary to other observations (Cadman et al. 1977; Canellos et al. 1975; Casciato and Scott 1979; Coleman et al. 1977; Valagussa et al. 1986). In the IDHD group 36% of deaths were induced by secondary leukemia. For the Milan group the absolute incidence is 35% and for the seminoma patients (Hellbardt et al. 1990) 17%. There is no reason evident for the lack of secondary leukemia in the Freiburg group.

Only some of the solid secondary malignancies occur within the directly irradiated area. In the Freiburg group 27% of the solid secondary malignancies developed in this area (Table 6). Similarily in the Milan group (Valagussa et al. 1980) a fraction of 30% is reported and in the group of patients with seminoma (Hellbardt et al. 1990) a fraction of 50%. In the Freiburg group the patients treated by radiation therapy alone have 31% solid secondary malignancies within the directly irradiated area, while for the patients who received radiation therapy and chemotherapy the proportion is 25%.

If the primary treatment or the overall treatment until occurrence of a secondary malignancy are taken as a basis for calculating the risk of secondary malignancy, the outcome differs markedly, as seen in Table 4a and 4b. Furthermore, different therapeutic modalities of the primary treatment or of the overall treatment modify the risk of a secondary malignancy (Table 4a,b). This is similar to the findings reported by Valagussa and coworkers for the Milan group (Table 8). It is remarkable that in both the Freiburg and the Milan series patients treated by radiation therapy and ABVD chemotherapy alone did not develop secondary malignancies. At highest risk for developing a secondary malignancy were those patients whose overall treatment was radiation therapy plus MOPP plus ABVD. This subgroup's cumulative risk of a secondary malignancy was 14% and 43% at 10 and 20 years, respectively. On the other hand, it should be mentioned that in this subgroup more than the half of the patients needed a second treatment because of relapses.

Table 8. Rate of secondary malignancies in Hodgkin's disease (n = 764) (Valagussa et al. 1980)

Treatment	n	Months after initial treatment		Secondary malignancies	% incidences within					
		Median	Range		3 years		5 years		10 years	
RT	236	47	3–182	Solid tumors,	1.1	(138)	2.6	(84)	14.9	(12)
				leukemia	0		0		0	
CT	36	24	3–85	Solid tumors,	0	(11)	0	(3)		
				leukemia	5.5		5.5			
RT + MOPP	147	40	5–183	Solid tumors,	0	(86)	0	(35)	0	(13)
				leukemia	2.9		5.4		5.4	
RT + MABOP	87	60	8–158	Solid tumors,	0	(65)	2.1	(43)	2.1	(10)
				leukemia	1.4		1.4		5.8	
RT + ABVD	55	45	5–186	Solid tumors,	0	(38)	0	(16)	0	(6)
				leukemia	0		0		0	
RT + other	203	46	5–175	Solid tumors,	0.7	(96)	1.7	(77)	12.0	(10)
				leukemia	0		0		2.9	

Numbers in brackets denote patient numbers for analysis CT, chemotherapy; RT, radiotherapy; MABOP, mustine + doxorubicin + bleomycin + vincristine + prednisone; MOPP and ABVD, see text

Conclusions

There is an increased risk of secondary malignancy following treatment for Hodgkin's disease. As a multifactorial etiology is postulated, we now cannot prove whether or to what extent a secondary malignancy is induced by the treatment. However, correlative analyses leave very little room for doubt that the risk of developing a secondary malignancy is increased markedly by escalating the treatment modalities. This has to be taken into account when planning study designs for the treatment of Hodgkin's disease.

References

Arseneau JC, Canellos GP, Johnson R, de Vita VT (1977) Risk of new cancers in patients with Hodgkin's disease. Cancer 40:1912–1916

Bizzozero OJ Jr, Johnson KG, Ciocco A (1966) Radiation-related leukemia in Hiroshima and Nagasaki, 1946–1964. I. Distribution, incidence and appearance time. N Engl J Med 274:1095–1101

Boice JD (1981) Cancer following medical irradiation. Cancer 47:1081–1090

Cadman EC, Capizzi RL, Bertino JR (1977) Acute non-lymphocytic leukemia: a delayed complication of Hodgkin's disease therapy. Analysis of 109 cases. Cancer 40:1280–1290

Canellos GP, de Vita VT, Arseneau JC, Whang Peng J, Johnson REC (1975) Second malignancies complicating Hodgkin's disease in remission. Lancet 1:947–949

Casciato DA, Scott JL (1979) Acute leukemia following prolonged cytotoxic agent therapy. Medicine (Baltimore) 59:32–47

Coleman CN, Williams CJ, Flint A, Glatstein EJ, Rosenberg SA, Kaplan HS (1977) Hematologic neoplasia in patients treated for Hodgkin's disease. N Engl J Med 297:1249–1254

Colemann CN (1982) Secondary neoplasms in patients treated for cancer: etiology and perspective. Radiat Res 92:188–200

Hellbardt A, Mirimanoff RO, Obradovic M, Mermillod B, Paunier JP (1990) The risk of second cancer (SC) in patients treated for testicular seminoma. Int J Radiat Oncol Biol Phys 18:1327–1331

Henry-Amar M, Somers R (1990) Survival outcome after Hodgkin's disease: a report from the International Data Base on Hodgkin's disease. Semin Oncol 17(6):758–768

Penn I (1982) Second neoplasms following radiotherapy or chemotherapy for cancer. Am J Clin Oncol 5:83–96

Seydel HG (1975) The risk of tumor induction in man following medical irradiation for malignant neoplasm. Cancer 35:1641–1645

Sieber SM, Adamson RH (1975) Toxicity of antineoplastic agents in man: chromosomal aberrations, antifertility effects, congenital malformations, and carcinogenic potential. Adv Cancer Res 22:57–155

Swelstad JA, Scanlon EF, Murphy ED (1977) Thyroid disease following irradiation for benign conditions. Arch Surg 112:380–385

Valagussa P, Santoro A, Kenda R, Fossati Bellani F, Franchi F, Banfi A, Rilke F, Bonadonna G (1980) Second malignancies in Hodgkin's disease: a complication of certain forms of treatment. Br Med J 280:216–219

Valagussa P, Santoro A, Fossati-Bellani F, Bianfi A, Bonadonna G (1986) Second acute leukemia and other malignancies following treatment for Hodgkin's disease. J Clin Oncol 4:830–837

Subject Index

MIX
Papier aus verantwortungsvollen Quellen
Paper from responsible sources
FSC® C105338
FSC
www.fsc.org

If you have any concerns about our products,
you can contact us on
ProductSafety@springernature.com

In case Publisher is established outside the EU,
the EU authorized representative is:
Springer Nature Customer Service Center GmbH
Europaplatz 3, 69115 Heidelberg, Germany

Printed by Libri Plureos GmbH
in Hamburg, Germany